AF342499

Yearbook of
Pediatric Endocrinology
2012

Endorsed by the European Society for Paediatric Endocrinology

Editors

Ken Ong
Ze'ev Hochberg

Associate Editors

Gary Butler
Evangelia Charmandari
Francesco Chiarelli
Stefano Cianfarani
Mehul Dattani
Nicolas De Roux
Helmuth-Günther Dörr
Outi Mäkitie
Orit Pinhas-Hamiel
Michel Polak
Olle Söder
Martin Wabitsch

KARGER

Sponsored by a grant from Pfizer Endocrine Care

© Copyright 2012 by S. Karger AG, P.O. Box, CH–4009 Basel (Switzerland)
www.karger.com
Printed in Switzerland on acid-free and non-aging paper (ISO 9706) by Reinhardt Druck, Basel
ISBN 978-3-318-02230-8
ISSN 1662-3391

Mehul T. Dattani

Developmental Endocrine Research Group
Clinical and Molecular Genetics Unit, Institute for Child Health
University College London
30 Guilford Street
London, WC1N 1EH, UK
Tel. +44 207 905 2657, Fax +44 207 404 6191, E-Mail m.dattani@ucl.ac.uk

Nicolas De Roux

INSERM U 690, Laboratoire d'Hormonologie, AP-HP
Hôpital Robert Debré, 48 Boulevard Sérurier
FR–75019 Paris, France
Tel. +33 1 40 03 19 85, Fax +33 1 40 40 91 95, E-Mail nicolas.deroux@inserm.fr

Helmuth-Günther Dörr

Pediatric Endocrinology, Department of Pediatrics
University of Erlangen, Loschgestr. 15
DE-91054 Erlangen, Germany
Tel. +49 9131 85 33732, Fax +49 9131 85 36131, E-Mail Helmuth-Guenther.Doerr@uk-erlangen.de

Outi Mäkitie

Pediatric Endocrinology and Metabolic Bone Diseases
Children's Hospital
Helsinki University Central Hospital and University of Helsinki
FI–00029 Helsinki, Finland
Tel. +358 9 4711, Fax +358 9 471 75888, E-Mail outi.makitie@helsinki.fi

Orit Pinhas-Hamiel

Pediatric Endocrine and Diabetes Unit
Safra Children's Hospital
Sheba Medical Center Ramat-Gan
IL–52621 Ramat-Gan, Israel
Tel. +972 3 5305015, Fax +972 3 5305055, E-Mail orit.hamiel@sheba.health.gov.il

Michel Polak

Paediatric Endocrinology, Gynecology and Diabetology INSERM U845
Université Paris Descartes
Hôpital Necker-Enfants Malades
149, rue de Sèvres
FR– 75015 Paris, France
Tel. +33 1 44 49 48 03/02, Fax +33 1 44 38 16 48, E-Mail michel.polak@nck.aphp.fr

Olle Söder

Pediatric Endocrinology Unit, Q2:08

Department of Woman and Child Health

Karolinska Institutet and University Hospital, Solna

SE–171 76 Stockholm, Sweden

Tel. +46 8 517 75124, Fax +46 8 517 75128, E-Mail olle.soder@ki.se

Martin Wabitsch

Division of Pediatric Endocrinology and Diabetes Endocrine Research Laboratory

Department of Pediatrics and Adolescent Medicine

University of Ulm, Eythstrasse 24

DE–89075 Ulm, Germany

Tel. +49 731 5005 7400, Fax +49 731 5005 7407, E-Mail martin.wabitsch@uniklinik-ulm.de

Table of Contents

Preface

The *2012 Yearbook of Pediatric Endocrinology* brings you summaries of the year's published breakthrough developments in the basic sciences and new evidence-based knowledge that are relevant to clinical practice in this field. This is the ninth edition and the Associate Editors will present their chapters at the European Society for Paediatric Endocrinology (ESPE) annual meeting in Leipzig 2012. This year, we introduce a new chapter on endocrine 'Oncology and Chronic Disease', while articles on population genetics are now distributed throughout the chapters.

This was another stimulating year (June 2011 to June 2012, when we submit the manuscripts to the publisher). New treatments tested include: insulin degludec and sensor-augmented pumps in type 1 diabetes; dual-release hydrocortisone in adrenal insufficiency; gefinitib and pasireotide in Cushing's disease; enzyme-replacement therapy in life-threatening hypophosphatasia; antenatal thyroid screening, and cholesterol-lowering foods in hyperlipidemia. In the basic sciences, (a) a new hormone 'irisin' was discovered, the first to be secreted by skeletal muscle, with beneficial effects on adipose tissue; (b) significant advance was made in laboratory culture of stem cells towards the goal of growing 'a pituitary in a dish'; (c) two separate whole-exome sequencing studies identified activating mutations in the PI3K/AKT/mTOR pathway as causes of overgrowth and insulin overactivity; (d) the Aboriginal Australian genomic sequence was found to represent one of the oldest continuous populations outside Africa, with no evidence of European admixture, and (e) the brain was identified as an evolutionary target; genes expressed in the neocortex arose soon after its morphological origin.

On 31 October, 2011, the world's population reached 7 billion, with 3 billion being children and the subjects of our care, as members of the world's pediatricians. Concerns over the expanding population seem to be abating, but the sheer number poses challenges for health and the environment. One billion people are hungry and the planet's resources are stretched thin. We all know what needs to be done: empower women in all aspects of life; reduce poverty as the root cause of hunger; distribute wealth more fairly; increase food production – through genetically engineered crops; develop renewable energy sources, and avoid further global warming. In October 2011, the UN Assembly recognized the needs of children with non-communicable diseases and, a month later, the Bill & Melinda Gates Foundation declared a scientific grand challenge on infant growth stunting. It seems that our plea to help children with endocrine and growth disorders is finally being recognized.

While considering our future, our history deserves to be remembered: 100 years ago, Harvey Cushing reported the 'polyglandular syndrome'. Case 45 (out of 47), a young Russian Jewess 'of extraordinary appearance', is believed to be the first description of Cushing's syndrome. The full article, written in 1910 and published in 1912, is reproduced online [http://www.grandrounds-e-med.com/articles/gr049003/cushingoriginal.pdf]. Another historical landmark is the first appearance in the medical literature of the term 'evidence-based medicine' twenty years ago in a paper by Guyatt et al. [Evidence-based medicine. A new approach to teaching the practice of medicine. JAMA 1992;268:2420–2425].

Considering our own history, we acknowledge the nine continuous years of generous support by Pfizer Ltd that makes the *Yearbook* possible. We thank again all the dedicated staff at our publisher, Karger, who have done a tremendous job to bring the *Yearbook* on time to the ESPE meeting with such a tight timeline. Our twelve Associate Editors and their coauthors have done an enormous work to select and highlight this year's advances, and provide their chapters in a timely fashion. Finally, we recognize Prof. Jean-Claude Carel's immense work and vision as the *Yearbook's* Joint Founding Editor during its first eight years.

Ze'ev Hochberg (Haifa)
Ken Ong (Cambridge)

Neuroendocrinology

Lukas Huijbregts, Lucie Chevrier and Nicolas de Roux

INSERM U676, Hôpital Robert-Debré and Université Paris Diderot, Paris, France

The literature on neuroendocrinology is highly diverse. Being scientists involved in endocrinology research, we naturally focused our attention on the central regulation of the endocrine axis. We have therefore selected papers proposing new concepts or new hypothalamic networks to explain these regulations. However, additional papers selected this year show that the hypothalamus cannot be restricted to its function in neuroendocrine regulations. Three points emerge from this selection: (1) It is well known that hypothalamic peptides that have a peripheral role, like oxytocin, may also have central effects. The improvement of in-vivo models of cellular activity has helped to characterize this concept. (2) Autophagy in peripheral tissues contributes to energy homeostasis. Autophagy in specific hypothalamic neurons also plays an important role in the neuroendocrine regulation of metabolism. (3) The role of the hypothalamus in the regulation of arterial tone. This function is highlighted by a paper showing the relation between dysfunctional proopiomelanocortin neurons and the occurrence of obesity-related hypertension. Such a role of hypothalamic neurons in obesity-related hypertension was suspected but not previously demonstrated.

New mechanism
Agouti-related protein and fertility in $Lep^{ob/ob}$ mice

Ablation of neurons expressing agouti-related protein, but not melanin-concentrating hormone, in leptin-deficient mice restores metabolic functions and fertility

Wu Q, Whiddon BB, Palmiter RD
Howard Hughes Medical Institute and Department of Biochemistry, University of Washington, Seattle, WA, USA
Proc Natl Acad Sci USA 2012;109:3155–3160

Background: Nonsense mutation in the leptin gene in mice ($Lep^{ob/ob}$ mice) induced obesity, hyperphagia, and infertility. A complex neuronal circuitry seems to be involved in this phenotype.
Methods: In $Lep^{ob/ob}$ mice treated with diphtheria toxin (DT), agouti-related protein (AgRP)- or melanin-concentrating hormone (MCH) neurons were selectively ablated due to specific expression of the human DT receptor in either AgRP or MCH neurons.
Results: Ablation of MCH neurons had no effect on food intake, body weight, fertility, but improved glucose tolerance in $Lep^{ob/ob}$ mice. Ablation of AgRP neurons in lean or severely obese $Lep^{ob/ob}$ mice induced a severe anorexia leading to moribund animals. However, moderately obese $Lep^{ob/ob}$ mice survived AgRP neuron ablation and became fertile.
Conclusion: AgRP neurons play a critical role in obesity and infertility of $Lep^{ob/ob}$ mice, whereas MCH neurons have only a minor effect.

Loss of leptin or its receptor leads to obesity, diabetes and infertility in humans and rodents. A complex neuronal circuit, including hypothalamic neurons expressing agouti-related protein (AgRP) and melanin-concentrating hormone (MCH), is involved in the body weight regulation and leptin signaling. Ablation of MCH-expressing neurons has a limited effect on metabolic functions in $Lep^{ob/ob}$ mice. However, ablation of AgRP neurons induces a severe anorexia in $Lep^{ob/ob}$ mice, suggesting that this anorexigenic effect is independent of MCH signaling. Anorexia induced by AgRP ablation is critical in lean and severely obese $Lep^{ob/ob}$ mice, while moderately obese $Lep^{ob/ob}$ mice survive and become fertile. It is difficult to determine if this differential effect in mice is modified by body weight or age, because body weight increased with the age of the animals (lean, moderate and severely obese mice were respectively 6, 8 and 10 weeks old). In older *Lep*^{ob/ob} mice, anorexia is accompanied by a severe decrease in body temperature linked to a decreased output of the sympathetic nervous system. Lethal anorexia induced by AgRP neuron ablation results from the loss of GABA signaling leading to a neuronal hyperactivity, which is compensated in moderate obese mice by an unknown mechanism. Restored fertility in *Lep*^{ob/ob} mice has already been observed in mice lacking NPY. AgRP neuron ablation does not affect all NPY neurons, indicating that restored fertility in *Lep*^{ob/ob} mice with ablation of AgRP neurons is not attributed to an NPY effect. This study highlights the critical role of AgRP neurons in metabolic function and fertility.

Concept revised
Kisspeptin release is developmentally regulated

Developmental increase in kisspeptin-54 release in vivo is independent of the pubertal increase in estradiol in female rhesus monkeys (*Macaca mulatta*)

Guerriero KA, Keen KL, Terasawa E
Wisconsin National Primate Research Center, University of Wisconsin-Madison, Madison, WI, USA
Endocrinology 2012;153:1887–1897

Background: The pulsatile release of kisspeptins, a potent stimulator of GnRH neurosecretion, is increased during pubertal maturation. The aim of this study was to determine if a developmental regulation of kisspeptin release exists in monkey.
Methods and Results: The pattern of release of Kp54 was measured in vivo in prepubertal and pubertal female monkeys. A developmental increase in mean Kp54 release, pulse frequency and pulse amplitude occurred between prepubertal and pubertal monkeys. Ovariectomy and estrogen administration had no effect on Kp54 in prepubertal animals. However, in pubertal animals, ovariectomy increased mean Kp54 release and pulse amplitude, an effect that was reversed by estrogen.
Conclusion: The pubertal increase of kisspeptin release occurs independently of circulating estrogen level. Kisspeptin release at the pubertal onset is unlikely to be responsible for the puberty onset, but seems to contribute later on to further increase the GnRH release during the progression of puberty.

Puberty is associated with an increased GnRH and kisspeptin pulsatile release. The developmental regulation of GnRH secretion is well understood, but few data are available concerning kisspeptin release. The present in-vivo study highlights a developmental regulation of kisspeptin release which coincides well with the developmental regulation of GnRH release. This strongly supports the role of kisspeptins in the regulation of pulsatile GnRH release during puberty, but also during the night. As for GnRH secretion, kisspeptin release in prepubertal monkeys does not depend on circulating estrogen level. This underscores differences between species. In fact, in prepubertal rodent, kisspeptin and GnRH signaling are regulated by estrogen. The fact that kisspeptin and GnRH release are not regulated by estrogen in prepubertal monkey is in accordance with the existence of a negative neuronal input by GABA on kisspeptin neurons. Altogether, it appears that in female monkey, kisspeptins do not play a critical role in triggering puberty onset, but contribute to the increase of pulsatile GnRH release during pubertal onset, illustrating the complex and species-specific mechanisms of pubertal onset.

Concept revised
The physiological link between kisspeptin and GABA

Tonic control of kisspeptin release in prepubertal monkeys: implications to the mechanism of puberty onset

Kurian JR, Keen KL, Guerriero KA, Terasawa E
Wisconsin National Primate Research Center (J.R.K., K.L.K., K.A.G., E.T.) and Department of Pediatrics (E.T.),
University of Wisconsin-Madison, Madison, WI, USA
Endocrinology 2012;153:3331–3336

Background: Reduction in γ-aminobutyric acid (GABA) inhibition is critical for the pubertal onset by increasing GnRH release. Kisspeptin release in the medial basal hypothalamus is low in prepubertal female monkeys. The authors hypothesized that the low levels of kisspeptin release in prepubertal monkey is due to the tonic GABA inhibition.
Methods: Kisspeptin release in the medial basal hypothalamus was studied by microdialysis in prepubertal and pubertal monkeys treated with bicuculline, a GABA(A) receptor antagonist.
Results: Infusion of bicuculline in prepubertal monkey induced a rapid effect on kisspeptin release. No effect was observed in midpubertal or pubertal monkeys. In a second series of experiments, the authors showed that the bicuculline-induced GnRH release was suppressed by a kisspeptin receptor antagonist.
Conclusion: The low kisspeptin release in the medial basal hypothalamus of prepubertal monkeys is due to a GABA inhibition on kisspeptin neurons.

The balance between inhibitory (GABA) and excitatory (glutamate) neurotransmitters is one mechanism that suppresses gonadotropic axis activity in prepubertal animals and allows activity at pubertal onset. Before pubertal onset, GABA was demonstrated to block GnRH release. At pubertal onset, this GABA inhibition is reduced, leading to an increase of GnRH release and then pubertal onset. This study proposes that the inhibitory effect of GABA on GnRH release is mediated by interneurons such as kisspeptin neurons. Again, this work shows that kisspeptin neurons are the main hypothalamic neurons where regulators of the gonadotrope axis converge. The difference between prepubertal and midpubertal monkeys may be explained by the reduced GABA release between these two stages. Several other regulators of GnRH release have a role in the juvenile period and in pubertal onset. Several of them act through kisspeptin neurons in association or not with GABA. This study adds an additional complexity in the network regulating pubertal onset.

New mechanism
GnIH is a switch between feeding and reproduction

Gonadotropin-inhibitory hormone is a hypothalamic peptide that provides a molecular switch between reproduction and feeding

Clarke IJ, Smith JT, Henry BA, Oldfield BJ, Stefanidis A, Millar RP, Sari IP, Chng K, Fabre-Nys C, Caraty A, Ang BT, Chan L, Fraley GS
Department of Physiology, Monash University, Clayton, Vic., Australia
Neuroendocrinology 2012;95:305–316

Background: Gonadotropin-inhibitory hormone-3 (GnIH-3) is a hypothalamic peptide that plays a role in the regulation of reproduction and feeding in mammals. However, reciprocal control of reproduction and feeding behavior is not known.
Methods and Results: In situ hybridization in ewes showed that GnIH-3 expression was low during the follicular phase, suggesting that it constitutes a permissive condition for the preovulatory LH surge. Infusion of GnIH-3 in different mammalian species (ewes, mouse, rat, monkey) had no effect on sexual

behavior, but increased food intake without modifying energy expenditure. Immunohistochemistry showed that GnIH-3 increased Fos expression in orexigenic neurons and also in anorexigenic neurons. *Conclusion:* GnIH-3 inhibits the reproductive system and concomitantly stimulates food intake in a range of mammalian species.

GnIH is a hypothalamic peptide that is known to inhibit GnRH neurons and gonadotropes, leading to suppression of reproductive capacity in mammals. GnIH has also stimulatory effects on feeding. The relationship between energy balance and reproduction is now well established, but the molecular mechanisms coupling them remain unclear. A high level of GnIH favors food intake over reproduction, while during the follicular phase, a low level of GnIH favors preovulatory LH pulse induced by estrogen and consequent reproductive function. GnIH does not affect sexual behavior, showing that in the brain, mechanisms controlling endocrine and behavioral actions of GnIH are distinct. The pituitary action of GnIH is controversial. However, in the present study, the parenteral administration of GnIH efficiently inhibited reproductive function in ewes without affecting sexual behavior, arguing for a pituitary action without any requirement to cross the blood-brain barrier. The fact that GnIH stimulates food intake without any effect on energy expenditure is of interest and indicates a potential role of this neuropeptide for the treatment of energy-restraint conditions. However, in absence of any genetic mutations in GnIH or physiological investigation, the function of this neuropeptide in humans remains a mystery.

New concerns
Endocrine disruptors in neuroendocrine homeostasis

Endocrine disruptors are of major interest in the field of neuroendocrinology. The two following studies concern two different endocrine disruptors: methylphenidate hydrochloride, a medication that delays puberty in males, and bisphenol A, a chemical compound of food packaging that leads to early puberty and masculinization in females. It is important to determine the mechanisms by which these substances alter pubertal onset in order to better assess their potential risks in humans and also to better understand the mechanisms of pubertal onset.

Pubertal delay in male non-human primates (*Macaca mulatta*) treated with methylphenidate

Mattison DR, Plant TM, Lin HM, Chen HC, Chen JJ, Twaddle NC, Doerge D, Slikker W, Jr, Patton RE, Hotchkiss CE, Callicott RJ, Schrader SM, Turner TW, Kesner JS, Vitiello B, Petibone DM, Morris SM
Epidemiology Branch, Division of Epidemiology, Statistics, and Prevention Research, The Eunice Kennedy Shriver National Institute for Child Health and Human Development, National Institutes of Health, Bethesda, MD, USA
mattisod@mail.nih.gov
Proc Natl Acad Sci USA 2011;108:16301–16306

Background: Methylphenidate hydrochloride (MPH) is one of the most widely prescribed medications in children. The aim of this study is to evaluate the impact of MPH on pubertal onset in non-human primate. *Methods:* Juvenile 2-year-old male rhesus monkeys were treated orally twice a day with vehicle (n = 10), 0.15 mg/kg of MPH increased to 2.5 mg/kg (low dose, n = 10), 1.5 mg/kg of MPH increased to 12.5 mg/kg for 14 months. Observations were made during 40 months. *Results:* Endocrine analyses indicate that serum testosterone level was decreased by MPH and that inhibin B level was increased. MPH reduced testicular volume and delayed testicular descent. However, differences between control and treated groups disappeared in adult monkeys. *Conclusion:* Pubertal onset is delayed by MPH in a non-human primate, but this effect is transient and no permanent deficit is seen in adult monkeys.

MPH is widely used as a chronic treatment for attention deficit hyperactivity disorder in children. The effect of this molecule on pubertal onset was interesting to investigate, as it is recognized as a potential modulator of the pubertal process. This study in juvenile male non-human primates indicates that MPH delayed the testicular development (testicular growth and descent), and decreased plasmatic testosterone level. However, no differences were observed in adult monkeys between control and treated animals. This observation of a transient effect of MPH is reassuring regarding the use of this medication in children. Additional studies must be undertaken to confirm this result in other animal models and in humans and to determine the molecular mechanisms by which MPH delays the pubertal onset in male.

Disrupted organization of RFamide pathways in the hypothalamus is associated with advanced puberty in female rats neonatally exposed to bisphenol A

Losa-Ward SM, Todd KL, McCaffrey KA, Tsutsui K, Patisaul HB
Department of Biology, North Carolina State University, Raleigh, NC, USA
Biol Reprod 2012;112:100826

Background: Neonatal exposure to bisphenol A (BPA) alters the timing of puberty onset in female rodents. Disrupted ontogeny of kisspeptin and RFamide-related peptide-3 (RFRP3), which are known to regulate GnRH neurons, could be a consequence of BPA exposure leading to premature puberty.
Methods: Transgenic female Wistar rats expressing enhanced green fluorescent protein (EGFP) in GnRH neurons were exposed to estradiol (E$_2$), a low dose of BPA (50 µg/kg) or a high dose of BPA (50 mg/kg) from postnatal day (PND) 0 through PND 3. Animals were sacrificed on PNDs 17, 21, 24, 28, and 33.
Results: Vaginal opening was advanced by E$_2$ and a low dose of BPA. On PND 28, E$_2$ and 50 mg/kg BPA-exposed females had decreased RFRP-3 fiber density and contacts on GnRH neurons. RFRP3 perikarya were also decreased in females exposed to 50 mg/kg BPA.
Conclusion: Premature puberty induced by neonatal BPA exposure seems to result from an accelerated decline of RFRP3 input on GnRH neurons.

Bisphenol A is an endocrine disrupting compound that advances female rodent puberty and induces persistent estrus by unknown cellular and molecular mechanisms. In this study, the authors hypothesize that BPA-induced puberty is linked to abnormal ontogeny of kisspeptins or FRFP3. Treatment with a low dose of BPA during the neonatal period (3 days after birth) induced an earlier vaginal opening associated with a decrease of RFRP3 fiber density, while a high dose of BPA decreased kisspeptin fibers in the arcuate nucleus. The nonmonotonic effect of BPA (a low dose leads to early puberty, while a high dose leads to masculinization) suggests that two distinct mechanisms coexist. E$_2$ treatment leads to a more advanced puberty than low-dose BPA, without affecting RFRP3 ontogeny. This observation suggests that BPA does not act as a classical estrogenic compound, or that BPA and E$_2$ act with a different kinetic. This study suggests a new mechanism by which a low dose of BPA modulates ontogeny of RFRP3 leading to advanced puberty. Now, it will be interesting to determine if other endocrine disrupting compounds have comparable effects.

Hypothalamic EAP1 (enhanced at puberty 1) is required for menstrual cyclicity in non-human primates

Dissen GA, Lomniczi A, Heger S, Neff TL, Ojeda SR
Division of Neuroscience, Oregon National Primate Research Center, Beaverton, CR, USA
disseng@ohsu.edu
Endocrinology 2012;153:350–361

Background: EAP1 was recently described as a transcriptional regulator playing a role in the hypothalamic control of female reproductive development and estrous cyclicity in rodents. The mechanism of this function is unknown. EAP1 probably interacts with specific transcription factors. EAP1 was shown to be highly expressed in the medial basal hypothalamus (MBH) of non-human primate. Here, Dissen et al. have studied the hypothalamic function of EAP1 in rhesus monkey.

Methods: Lentiviral-mediated delivery of small interfering (si)RNA directed against EAP1 was used to reduce EAP1 mRNA levels in the mediobasal hypothalamus. The hypothalamic region of the injection was controlled by a MRI-assisted stereotactic procedure. Green fluorescent protein directed by the cytomegalovirus promoter was used to follow transduced cells in the hypothalamus.

Results: Lentivirus-mediated siRNA against EAP1 in the mediobasal hypothalamus resulted in knock-down of EAP1 and in cessation of menstrual cyclicity in female rhesus monkeys undergoing regular menstrual cycles. Neither lentiviruses encoding an unrelated siRNA nor the placement of viral particles carrying EAP1 siRNA outside the mediobasal hypothalamus-arcuate nucleus region affected menstrual cycles.

Conclusion: The region-specific expression of EAP1 in the hypothalamus is required for menstrual cyclicity in higher primates. EAP1 is thus an integral component of a powerful transcriptional-repressive complex which may control reproductive cyclicity by inhibiting downstream repressor genes involved in the neuroendocrine control of reproductive function.

The understanding of the hypothalamic network regulating estrous cyclicity has been recently improved by several original studies. Most of these proteins are receptors, neuropeptides or neurotransmitters. The analysis of EAP1 in the neuroendocrine control of female cyclicity may open new perspectives to understand this very complex process. This study showed that cessation of menstrual cyclicity did not disturb the distribution and the number of GnRH neurons as well as kisspeptin neurons. Thus, other mechanisms must be evocated. The authors proposed that EAP1 silencing probably enhanced activity of neurons involved in the inhibitory control of the estrous cyclicity. Some of EAP1 target genes may be proapoptotic. The silencing of EAP1 may thus result in an increased apoptosis in the hypothalamus. This possible association between apoptosis and gonadotropic deficiency is interesting and should be further characterized.

New mechanism
How steroid hormones control behaviors

During early development, sex steroids have a dramatic impact on the establishment of sexually dimorphic brain regions that will further determine typical male or female behaviors. The following article by Xu et al. brings major findings and novel directions on genetic determinisms of sexually dimorphic behaviors whereas the article by Lombardo et al. is the first study to show that in humans, fetal testosterone has an organizing impact on the adult sexually dimorphic brain.

Modular genetic control of sexually dimorphic behaviors

Xu X, Coats JK, Yang CF, Wang A, Ahmed OM, Alvarado M, Izumi T, Shah NM
Department of Anatomy, University of California, San Francisco, San Francisco, CA, USA
Cell 2012;148:596–607

Background: It is well known that the development of sexually dimorphic behaviors in vertebrates highly depends on sexual hormones such as estrogen and testosterone. However, the molecular mechanisms responsible for the establishment of the underlying neural circuitry that drives such behaviors still remain to be clearly defined.

Methods and Results: To bring further understanding in these mechanisms, the authors used dual color microarray on adult mouse hypothalamus and amygdala to define sexually dimorphic gene expression patterns between males and females. Further in-situ hybridization analysis of candidate genes revealed sex- and region-specific expressions of hormonally regulated genes. Moreover, among these genes, four were shown to alter distinct sexually dimorphic behavior when individually disrupted (Brs3, Cckar, Irs4 and Sytl4).

Conclusion: These results suggest that sexually dimorphic behaviors such as sexual behavior, male aggression or maternal care are governed by separable genetic programs.

This study is extremely important because it brings further insight in the complex and poorly understood mechanism of how sexual hormones have such a dramatic impact on the organization of the brain. Here, the authors identified 16 dimorphically expressed genes, among which the already known esr1 encoding estrogen receptor-α, but also novel genes whose functions in sexual behaviors are unknown. Furthermore, the authors used knockout animals to show that specific disruption of some of these genes have very specific impact on sexual behavior. This impact is also different depending on whether the disruption occurs in males or females. For instance, loss of Cckar or Irs4 had no impact on behavior in males but in females, Irs4 participates in maternal behavior whereas Cckar is important for sexual behavior. This study therefore opens novel leads to understand how the environment may alter dimorphic behaviors, for instance through epigenetic modification of such genes. It may also account for subtle behavioral differences between individuals based on polymorphisms or mutations in the target genes. Finally, the microarray used by the authors did not identify several well-described sexual dimorphic genes such as *Kiss1*, androgen receptor or aromatase, showing the limits of such approach but also emphasizing the need of combining different high throughput strategies for the identification of sexual dimorphic genes.

Fetal testosterone influences sexually dimorphic gray matter in the human brain

Lombardo MV, Ashwin E, Auyeung B, Chakrabarti B, Taylor K, Hackett G, Bullmore ET, Baron-Cohen S
Autism Research Centre, Department of Psychiatry, University of Cambridge, Cambridge, UK
ml437@cam.ac.uk
J Neurosci 2012;32:674–680

Background: It is well established that during early development of non-human species, testosterone has a major organizing effect on the adult sexually dimorphic brain. However, if such mechanism also occurs in the sexual differentiation of the human brain remains unclear.
Methods and Results: To assess this question, the authors used magnetic resonance imaging in human prepubertal males (aged 8–11) and show that fetal testosterone (FT) levels correlate with the local gray matter volume of specific brain regions such as the right temporoparietal junction/posterior superior temporal sulcus (RTPJ/pSTS), the planum temporal/parietal operculum (PT/PO) and the posterior lateral orbitofrontal cortex (plOFC). Indeed, FT levels positively correlated with the size of RTPJ/pSTS which was therefore bigger in males than females, whereas PT/PO and plOFC size negatively correlated with FT and was smaller in males than in females. Other sexually dimorphic regions such as the hypothalamus and the amygdala were unrelated to FT levels although FT positively predicted the size of a nonsexually dimorphic region of the amygdala.
Conclusion: Fetal testosterone appears to act as an organizing mechanism for the sexual differentiation of the human brain.

This is the first study to bring evidence that, in humans, there is a direct correlation between fetal testosterone levels and the gray matter volumes of sexually dimorphic parts of the brain in males. Indeed, by comparing fetal testosterone levels (measured from amniotic fluid samples) to the volume of brain regions in the corresponding prepubertal boys, they observed that FT was likely to organize some specific sexually dimorphic regions of the brain. However, some other well-known sexually dimorphic regions did not seem to be correlated with FT levels, raising the possibility that FT is not the only organizer of the sexually dimorphic brain. Unfortunately, such observational studies are limited, for example one cannot exclude the possibility that FT levels are also correlated to testosterone levels at later stages of development.

FT levels may also not solely account for differences between males and females, but unfortunately, the study is based on only male samples of FT. Then it would be interesting to assess how differences between males and females take place and whether similar correlation between fetal sex steroids levels and local brain regions size is true in females. How FT influences the size of discrete parts of the adult brain remains an open question, especially which are the targeted genes downstream of the FT signaling that are transcriptionnally activated or inhibited.

Autophagy is a cellular mechanism that participates in the cellular homeostasis and viability by removing deficient organelles and supplying energy. Recent studies have shown that autophagy contributes to energy homeostasis in the liver, pancreas and adipocytes. However, the role of autophagy in the arcuate nucleus, which integrates all the metabolic signals, remains unknown. Therefore, the three following studies share the same prospect, to show and understand if autophagy participates in the energy balance and metabolism regulation by hypothalamic neurons.

Autophagy in hypothalamic AgRP neurons regulates food intake and energy balance

Kaushik S, Rodriguez-Navarro JA, Arias E, Kiffin R, Sahu S, Schwartz GJ, Cuervo AM, Singh R
Department of Medicine, Albert Einstein College of Medicine, Bronx, NY, USA
Cell Metab 2011;14:173–183

Background: Along with proopiomelanocortin (POMC) neurons, agouti-related peptide (AgRP)-expressing neurons belong to the complex neuronal system that integrates nutritional and metabolic signals in the hypothalamus. Therefore, the authors tested the hypothesis that altered autophagy in AgRP neurons may have a critical impact on the regulation of food intake and energy balance.

Methods and Results: The authors first showed that autophagy was induced in the hypothalamus of starved animals and led to an increase of AgRP expression. Functional studies in the hypothalamic cell line GT1-7 showed that the regulation of AgRP levels is due to an increase of free fatty acids generated by the degradation of endogenous lipids. The authors next generated a mouse line selectively lacking expression of the autophagy gene *Atg7* in AgRP neurons and showed they had impaired feeding and energy balance. Indeed, these mice had reduced body weight and total fat mass without modification of food intake. They further showed that altered autophagy led to a downregulation of *AgRP* in response to starvation whereas *POMC* was upregulated.

Conclusion: This study demonstrates that autophagy participates in the neuropeptide response to metabolic status and brings important functional insight into how such mechanisms may occur.

Autophagy was long thought to be induced in almost all tissues, but not in the brain. In this study, Kaushik et al. clearly demonstrate that starvation activates autophagy in the hypothalamus. By using in-vivo and in-vitro models, the authors first show that starvation induced autophagy in the AgRP neurons, mobilizing lipid droplets that stimulate *AgRP* expression, a neuropeptide that controls appetite. When autophagy was blocked, *AgRP* mRNA levels failed to rise upon starvation and α-*MSH* mRNA levels, a cleavage product of POMC, increased. This resulted in decreased animal body weight and total fat mass. Therefore, a high fat diet might trigger a vicious circle of overfeeding, as it might modify lipid metabolism in AgRP neurons. Finally, this study brings novel therapeutic targets for the treatment of obesity.

Loss of autophagy in proopiomelanocortin neurons perturbs axon growth and causes metabolic dysregulation

Coupe B, Ishii Y, Dietrich MO, Komatsu M, Horvath TL, Bouret SG
The Saban Research Institute, Neuroscience Program, Children's Hospital Los Angeles, University of Southern California, Los Angeles, CA, USA
Cell Metab 2012;15:247–255

Background: The neurons that produce the proopiomelanocortin (POMC)-derived peptides are part of the hypothalamic melanocortin system, which is a major negative regulator of energy balance. These neurons develop their unique features during neonatal life and begin to form functional neural systems through complex mechanisms such as autophagy, which is a major intracellular mechanism involved in the degradation of proteins and organelles which was recently shown to participate in the energy homeostasis.

Methods and Results: The authors tested the hypothesis that the autophagy-related gene, *Atg7*, a major autophagy gene, is essential to maturation of POMC neurons. Specific deletion of *Atg7* in POMC neurons resulted in higher postweaning body weight, increased adiposity and glucose intolerance. It also caused an age-dependent accumulation of ubiquitin and p62 aggregates in the arcuate nucleus as well as an abnormal development of POMC neuronal projections.

Conclusion: This study brings strong evidence that abnormal autophagy in the hypothalamus can lead to the pathogenesis of obesity and that the expression of Atg7 in POMC neurons is important for normal metabolic regulation and neurogenesis.

Role of hypothalamic proopiomelanocortin neuron autophagy in the control of appetite and leptin response

Quan W, Kim HK, Moon EY, Kim SS, Choi CS, Komatsu M, Jeong YT, Lee MK, Kim KW, Kim MS, Lee MS
Department of Medicine, Samsung Medical Center, Sungkyunkwan University School of Medicine, Seoul, Korea
Endocrinology 2012;153:1817–1826

Background: Autophagy has been described as a key cellular mechanism involved in body metabolism in many different tissues. However, its role in POMC neurons, which are key regulators of energy balance, remains unclear.

Methods and Results: This study aimed to examine the role of autophagy in leptin sensitivity, which is critical for the control of body weight. The authors generated a specific mouse line Atg7$^{\Delta POMC}$ in which the autophagy-related gene, *Atg7*, is specifically deleted in POMC neurons. Autophagy substrate, p62, was found to accumulate in POMC neurons and colocalized with ubiquitin. Atg7$^{\Delta POMC}$ were obese due to increased food intake and decreased exercise, and were unresponsive to leptin. The loss of Atg7 did not alter POMC neuron number but caused a reduced STAT3 phosphorylation upon leptin challenge.

Conclusion: Overall, these findings show that autophagy in POMC neurons is critical for the control of energy homeostasis and leptin signaling.

These two separate studies used the same experimental strategy to show that autophagy plays a key role in POMC neurons to regulate feeding and energy balance. Targeted deletion of the autophagy gene Atg7 (encoding ubiquitin E1-like ligase) in POMC neurons led to impaired autophagy in these neurons only and resulted in increased body weight and adiposity as well as perturbations in glucose homeostasis. Altogether, these two studies underline the importance of autophagy in the control of energy balance by POMC neurons processes. POMC neurons are major intermediates in leptin signaling, and both Coupé et al. and Quan et al. show that impaired energy balance is probably due to leptin unresponsiveness in *Atg7*-deleted POMC neurons. Coupé et al. also show that loss of autophagy impairs the ability of POMC neurons to send projections to their target nuclei, showing that autophagy participates in the complex neuronal network that regulates energy homeostasis. *Atg7* is a major autophagy gene, therefore the authors conclude that it is autophagy impairment that leads to energy homeostasis alterations. However, it is unlikely that Atg7 participates in a single cellular mechanism, as it was shown for other autophagy genes. Moreover, both studies show an increase of p62 accumulation in POMC neurons, and as p62 is involved in many intracellular signal transduction pathways, leptin unresponsiveness might be the result of several impairments of the global intracellular network. The authors focused their study on the arcuate nucleus of the hypothalamus but POMC is also expressed in corticotroph cells of the pituitary and in the hindbrain. Although Quan et al. bring evidence that cortisol levels are not altered in Atg7$^{\Delta POMC}$, one cannot rule out that loss of autophagy in these cells does not impact on the phenotype. Altogether, these two complementary articles bring a major advance in the understanding of the central control of energy balance and underline the importance of autophagy in metabolism regulation.

Uncoupling the mechanisms of obesity and hypertension by targeting hypothalamic IKK-β and NF-κB

Purkayastha S, Zhang G, Cai D
Department of Molecular Pharmacology, Albert Einstein College of Medicine, New York, NY, USA
Nat Med 2011;17:883–887

Background: Recent research on the pathophysiology of obesity has implicated a role for the hypothalamus. However, it remains unknown whether the often-seen coupling of hypertension with obesity can also be explained by hypothalamic dysfunction.
Methods and Results: Overexpression of a constitutively active IKK-β to activate NF-κB in the mediobasal hypothalamus elevated blood pressure in mice independently of obesity. This form of hypothalamic inflammation-induced hypertension was reversed by sympathetic suppression. Loss-of-function studies further showed that NF-κB inhibition in the mediobasal hypothalamus counteracted obesity-related hypertension in a manner that was dissociable from changes in body weight. The authors found that proopiomelanocortin (POMC) neurons were crucial for the hypertensive effects of the activation of hypothalamic IKK-β and NF-κB.
Conclusion: Obesity-associated activation of IKK-β and NF-κB in the mediobasal hypothalamus in the hypothalamic POMC neurons is a primary pathogenic link between obesity and hypertension. The treatment of hypothalamic inflammation is therefore a new avenue to control and prevent obesity-related hypertension.

Obesity-related hypertension in children is becoming more prevalent around the world as a consequence of widespread childhood obesity. Epidemiologic studies have shown that early hypertension in childhood increases the risk of developing hypertension later in life and an early treatment is important to reduce cardiovascular risk. Endocrine mechanisms, cytokine-related mechanisms as well as neuronal mechanisms have been proposed to explain obesity-related hypertension. In this study, the authors have showed the role of the sympathetic system in the occurrence of obesity-related hypertension in obese mouse fed with a high-fat diet. It is clear that obesity-related hypertension is not only due to one mechanism but their results indicate that treatment oriented toward the NF-κB system in POMC hypothalamic neurons may represent an original avenue to control obesity-related hypertension.

Evoked axonal oxytocin release in the central amygdala attenuates fear response

Knobloch HS, Charlet A, Hoffmann LC, Eliava M, Khrulev S, Cetin AH, Osten P, Schwarz MK, Seeburg PH, Stoop R, Grinevich V
Department of Molecular Neurobiology, Max Planck Institute for Medical Research, Heidelberg, Germany
Neuron 2012;73:553–566

Background: Recently, oxytocin (OT) received increasing attention for its effects on social behaviors. The mechanism of this effect and specifically how it reaches central brain regions is still unclear. In this study, the authors used a very recent and promising in-vivo strategy, the optogenetic model, to analyze this mechanism.
Methods: The authors used recombinant viruses to selectively express channel rhodopsin 2 (ChR2) in OT neurons and then activated ChR2 by blue light to locally induce the release of OT at the exon terminals of OT neurons.
Results: The authors initially validated the optogenetic model using fluorescent markers. Subsequently, they showed projection of OT axons in the central amygdala, a structure involved in OT-mediated fear suppression. Local blue-light induced an endogenous OT release in the central amygdala and decreased freezing responses in fear-conditioned rats.
Conclusion: This study shows the widespread central projections of hypothalamic OT neurons and demonstrates that OT release from local axonal endings can specifically control region-associated behaviors at distance from the hypothalamus.

This study is interesting for two mains reasons. The first reason is a strategic one, as it illustrates the optogenetic technique to specifically control neuropeptide release by axonal endings in a specific region of the brain. Optogenetics was declared by *Nature Methods* as the Method of the Year 2010 [Deisseroth K: Optogenetics. Nat Methods 2011;8:26–29]. This method is based on the idea that light may be used to experimentally control cell activity by expressing genetically encoded light-sensitive proteins in highly selected cell types. It offers the capacity to control neuronal activity at timescales relevant to the brain's in-vivo physiology. In this study, the authors adapted the method to study OT neuronal effects distal to the hypothalamus. Using virus-directed gene expression, they specifically expressed ChR2 in all hypothalamic OT neurons and at axon endings outside the hypothalamus. As blue-light activation was able to induce OT release, they were able to specifically analyze the effect of OT in the central amygdala. This is the second reason of the interest of this study. The authors showed that endogenous OT has an inhibitory effect in the central amygdala. This effect controls the fear response in fear-conditioned rats. The function of OT in the control of fear response is not new, but this study showed for the first time that this effect is mediated via OT neurons originated from the hypothalamus.

The development of optogenetics is going to completely change our in-vivo approach. It is now possible to specifically control cell activity and therefore should be very helpful to delineate the very complex hypothalamic regulation of the endocrine axis.

Pituitary

Evelien F. Gevers[a,b], Carles Gaston-Massuet[a] and Mehul T. Dattani[a]

[a]Developmental Endocrine Research Group, Clinical and Molecular Genetics Unit, Institute for Child Health, London, UK
[b]Great Ormond Street Hospital for Children, Department of Endocrinology, London, UK

Major breakthroughs were made in the field of pituitary research during the last year. A paper by Levkowitz's group shows that oxytocin itself is involved in hypothalamo-pituitary development and functions as a guidance molecule to form the neurovascular interface of the hypothalamo-neurohypophyseal system. Using several fluorescent tags, the vasculature was beautifully visualized in translucent fish so that development could be tracked. The second breakthrough was the accomplishment of the growth from embryonic stem cells in vitro of tissue that was similar to Rathke's pouch and developed into functioning pituitary cells. This development may open the way to future stem cell treatment for a variety of pituitary disorders. Further promising developments regard new treatments for Cushing's disease: the first using a tyrosine kinase inhibitor that targets the EGF receptor, and the second using pasireotide, a somatostatin agonist targeting the somatostatin receptor subtype 5, and further understanding of the pathogenesis of craniopharyngioma. Important for clinical endocrinology is a paper suggesting that permanent hypopituitarism is rare after traumatic brain injury, a paper describing a new association between ACTH deficiency and immune deficiency (DAVID) and the description of the largest cohort so far of isolated ACTH deficiency. Finally, a plethora of papers describing functional cell networks in the pituitary has been published this year.

Mechanism of the year

The hypothalamic neuropeptide oxytocin is required for formation of the neurovascular interface of the pituitary

Gutnick A, Blechman J, Kaslin J, Herwig L, Belting HG, Affolter M, Bonkowsky JL, Levkowitz G
Department of Molecular Cell Biology, Weizmann Institute of Science, Rehovot, Israel
Dev Cell 2011;21:642–654

Background: The neuropeptides oxytocin and arginine vasopressin are secreted directly into the circulation by the hypothalamus-neurohypophyseal system. These neuropeptides are synthesized by the magnocellular neurons from the hypothalamus and are transported to the neurohypophysis by axonal projections that meet the neurohypophyseal blood vessels. The connection between neurohypophyseal axons and the blood vessels form a congruent neurovascular interface. The development of this congruence and the molecular mechanisms underlying it are poorly understood.
Methods: To dissect the role of hypothalamic neurons in the formation of the neurovascular interface, transgenic zebrafish reporter lines were generated to allow the visualization of these neurons. Visualization of hypothalamic oxytocinergic cell bodies was accomplished by linking GFP to the regulatory region of the zebrafish oxytocin gene *oxtl* creating a *Oxtl:EGFP* transgenic line. Visualization of hypophyseal vasculature was accomplished by using a *vegfr2-Cherry* line. Generation of a double transgenic lines *Oxtl:EGFP;vegfr2-Cherry* allowed visualization of both oxytocinergic axons and blood vessels. Furthermore, conditional genetic ablation of oxytocinergic neurons was accomplished by the creation of a triple transgenic line *otpb:Gal4;UAS:NTRCherry;vegfr2:EGFP*. This transgenic line allows ablation of cells that express nitroreductase (NTR), an enzyme that converts the prodrug metronidazole into a potent cytotoxic agent. Since NTR is only expressed by the hypothalamic oxytocinergic neurons, cell-specific ablation is accomplished.
Results: Visualization of hypothalamic oxytocinergic neurons using the double zebrafish transgenic line *Oxtl:EGFP:vegfr2:Cherry* showed that axonal projections colonize the neurohypophysis before the vessels form. These hypothalamic projections into the neurohypophysis are independent of vessel formation, since *Cloche* mutants, that lack head vasculature, exhibit normal axonal innervation of the neurohypo-

physis. In order to assess if newly arrived neurohypophyseal axons are required for endothelial cells to form vessels, ablation of oxytocin neurons was performed using the triple transgenic line *otpb:Gal4;UAS:NTRCherry;vegfr2:EGFP*. Ablation of these neurons resulted in impaired hypophyseal vasculature indicating that neurohypophyseal axons are required for the formation of the neurovasculature interface.

Conclusion: Oxytocin functions as a guidance cue for endothelial cells to form the neurohypophyseal vasculature.

Although many molecules and pathways have been identified that direct neurovascular development, such as VEGF [1], class 3 semaphorins [2] and Eph:Ephrin signaling [3], the mechanisms that dictate neurovascular function in the secretory endocrine system is largely unknown. In this elegant article, Levkowitz and colleagues show a novel mechanism by which oxytocin-producing neurons signal to endothelial cells to form a congruent neurovascular interface. This neurovascular interface is required for the proper secretion of the hypothalamic neuropeptides into the bloodstream and the anterior pituitary, and therefore it is key to its proper endocrine function. Oxytocin has been reported to stimulate the migration and sprouting of human endothelial cells that express oxytocin receptor [4, 5]. Levkowitz and colleagues identify for the first time a molecular mechanism by which oxytocin functions as a vascular guidance cue to promote blood vessel formation. By using transgenic tools in the optically transparent zebrafish embryo, the authors visualized the formation of the neurovascular interface in the neurohypophysis. Genetic ablation of oxytocin-producing cells results in abnormal vascularization. As is the case for all very good articles, new questions arise from this work: Does oxytocin function as a vascular cue in other organs? Are other hypothalamic releasing factors important in the formation of the portal system that connects the anterior pituitary in mammals? Do other hypothalamic neuropeptides work in a similar fashion to oxytocin in attracting endothelial cells for their contact? Answers to these questions will emerge from future studies, but at present, this work sets the path towards understanding how the intricate congruence between the axonal projections and vessels is established in the pituitary.

New hope

Self-formation of functional adenohypophysis in three-dimensional culture

Suga H, Kadoshima T, Minaguchi M, Ohgushi M, Soen M, Nakano T, Takata N, Wataya T, Muguruma K, Miyoshi H, Yonemura S, Oiso Y, Sasai Y

Neurogenesis and Organogenesis Group, RIKEN Center for Developmental Biology, Kobe, Japan
Nature 2011;480:57–62

Background: No efficient stem cell culture for the generation of anterior pituitary cells is available, due to insufficient knowledge about induction of pituitary primordium (Rathke's pouch) in the embryonic head ectoderm. In this paper, efficient self-formation of three-dimensional anterior pituitary tissue in an aggregate culture of mouse embryonic stem (ES) cells was achieved.

Methods: ES cells were stimulated to differentiate into nonneural head ectoderm and hypothalamic neuroectoderm in adjacent layers within the aggregate, and treated with agonists of hedgehog signaling.

Results: Self-organization of Rathke's pouch-like three-dimensional structures occurred at the interface of these two epithelia. Various endocrine cells were subsequently produced and these cells were able to respond to trophic hormones.

Conclusion: Functional anterior pituitary tissue self-forms in culture after manipulation of ES cells, recapitulating local tissue interactions.

Growing pituitary spheres with hormone-producing cells from adult pituitary progenitors has been achieved [6] but rebuilding the pituitary from ES cells is a more complicated task. Relatively little is known about the formation of Rathke's pouch, knowledge needed to form a pituitary in a dish. The head ectoderm forms the outer parts of the head including the ears and eyes, and part of the ectoderm develops into Rathke's pouch. Interaction with the adjacent neuroepithelial cell layers that will form the hypothalamus is necessary for the formation of Rathke's pouch. In this paper, the authors succeeded in growing hormone-producing cells from ES cells within 3 weeks. They used specific conditions for ES cells to develop into hypothalamic like neuroepithelium and developed conditions in which ES cells formed rostral head ectoderm simultaneously. These aggregates expressed markers of neuroepithelium and head ectoderm adjacently. Hedgehog/BMPs and FGFs (FGF8, FGF10) play a vital role in midline brain development, and Rathke's pouch formation is disrupted in the absence of these factors [7]. The authors found that Sonic hedgehog agonist treatment of the cultures increased the Rathke's pouch marker Lhx3. The resulting 3D structures had a central cavity and the resemblance to Rathke's pouch was striking, as was the topographical location between the neuroepithelium and the rostral head-like ectoderm. The juxtaposition of the two tissues, mimicking the spatial organization in embryonic development, was indeed critical as Rathke's pouch-like vesicles did not develop when neuroepithelial tissue was not present.

One wonders whether this is the first step towards stem cell treatment for pituitary disorders. ACTH-expressing cells developed from the vesicle-like structures and activation of Wnt signaling led to expression of Pit1, GH and prolactin. LH/FSH/TSH expression was also achieved albeit after more intense manipulation of the culture conditions. When ES-derived cell aggregates were implanted under the kidney capsule in hypophysectomized mice, corticosterone was produced. The first step towards stem cell treatment may therefore indeed have been taken.

Another important aspect of this work is that it shows that processes taking place in the embryo with complex movements of structures, can be recapitulated in a dish and that induction of a tissue by adjacent tissue is possible in vitro. This is promising for the formation of other complex tissues in vitro, as noted by others [8].

It is amazing how small a tool kit of growth factors was required for the development of a complex structure like the pituitary from ES cells. The next paper shows that it takes even less to disrupt normal pituitary development and morphogenesis.

New mechanism – and new hope!

Increased wingless (Wnt) signaling in pituitary progenitor/stem cells gives rise to pituitary tumors in mice and humans

Gaston-Massuet C*, Andoniadou CL*, Signore M, Jayakody SA, Charolidi N, Kyeyune R, Vernay B, Jacques TS, Taketo MM, Le Tissier P, Dattani MT, Martinez-Barbera JP
Neural Development Unit, University College London Institute of Child Health, London, UK

Proc Natl Acad Sci USA 2011;108:11482–11487

Background: Adamantinomatous craniopharyngiomas are pediatric tumors located within the sellar/suprasellar region that often invade nearby structures in the brain and optic nerves. Craniopharyngiomas arise from the pituitary gland and account for 5–10% of all pediatric nonneural intracranial tumors. Mutations in the Wnt signaling effector β-catenin (*CTNNB1*, gene) have been identified in human craniopharyngioma, however neither a causative role for mutations in β-catenin, the cellular origin nor the pathogenesis of these tumors has been firmly established.

Methods: This work used transgenic mice to conditionally ablate exon3 of the β-catenin gene (*Ctnnb1-lox(ex3)*) in *Hesx1*-expressing Rathke's pouch progenitors. Deletion of exon3 (*Hesx1$^{Cre/+}$;Ctnnb1$^{+/lox(ex3)}$*) renders a degradation-resistant form of β-catenin, which results in the constitutive activation of the Wnt pathway in undifferentiated precursors of the pituitary gland.

Results: Activation of the Wnt/β-catenin pathway in the developing pituitary gland leads to craniopharyngioma-like pituitary tumors that express diagnostic markers of craniopharyngioma, such as β-catenin in cell clusters, cytokeratin 8 and 18, and fail to express hormones. Although all cells of the developing pituitary have mutated β-catenin, only a proportion of precursor cells were responsive to β-catenin mutations and formed tumor lesions. When mutated β-catenin was expressed in differentiated cells, no tumors developed indicating an undifferentiated pituitary precursor origin for craniopharyngioma. The cells responsive to mutated β-catenin were Sox2^{+ve}, p27Kip2^{+ve} Sox9^{-ve} and were quiescent in vivo, all characteristics of pituitary stem cells. Furthermore, the craniopharyngioma-mouse model contains an increased number of pituitary progenitor/stem cells, with a double rate of proliferation that underlies the formation of these tumors.

Conclusion: These results show a causative role for activating mutations in β-catenin in the genesis of craniopharyngioma. Furthermore, the cellular origin of these tumors are pituitary progenitors/stem cells, indicating that, like many other tumors, Wnt/β-catenin can influence the pituitary progenitor/stem cell pool and that activation of this pathway leads to tumors in mouse and humans.

In this article, Martinez-Barbera and co-workers identify for the first time a causative role of activating β-catenin mutations in the formation of adamantinomatous craniopharyngioma tumors. Although an association between mutations in β-catenin and craniopharyngioma had been reported previously [9, 10], a causative role had been elusive. Moreover, little was known about the etiology and cell origin of the tumors, and further research into these areas was hampered by the lack of an appropriate animal model. In this work, the authors have generated a valuable craniopharyngioma-mouse model that enabled them to perform important experiments indicating that only undifferentiated pituitary progenitors/stem cells are responsive to mutated β-catenin. Thus a previously unknown embryonic and stem cell origin of this tumor is established in this work. Moreover, this mouse model offers the possibility to identify pathways important in progression of craniopharyngioma. In fact, a recent paper by Andoniadou et al. [11] uses this mouse model to show differences in expression profiles of purified β-catenin-accumulating cells, suggesting that deregulation of pathways such as SHH, BMP and FGF are implicated in both mouse and human ACPs. Furthermore, this novel mouse model will be a very useful tool to test chemical compounds for their therapeutic effect in order to identify much needed medical treatment for craniopharyngiomas.

FGF-dependent midline-derived progenitor cells in hypothalamic infundibular development

Pearson CA, Ohyama K, Manning L, Aghamohammadzadeh S, Sang H, Placzek M
MRC Centre for Developmental and Biomedical Genetics and Department of Biomedical Science, University of Sheffield, Sheffield, UK
Development 2011;138:2613–2624

Background: Control of body homeostasis is accomplished by the hypothalamic-pituitary axis. The infundibulum, derived from the ventral diencephalon, is devoid of hormone-producing cells but contains the hypothalamic axonal projection that links the nervous and endocrine systems. Signals from the infundibulum are critical for the development and patterning of the underlying pituitary tissue. Despite its importance, very little is known about the development and cell origin of this critical embryonic structure.
Methods: This paper uses DiI/DiO labeling techniques in chick embryos to fate map cells to establish the origin of cells of the infundibulum. It uses a range of transplantation, immunostaining and in-situ hybridization techniques to identify different molecular profiles of the FP subpopulations.
Results: The infundibulum has a dual cell origin and comes from two different cell populations that reside in the ventral floor plate region of the forebrain, a region known to be involved in formation of the infundibulum. One population of cells forms the definitive infundibulum whilst the second population forms the so-called 'collar zone' that surrounds the infundibulum. These two distinct cell populations have differential gene expression. Collar zone cells can colonize the infundibulum over time and contain undifferentiated precursors/stem cells that can differentiate into multiple hypothalamic infundibular cell types.
Conclusion: The infundibulum is formed by two separate populations of cells that are derived from different forebrain floor plate cells. One distinct population, the collar cells, which are Fgf3+ Sox3+ are required for growth of the infundibulum.

The role of the infundibulum as a signaling center that controls the underlying Rathke's pouch development has been firmly studied. For instance, absence of infundibulum in the *Nkx2.1* null embryos results in failure of Rathke's pouch and anterior pituitary gland formation [12]. However, how the infundibulum develops into this separate anatomical structure remains poorly understood. Placzek and colleagues nicely described by using fate mapping and classical embryology techniques that infundibulum cells come from two forebrain floor plate cell populations. These two populations form two distinct structures, the infundibulum proper and the collar zone surrounding the infundibulum. This newly identified structure differentially expresses *Ffg3* and *Sox3*, and it promotes the maintenance and proliferation of the infundibulum through expression of FGF signals. This adds valuable information to our understanding of the infundibulum structure and raises questions about the requirement or sufficiency of the collar zone cells in infundibulum development. Future ablation experiments of the collar zone cells will provide further information on the exact specific requirement of these cells in infundibulum development.

Old genes – new knowledge

Phenotypic homogeneity and genotypic variability in a large series of congenital isolated ACTH-deficiency patients with TPIT gene mutations

Couture C, Saveanu A, Barlier A, Carel JC, Fassnacht M, Fluck CE, Houang M, Maes M, Fhan-Hug F, Enjalbert A, Drouin J, Brue T, Vallette S
Institut de Recherches Cliniques de Montreal, Montreal, Que., Canada
J Clin Endocrinol Metab 2012;97:E486–495

Background: TPIT, a T-box transcription factor, is restricted to POMC-expressing cells in the pituitary and essential for both POMC gene transcription and terminal differentiation of POMC-expressing cells. Congenital isolated ACTH deficiency was poorly defined before *TPIT* mutations were identified as its principal molecular cause. The authors enlarged their series of patients with isolated ACTH deficiency to better characterize the phenotype and the genotype of this rare disorder.

Methods: *TPIT* gene exons and exon/intron boundaries were sequenced in these patients. A functional analysis of each new *TPIT* mutation was performed. Clinical information of all 91 patients was collected.

Results: Three distinct groups were identified in the cohort: neonatal-onset complete or partial isolated ACTH deficiency or late-onset isolated ACTH deficiency. No *TPIT* mutations were detected in patients with partial or late-onset ACTH deficiency but *TPIT* mutations were found in 65% of patients with neonatal-onset complete ACTH deficiency. Nine new mutations were detected: four missense, one single nucleotide deletion, three splice-site mutations, and one large deletion. Different mechanisms lead to loss of function of TPIT, such as nonsense-mediated mRNA decay, abnormal mRNA splicing, loss of TPIT DNA binding or protein-protein interaction defects.

Conclusion: Two thirds of patients with neonatal-onset complete isolated ACTH deficiency have *TPIT* mutations but none of the patients with partial- or late-onset isolated ACTH deficiency had mutations in the gene.

This paper adds to our knowledge of adrenal insufficiency and also emphasizes the need to recognize the condition early. These authors have shown in the past that *TPIT* mutations are responsible for 60% of neonatal isolated ACTH deficiency. They now describe the largest cohort so far, consisting of 91 patients with isolated ACTH deficiency. This gives valuable information about this rare disorder that still results in neonatal deaths, in 25% of the families in this and the previous cohort [13]. *TPIT* mutations were found in 65% of patients with severe neonatal adrenal insufficiency, and in none of those with partial- or late-onset adrenal insufficiency. All patients with identified mutations had extremely severe adrenal insufficiency with very low cortisol concentrations (24 ± 6 nmol/l) from birth and absent or a weak response to intravenous CRH. All presented with severe hypoglycemia, 53% had associated seizures and 64% had cholestatic jaundice, which still is often unrecognized as a sign of hypocortisolism. An impressive 64% of the cases with *TPIT* mutations were familial and consanguinity was observed in 42%. Most mutations (35/37) were homozygous or compound heterozygous; heterozygous parents were unaffected. Mutations were distributed throughout the *TPIT* gene, but mainly in the T box, affecting DNA binding.

Of interest is the fact that, consistent with previous reports, *TPIT* mutations were not responsible for partial- or late-onset isolated ACTH deficiency. Mutations in regulatory sequences of *TPIT* could be responsible for less severe adrenal insufficiency, but these have yet to be identified.

Related pituitary cell lineages develop into interdigitated 3D cell networks

Budry L, Lafont C, El Yandouzi T, Chauvet N, Conejero G, Drouin J, Mollard P
Laboratory of Molecular Genetics, Institut de Recherches Cliniques de Montreal, Montreal, Que., Canada
Proc Natl Acad Sci USA 2011;108:12515–12520

Background: Terminally differentiated secreting cells are not distributed randomly in a patchwork-like fashion throughout the pituitary gland. Instead, data suggest that these cells organize themselves in homotypic networks. This was first shown by Bonnefont et al. when growth hormone (GH)-secreting cells were visualized in pituitary slices using high-resolution imaging [14]. The connectivity between the cells of this network is important for the delivery of coordinated secretory pulses of hormones to their target tissues. The current article addresses the question of whether the two least abundant pituitary cell types, corticotrophs and gonadotrophs, are also organized in homotypic cell networks and if the interaction between these cells within the networks is important for their development and function.

Methods: High-resolution multiphoton imaging and confocal reconstruction was used to visualize corticotrophs and gonadotrophs in 3D throughout pituitary development. POMC-GFP and LH-Cer (cerulean fluorescence) transgenic mice were used to specifically detect corticotrophs and gonadotrophs throughout their ontogeny in the pituitary gland.

Results: Like the GH cells, corticotrophs and gonadotrophs also form homotypic cell networks during development. The Pit1-independent cell lineage networks may function in a similar way to the Pit1-dependent somatotroph network to better integrate and propagate cell responses. Structural differences between corticotroph and gonadotroph cell networks exist at the cellular level. Gonadotrophs are in close proximity to microvasculature, whilst the corticotroph network is established away from microvasculature and hence, corticotrophs extend processes or cytonemes. Furthermore, heterotypic interactions occur during development, such that the gonadotroph network depends on differentiated corticotrophs that act as a scaffold.

Conclusion: Pituitary scale-3D high-resolution imaging has identified cell networks of corticotrophs and gonadotrophs. These networks develop specific cell-cell interactions that lead to ordered positioning of pituitary cells.

Existence of long-lasting experience-dependent plasticity in endocrine cell networks

Hodson DJ, Schaeffer M, Romano N, Fontanaud P, Lafont C, Birkenstock J, Molino F, Christian H, Lockey J, Carmignac D, Fernandez-Fuente M, Le Tissier P, Mollard P
Centre National de la Recherche Scientifique, Institut de Génomique Fonctionnelle, Montpellier, France
Nat Commun 2012;3:605

Background: Hormone-producing cells in the pituitary are organized in homotypic cell networks rather than randomly placed through the pituitary gland. In some biological systems that are organized into networks, an experience-dependent plasticity exists that confers adaptive advantage to physiological changes. For instance in the nervous system, continuous stimulation leads to changes in the wiring and number of synaptic contacts. This article explores a potential role for experience-dependent plasticity in the organized cell networks of the pituitary gland.

Methods: Transgenic mice expressing DsRed under the *Prl* promoter were used throughout this work. Moreover, a multibeam two-photon high-resolution calcium imaging system was utilized to analyze changes in cytosolic Ca^{2+} as well as visualization of prolactin cells in vivo.

Results: By using lactation to repeatedly stimulate the lactotroph cell network, the authors show that the lactotroph cell network undergoes functional plasticity in response to stimuli. Upon lactation, this cell population establishes a functional connectivity template. This is mediated through cell morphological changes and gap junctions and establishes a long-lasting pattern that results in a long-term experience-dependent plasticity.

Conclusion: The pituitary lactotrophs arrange themselves in homotypic cellular network that have long-term experience-dependent responses to physiological changes. This allows for better functional adaptation to physiological changes to mount homeostatic responses.

Influence of estrogens on GH-cell network dynamics in females: a live in-situ imaging approach

Schaeffer M, Hodson DJ, Meunier AC, Lafont C, Birkenstock J, Carmignac D, Murray JF, Gavois E, Robinson IC, Le Tissier P, Mollard P
Centre National de la Recherche Scientifique, Institute of Functional Genomics, Institut National de la Sante et de la Recherche Médicale, Montpellier, France
Endocrinology 2011;152:4789–4799

Background: Pituitary hormone production is tightly regulated and adapts to changing physiological status and environmental stimuli. The pituitary gland must therefore undergo marked structural and functional plasticity. This is thought to primarily rely on changes in cell proliferation and size. This study investigated whether cell motility, important for organ development during embryogenesis, represents an additional mechanism to promote plasticity within the adult pituitary gland.
Methods: Multiphoton time-lapse imaging methods were used to track cell dynamics over a period of 12 h in GH-eGFP transgenic mice to assess adaptation of the GH axis to varying gonadal steroid environments.
Results: Ovariectomy induced a dramatic increase in cell motility associated with GH-cell network remodeling. Estradiol treatment after ovariectomy prevented these changes. Estradiol also increased coordinated GH-cell activity during multicellular calcium recordings, suggesting enhanced network connectivity. Male castration did not result in similar alterations.
Conclusion: GH-cell motility is involved in the structural and functional pituitary plasticity in response to changing estradiol concentrations in the female.

These three articles, by Chauvet, Hodson and Schaeffer from Mollard's laboratory elegantly show that terminally differentiated hormone-producing cells of the pituitary are organized in homotypic cell networks and that these cellular networks generate experience-dependent responses. Previous work by Bennefont et al. refuted the previous dogma of pituitary cells being organized in a random patchwork fashion, and showed that GH cells form a three-dimensional network of cadherin-linked cells [14]. This somatotroph network exhibits a large-scale coordinated increase in intracellular calcium associated with hormone pulses. This distribution of cells into networks facilitates the coordinated physiological responses to stimuli. This article raised the question of whether other pituitary cell types exhibited a specific cell network distribution. Making use of powerful 3D two photon high-resolution imaging techniques combined with mouse transgenics, Chauvet and colleagues now demonstrate that two other pituitary cell types, corticotrophs (POMC-EGFP) and gonadotrophs (LH-Cer), are organized in distinct homotypic cell networks that are intertwined. Interestingly, heterotypic interactions between the corticotroph and the gonadotroph networks exist, as shown by hyperplasia of the gonadotroph network in the *Tpit* null mice that lack POMC cells. Moreover, the corticotroph network acts as a scaffold to gonadotrophs during development, further indicating the interdependence of these two cell networks. Impressive work from Hodson et al., delves deeper into the function of these networks, and identifies for the first time the important phenomenon of experience-dependent plasticity within the lactotroph network. Hodson and co-workers utilize system biology with high-resolution imaging and physiology to understand the impact on the lactotroph network upon continuous stimulation (lactation). Interestingly, a pattern/template is established by cell-cell communication during lactation which may improve cell population responses to future lactation. These exciting studies not only offer novel insights into our understanding of pituitary physiology, but also suggest new tools and methods to further characterize pituitary phenotypes in mutant mouse strains. Previous work in the pituitary development area has mostly centered on a two-dimensional analysis of the pituitary gland, and by doing so, important information on how genes affect cell network formation or function, and thus pituitary function, has been overlooked.

Pulsatile patterns of pituitary hormone gene expression change during development

Featherstone K, Harper CV, McNamara A, Semprini S, Spiller DG, McNeilly J, McNeilly AS, Mullins JJ, White MR, Davis JR
Developmental Biomedicine Research Group, Faculty of Medical and Human Sciences, University of Manchester, Manchester, UK
J Cell Sci 2011;124:3484–3491

Background: Recent research has attempted to investigate the important issue of the timing of transcription in living cells. Studies on clonal cell lines have shown that transcription is often pulsatile and stochastic, with implications for cellular differentiation. However, few studies have investigated changes in transcriptional activity during development at cellular resolution within a physiological context. In this study, the authors aimed to study the transcription of the gene encoding prolactin at various developmental stages.

Methods: To investigate single-cell transcriptional activity in real-time in living tissue, the authors used bioluminescence imaging of pituitary tissue from transgenic rats in which luciferase gene expression is driven by the prolactin (*Prl*) promoter. The authors studied both fetal and neonatal pituitary tissue to assess whether dynamic patterns of transcription change during tissue development.

Results: The authors report that gene expression in single cells is highly pulsatile and rapidly turns on and off at the time lactotrophs first appear during murine fetal development (E16.5); later on *Prl* gene expression levels increase but become stabilized as the tissue develops in early neonatal life. Since isolated cells, generated from enzymatic dispersion of pituitary tissue, display pulsatile luminescence, the stabilized transcription pattern might depend upon tissue architecture or paracrine signaling. Nascent cells in embryonic tissue also showed coordinated transcription activity over short distances, further indicating that cellular context is important for transcription activity.

Conclusion: These data show that transcriptional activity is a dynamic process, and cells alter their patterns of gene expression according to their context and developmental stage, with important implications for cellular differentiation.

This is an important study using a combination of transgenesis and single cell transcriptional assays. The authors show that prolactin gene expression is dynamic from an early stage. During embryogenesis, from E16.5 in the rat embryo, lactotrophs show pulsatile transcriptional responses of prolactin gene expression. As gestation progresses, the transcriptional activity is more stable. Hence, lactotrophs alter their transcription pattern depending on their developmental context. These data suggest the importance of transcriptional patterns on cell differentiation. The authors suggest that pulsatile gene expression early in tissue development may occur before lineage commitment, when numerous genes might exist in a poised state and can be transcribed at low levels. Commitment to a cell lineage leads to higher expression of the required genes and silencing of other genes. This hypothesis is supported by observations that chromatin structure exists in a globally open and plastic conformation in embryonic stem cells and adopts a more closed structure upon cell differentiation. The authors also show that the stable transcriptional activity of neonatal lactotroph cells switches to a pulsatile pattern when the pituitary tissue is enzymatically dispersed. Hence, the architecture of the tissue in which the cells are located is also critical in determining patterns of gene expression. These studies have wider applications, and suggest that gene transcription may vary according to developmental stage and the cellular context. Paracrine cell signaling may be critical for normal gene expression, and it is important to note that transcriptional activity may differ in isolated cells in vitro and in vivo.

Disruption of SoxB1-dependent Sonic hedgehog expression in the hypothalamus causes septo-optic dysplasia

Zhao L, Zevallos SE, Rizzoti K, Jeong Y, Lovell-Badge R, Epstein DJ
Department of Genetics, Perelman School of Medicine, University of Pennsylvania, Philadelphia, PA, USA
Dev Cell 2012;22:585–596

Background: The congenital birth defect septo-optic dysplasia (SOD) is characterized by optic nerve, midline forebrain and/or pituitary gland abnormalities. Only a few genes that cause SOD have been identified, amongst others *Hesx1*, *Sox2* and *Sox3* are implicated. The precise role of other genes in the etiology of SOD is poorly understood. *Sonic hedgehog* (*Shh*) is an important gene that regulates early formation and patterning of the central nervous system. Its haploinsufficiency in humans causes holoprosencephaly (HPE). *SHH* is crucial for the formation of the hypothalamus and HPE patients can exhibit a compromised hypothalamic-pituitary axis. However, studies into the role of *Shh* in murine hypothalamic development have been hampered by the severe phenotype of the *Shh* null embryos. In this paper, using a conditional gene targeting approach, the requirement of the hypothalamus for *Shh* is unraveled.
Methods: Use of a transgenic approach to achieve specific ventral-diencephalic (VD) deletion of *Shh* by crossing a *Shh^{loxp/loxp}* to the *SBE:Cre* line (where Cre is expressed under the *Shh*-brain enhancer-2 *SBE2*). This transgenic line (*Shh^{Δhyp}*) results in deletion of Shh in the VD whilst expression of Shh in other parts of the brain remains uncompromised, allowing the study of the role of Shh in the hypothalamus and in the phenotype of SOD.
Results: Expression of Shh in the VD is required for proper patterning of the prospective hypothalamic region. Absence of Shh in *Shh^{Δhyp}* embryos leads to hypoplasia of the pituitary gland and abnormal early patterning and positioning of the hypothalamus. Moreover, *Shh* morphogen activity from the VD is required for the proper patterning of the retina and for optic disc formation. The *SBE2* enhancer that directs expression of *Shh* in the hypothalamus contains highly conserved SOXB1-binding sites and Sox2 and Sox3 directly regulate Shh expression by binding to the SBE2 enhancer.
Conclusion: Ventral diencephalic expression of *Shh* is regulated by Sox2 and Sox3, and the absence of *Shh* signaling causes SOD-like features in the mouse.

This article describes, for the first time, the requirement of Shh signaling from the embryonic prospective hypothalamic region in the formation of the hypothalamic-pituitary axis and eye development. A role for oral ectoderm-Shh-derived signaling has been described to be important for pituitary formation, and the lack of Shh in the oral ectoderm results in the absence of ventral pituitary cell types [3, 7]. However, the role of SHH emanating from other sources such as the ventral diencephalon in the formation of the hypothalamus was unknown. Absence of *Shh* from the prechordal plate causes HPE; the telencephalic vesicles fail to divide, resulting in cyclopic embryos. Due to this severe phenotype the study of *Shh*-associated phenotypes was hampered. Epstein and colleagues ablated *Shh* from the ventral diencephalon (the prospective hypothalamic region) by using a neat conditional transgenic line that expresses Cre under the Shh-ventral diencephalon-specific enhancer (*SEB2:Cre*) [15]. This method allows expression of Shh to be normal in the prechordal plate, thereby bypassing the severe Shh-HPE phenotype. Interestingly, Shh expression from the ventral diencephalon is required for both eye disc formation and hypothalamic-pituitary development. In the absence of *Shh* signaling the pituitary is hypoplastic and the hypothalamic region displays patterning defects, reminiscent of SOD. The authors go one step further and identify SoxB1-binding sites in the Shh-ventral diencephalon enhancer and show with biochemical assays that *SOX2* and *SOX3* regulate *Shh* expression in the VD. As SOX2 and SOX3 have been shown to be involved in SOD, these phenotypes could be linked to the lack of early Shh expression from the prospective hypothalamus. Thus, understanding how these genes regulate transcriptional cascades will provide a further explanation for a congenital malformation such as SOD.

EGFR as a therapeutic target for human, canine, and mouse ACTH-secreting pituitary adenomas

Fukuoka H, Cooper O, Ben-Shlomo A, Mamelak A, Ren SG, Bruyette D, Melmed S
Pituitary Center, Department of Medicine, Cedars-Sinai Medical Center, Los Angeles, CA, USA
J Clin Invest 2011;121:4712–4721

Background: Cushing's disease is a condition in which the pituitary gland releases excessive adrenocorticotropic hormone (ACTH) as a result of an adenoma arising from ACTH-secreting cells. Optimal therapy currently entails surgical adenoma resection, with initial remission rates of 65–90% for microadenomas and <65% for macroadenomas. However, 10-year recurrence rates are 10–20% for microadenomas and up to 45% for macroadenomas. Pituitary-directed medical therapies are mostly ineffective, and new treatment options are needed. As these tumors express EGFR, the authors tested whether EGFR might provide a therapeutic target for Cushing's disease.

Methods: The effect of gefitinib, a tyrosine kinase inhibitor (TKI) that targets the EGFR, was tested on human corticotroph adenoma cells that express EGFR, and on ACTH-producing canine pituitary tumor cells. Additionally, the drug was tested on a murine corticotroph adenoma, investigating both cell proliferation and apoptosis.

Results: The authors show that in surgically resected human and canine corticotroph cultured tumors, blocking EGFR with gefitinib suppressed expression of proopiomelanocortin (POMC) as well as ACTH secretion. In mouse corticotroph EGFR transfectants, ACTH secretion was enhanced, and EGF increased Pomc promoter activity, an effect that was MAPK-dependent. Blocking EGFR activity with gefitinib attenuated Pomc expression, inhibited corticotroph tumor cell proliferation, and induced apoptosis. As predominantly nuclear EGFR expression was observed in canine and human corticotroph tumors, EGFR was preferentially targeted to mouse corticotroph cell nuclei, which resulted in higher Pomc expression and ACTH secretion, both of which were inhibited by gefitinib. In athymic nude mice, EGFR overexpression enhanced the growth of explanted ACTH-secreting tumors and further elevated serum corticosterone concentrations. Gefitinib treatment decreased both tumor size and corticosterone concentrations; it also reversed signs of hypercortisolemia, including elevated glucose concentrations and excess omental fat.

Conclusions: These results suggest that inhibition of EGFR signaling may be a novel strategy for treating Cushing's disease, and gefinitib may be a potential therapeutic agent in Cushing's disease.

A 12-month phase 3 study of pasireotide in Cushing's disease

Colao A, Petersenn S, Newell-Price J, Findling JW, Gu F, Maldonado M, Schoenherr U, Mills D, Salgado LR, Biller BM
Department of Molecular and Clinical Endocrinology and Oncology, Section of Endocrinology, University of Naples Federico II, Naples, Italy
N Engl J Med 2012;366:914–924

Background: Cushing's disease is associated with high morbidity and mortality. Therapy is challenging, with relapse in up to 30% of patients. Corticotroph adenomas express somatostatin receptors, predominantly somatostatin-receptor subtype 5. A novel potential therapy, pasireotide, has a unique, broad somatostatin-receptor-binding profile, with high binding affinity for somatostatin-receptor subtype 5.

Methods: In this double-blind, phase 3 study, 162 adults with Cushing's disease and a urinary-free cortisol level of at least 1.5 times the upper limit of the normal range were randomly assigned to receive subcutaneous pasireotide at a dose of 600 μg (82 patients) or 900 μg (80 patients) twice daily. Patients with urinary-free cortisol not exceeding 2 times the upper limit of the normal range (ULN) and not exceeding the baseline level at month 3 continued to receive their randomly assigned dose; all others received an additional 300 μg twice daily. Primary endpoint: a urinary-free cortisol level at or below the upper limit of the normal range at month 6 without an increased dose. Open-label treatment continued through month 12.

Results: Twelve of 82 patients in the 600-μg group and 21 of 80 patients in the 900-μg group met the primary endpoint. The median urinary-free cortisol level decreased by approximately 50% by month 2 and remained stable in both groups. A normal urinary-free cortisol level was achieved more frequently in patients with baseline levels not exceeding 5 times the ULN range than in patients with higher baseline levels. Serum and salivary cortisol and plasma corticotropin levels decreased, and clinical signs and symptoms of Cushing's disease diminished. Pasireotide was associated with hyperglycemia-related adverse events in 118 of 162 patients; other adverse events were similar to those associated with other somatostatin analogues. Despite reductions in cortisol concentrations, blood glucose and glycated hemoglobin concentrations increased soon after treatment initiation and then stabilized; treatment with a glucose-lowering medication was initiated in 74 of 162 patients.

Conclusion: The significant decrease in cortisol concentrations in patients with Cushing's disease who received pasireotide supports its potential use as a targeted treatment for corticotropin-secreting pituitary adenomas.

These two papers tackle the thorny issue of Cushing's disease, a condition that can be challenging to treat. In children and adolescents with Cushing's disease, 80–85% have surgically identifiable microadenomas; 20% relapse post-surgery with a net cure rate of 70–75%. Radiotherapy is used if surgery is unsuccessful; children respond more rapidly, with a cure rate of 92%. However, GHD is common and other pituitary hormone deficiencies may occur, although with a lower frequency.

Recent advances have revealed a role for novel signaling pathways in the etiology of Cushing's disease, one of which is the EGFR signaling pathway. The paper by Fukuoka et al. has utilized this pathway to identify novel medical therapies; EGFR led to increased *POMC* promoter activity with an increase in ACTH secretion. The authors then used a tyrosine kinase inhibitor, gefitinib, to block EGFR signaling and found that corticotroph tumor cell proliferation was reduced and apoptosis induced. In mice, in vivo studies revealed that Gefitinib treatment decreased both tumor size and corticosterone concentrations; it also reversed signs of hypercortisolemia. These data are promising, but whether they will translate to human patients with Cushing's disease remains to be seen. In particular, the interruption of the EGFR signaling pathway in other organs may lead to a number of unwanted effects.

In the second study, Colao and colleagues have used a somatostatin receptor subtype 5 agonist, pasireotide, for the treatment of Cushing's disease. The results are promising, with a reduction in cortisol secretion and improvement in clinical features such as hypertension. However, there is a significant increase in the degree of hyperglycemia, with adverse events due to elevated blood glucose concentrations being documented in 118/162 patients. Currently, the potential indication for this drug would appear to be in resistant cases of Cushing's disease.

Concepts revised

Permanent hypopituitarism is rare after structural traumatic brain injury in early childhood

Heather NL, Jefferies C, Hofman PL, Derraik JG, Brennan C, Kelly P, Hamill JK, Jones RG, Rowe DL, Cutfield WS
Liggins Institute, University of Auckland, Auckland, New Zealand
J Clin Endocrinol Metab 2012;97:599–604

Background: Hypopituitarism or isolated GH deficiency can occur after traumatic brain injury. This study aimed to determine the incidence of permanent hypopituitarism in a group of young children after structural traumatic brain injury (TBI).
Methods: This is a cross-sectional study with longitudinal follow-up. Pituitary function was dynamically tested in all subjects. Diagnosis of GH deficiency was based on assessment of stimulated GH peak (<5 µg/l), IGF-I, and growth pattern. ACTH deficiency was diagnosed if there was a subnormal response to two serial Synacthen tests (peak cortisol <500 nmol/l) and a Metyrapone test.
Results: 198 survivors of structural TBI sustained at an early age (1.7 ± 1.5 years) were studied 6.5 ± 3.2 years after injury. Brain injury was inflicted in 33% and accidental in 68%. Precocious puberty occurred in 2 patients, just within the expected rate for the normal population. Peak stimulated GH was <5 µg/l in 16 participants (8%), but these children had normal IGF-I and normal growth. Stimulated peak

cortisol was low in 17 (8%), but all had normal ACTH function on Metyrapone testing. One participant had a transient low serum T_4.

Conclusion: Permanent hypopituitarism is rare after both inflicted and accidental TBI in early childhood. Precocious puberty was the only pituitary hormone abnormality found, but the prevalence did not exceed that of the normal population.

This is an important study that gives insight into the incidence of pituitary dysfunction after brain injury, which may develop probably as a result of injury to portal vessels. Many reports over the last decade have emphasized the occurrence of such pituitary insufficiency, and a recent meta-analysis in adults reported the rate of hypopituitarism in traumatic brain injury being as high as 30%. Studies in children show a highly variable rate of hypopituitarism (5–60%), possibly due to the variable severity of brain injury, small cohort size and nonstandardized methodology. This study by Heather et al. stands out because of its large homogeneous cohort of patients with severe brain injury leading to structural abnormalities (198 patients, 40% intensive care treatment, 66% intracerebral hemorrhage, 66% cerebral injury and 70% skull fractures) and its thorough analysis of pituitary function.

In contrast to other studies, none of the patients had permanent hypopituitarism, despite the severe degree of brain injury. Precocious puberty was the only endocrine abnormality found although, despite the large size of the group, the rate was too low to know whether this was due to brain injury. Low GH responses to GH testing were noted (33% had a GH peak <10 µg/l) but, in contrast to other studies and following national guidelines, a diagnosis of GH deficiency was only made if there was a combination of low GH peak (<5 µg/l) on two stimulation tests, low IGF-1 concentration and poor growth. The authors show biochemical and growth details of the patients with GH peaks <5 µg/l, supporting the absence of GHD although growth charts were not shown. Of note is the presence of obesity in all of these children (BMI +2 to 3 SD); the authors suggest that this may be the reason for their low GH peak concentration. Similarly, a diagnosis of ACTH deficiency was only made if both Synacthen and Metyrapone tests were abnormal, but this occurred in none of the patients.

In conclusion, permanent hypopituitarism is uncommon after severe brain injury in young children when stringent clinical criteria for pituitary insufficiency are used. Routine testing of pituitary function, as suggested for adults, may not be necessary in children and will lead to a high number of abnormal test results, the significance of which is unknown.

Concepts (not) revised

Aged PROP1-deficient dwarf mice maintain ACTH production

Nasonkin IO, Ward RD, Bavers DL, Beuschlein F, Mortensen AH, Keegan CE, Hammer GD, Camper SA
Department of Human Genetics, University of Michigan, Ann Arbor, MI, USA
PLoS One 2011;6:e28355

Background: *PROP1* mutations in humans are associated with the phenotype of multiple pituitary hormone deficiencies (MPHD) that typically progress from growth deficiency/insufficiency (GHD/GHI) diagnosed in infancy to include other hormone (GH) deficiencies including TSH, prolactin and gonadotrophin deficiencies. This progressive reduction in other anterior pituitary hormones eventually includes ACTH deficiency. It is therefore critically important to test the hypothalamo-pituitary-adrenal (HPA) axis regularly in order to detect evolving ACTH deficiency at a pre-symptomatic stage. Congenital deficiencies of GH, prolactin, and thyroid stimulating hormone have been reported in the *Prop1*(null) (*Prop1*(–/–)) and the Ames dwarf (*Prop1*(*df/df*)) mouse models, but corticotroph and pituitary adrenal axis function have not been thoroughly investigated in these murine models.

Methods: *Prop1* null mutants were generated on the N4 B6 background. Corticosterone, ACTH and blood glucose concentrations were measured basally and in response to restraint stress. Adrenal glands were weighed.

Results: The N4 B6 background results in a wasting phenotype in the mutant mice that is associated with severe hypoglycemia and lethality in approximately one third of the mice, between weaning and adulthood; remaining homozygotes live with no signs of illness. Circulating ACTH and corticosterone levels are elevated in juvenile and aged *Prop1* mutants, indicating activation of the pituitary-adrenal axis. Despite this, young adult Prop1-deficient mice are capable of responding to restraint stress with further elevation of ACTH and corticosterone. The elevation in ACTH and corticosterone concentrations, which is present basally, is likely due to low blood glucose concentrations, which in turn is possibly due to GH deficiency. In keeping with the chronically elevated ACTH and corticosterone concentrations, the ratio of adrenal weight to body weight was elevated in *Prop1*$^{-/-}$ males compared to wild type animals.

Conclusion: The Prop1-deficient mouse model differs from the human patients who display progressive hormone loss and hypocortisolism. The underlying reason for the ACTH deficiency in humans remains unknown.

Mutations in the gene *PROP1* are not infrequently identified in patients with familial MPHD. The phenotype includes GH, TSH, prolactin and gonadotrophin deficiencies and can be highly variable. In particular, the TSH and gonadotrophin deficiencies can develop later, with puberty commencing spontaneously in a number of cases but then failing to progress. Two clinical features of human PROP1 deficiency are particularly perplexing; namely the later evolution of ACTH deficiency with hypocortisolemia and an enlarged pituitary gland that then involutes. For neither phenomenon has a satisfactory explanation been advanced to date. This paper has attempted to answer the first of these questions. However, the authors clearly show that murine Prop1 mutants manifest increased lethality, but this is not related to ACTH or corticosterone deficiency. In fact, the mutant mice have elevated ACTH and corticosterone concentrations, and these chronically elevated measurements are probably related to GH deficiency. In keeping with these data, the adrenals were relatively enlarged in the affected mice. Hence these data suggest important differences between mice and humans in terms of the HPA axis.

Deficit in anterior pituitary function and variable immune deficiency (DAVID) in children presenting with adrenocorticotropin deficiency and severe infections

Quentien MH, Delemer B, Papadimitriou DT, Souchon PF, Jaussaud R, Pagnier A, Munzer M, Jullien N, Reynaud R, Galon-Faure N, Enjalbert A, Barlier A, Brue T
Centre de Recherche en Neurobiologie et Neurophysiologie de Marseille, Aix-Marseille Universite, Marseille, France
J Clin Endocrinol Metab 2012;97:E121–128

Background: The French GENHYPOPIT network contained 21 patients with isolated ACTH deficiency without a TPIT mutation. Three of those (13.6%) displayed common variable immunodeficiency (CVID). The authors present this previously unrecognized disease association.

Methods: The hypothesis of ACTH deficiency being associated with antipituitary autoimmunity or lymphocytic hypophysitis was tested using assays for pituitary auto-antibodies. A candidate gene approach and sequence analysis was used to detect a common underlying gene alteration.

Results: All patients including a pedigree with two affected siblings had ACTH deficit diagnosed from 5 to 15 years, and CVID diagnosed from 2 to 8 years revealed by recurrent infections. Three of the four patients had a hypoplastic pituitary. One patient had low IGF-I and subnormal GH response to stimulation, suggesting that secretion of other pituitary hormones may also be affected. All patients proved negative for pituitary autoantibodies and had no alteration in the genes *LIF, IKAROS* or *EOS*.

Conclusions: The remarkable association of two rare disorders affecting two functionally related systems in four patients from three independent pedigrees, including a familial case, provides strong evidence of the existence of a disease association: deficit in anterior pituitary function and variable immune deficiency, or DAVID.

The paper shows the importance of maintaining databases for the detection and understanding of rare diseases. The GENHYPOPIT database is a clinical research network in France that contains approx. 700 index cases with CPHD. The authors recognized that of 31 patients with isolated ACTH deficiency, 4 patients (both male and female) from 3 separate families also had Common Variable Immune Deficiency. Most patients showed anterior pituitary hypoplasia on MRI but no other anatomical abnormalities. CVID is a hugely heterogeneous disorder but all patients suffered from the same type of CVID supporting the notion that this is a previously unrecognized disease association that the authors named 'Deficit in Anterior pituitary function and Variable Immune Deficiency', or DAVID. A candidate gene approach was not sufficient to pinpoint the underlying genetic aetiology, but next generation sequencing is what is really needed to establish the cause of this new disease association.

Important for clinical practice

Symptomatic heterozygotes and prenatal diagnoses in a nonconsanguineous family with syndromic combined pituitary hormone deficiency resulting from two novel LHX3 mutations

Sobrier ML, Brachet C, Vie-Luton MP, Perez C, Copin B, Legendre M, Heinrichs C, Amselem S
Institut National de la Sante et de la Recherche Medicale Unite 933, Universite Pierre et Marie Curie-Paris 6, Hopital Armand Trousseau, Paris, France
marie-laure.sobrier@inserm.fr
J Clin Endocrinol Metab 2012;97:E503–509

Background: LHX3 is a member of the LIM family of transcription factors that has been shown to be important for the normal development of the anterior pituitary gland and motor neurons. To date, 11 mutations have been reported in *LHX3*; all patients were homozygous from consanguineous pedigrees, with various syndromic forms of combined pituitary hormone deficiency (CPHD), including limited rotation of the neck and sensorineural hearing loss.

Methods: The authors aimed to report the family history and the molecular basis of a nonconsanguineous patient with syndromic CPHD, limited neck rotation, severe scoliosis, but normal intelligence. His father and paternal grandmother displayed limited head rotation. In view of this, the authors sequenced the *LHX3* gene. Novel mutations were then inserted into plasmids and functional studies were performed using transcriptional activation assays with the human PRL promoter.

Results: Two new *LHX3* mutations were identified. The paternally inherited c.252-3C>G mutation, which disrupts an acceptor splice site, led to severely truncated proteins containing a single LIM domain, resembling LIM-only proteins. Co-expression studies revealed a dominant-negative effect of this LIM-only protein over the wild-type LHX3. The maternally inherited p.Cys118Tyr mutation resulted in partial loss of transcriptional activity and synergy with POU1F1. Given the severity of the patient's phenotype, prenatal diagnoses were performed on two occasions: the first led to termination of the pregnancy whilst the second resulted in the birth of a healthy boy.

Conclusion: This study reports the first nonconsanguineous patient with *LHX3* mutations and supports the pleiotropic roles of LHX3 during development and its involvement in a complex disease phenotype. Isolated limitation of head rotation may exist in heterozygous carriers and may result from a dominant-negative effect. These data allowed the first published description of prenatal diagnoses of this severe condition.

Mutations within the early transcription factors and signaling molecules involved in anterior pituitary gland formation are often associated with complex syndromic phenotypes in association with hypopituitarism. Initially, mutations in *LHX3* were identified in patients with hypopituitarism associated with limited neck rotation. It was felt that corticotrophs were spared and ACTH deficiency was not a feature of the syndrome. Subsequently, patients with *LHX3* mutations were noted to be ACTH-deficient, and in patients with mutations in the C-terminus of the protein, neck rotation was normal. Additionally, hearing impairment is now recognized as a consistent feature of the LHX3-deficient phenotype.

In this paper, Sobrier et al. confirm the association of hypopituitarism, hearing impairment and skeletal abnormalities in patients with LHX3 deficiency. However, they also show a dominant negative effect for the splicing mutation identified in this family. Importantly, the proband's father and paternal grandmother, both of whom carry the splicing mutation, have a mild phenotype characterized by limited neck rotation. It would therefore be important to screen heterozygous carriers of *LHX3* mutations for milder phenotypes; the existence of both dominant and recessive mutations has already been identified in the *POU1F1* and *HESX1* genes. These studies further emphasize the importance of functional characterization of genetic mutations.

Food for thought

Dwarfism in mice lacking collagen-binding integrins $\alpha_2\beta_1$ and $\alpha_{11}\beta_1$ is caused by severely diminished IGF-1 levels

Blumbach K, Niehoff A, Belgardt BF, Ehlen HW, Schmitz M, Hallinger R, Schulz JN, Bruning JC, Krieg T, Schubert M, Gullberg D, Eckes B
Department of Dermatology, University of Cologne, Cologne, Germany
J Biol Chem 2012;287:6431–6440

Background: $\alpha_2\beta_1$ and $\alpha_{11}\beta_1$ integrins are the major receptors for collagen I. Collagen I is the major collagen of bone and $\alpha_{11}\beta_1$ integrin is thought to have an important role in bone turnover, in contrast to $\alpha_2\beta_1$.
Methods: Integrin $\alpha_2\beta_1$-deficient mice and integrin $\alpha_{11}\beta_1$-deficient mice were bred to generate mice deficient in both integrins.
Results: These mice have a normal size at birth but develop dwarfism within the first 4 weeks of life. They have shorter, less mineralized, and functionally weaker bones but there are no growth plate abnormalities or osteoblast dysfunction. All organs are proportionally smaller, suggesting a systemic cause for the overall size reduction. Serum IGF-1 concentrations of mice lacking either $\alpha_2\beta_1$ or $\alpha_{11}\beta_1$ or both integrins were reduced by 39, 64, or 81% respectively. Growth hormone-releasing hormone expression in the hypothalamus and growth hormone gene expression in the pituitary glands were also reduced in these mice.
Conclusion: Collagen-binding integrin receptors are involved in the control of the growth hormone/IGF-1 axis. Thus, coupling hormone secretion to extracellular matrix signaling via integrins represents a novel concept in the control of endocrine homeostasis.

This is an interesting paper that convincingly shows that mice lacking $\alpha_2\beta_1$ and $\alpha_{11}\beta_1$ integrins, the major receptors for collagen 1, develop dwarfism with a proportional reduction in size of all organs in the first month of life. They have a reduction of serum IGF-1 concentrations, pituitary GH content and hypothalamic GHRH content without evidence of other pituitary hormone deficiencies. Intrinsic bone metabolism and bone development is normal and the authors therefore argue that the dwarfism is due to GH and IGF-1 deficiency. This uncovers a novel mechanism for growth regulation and suggests a feedback loop from extracellular matrix in the bone to the hypothalamus-pituitary involving collagen I. Feedback regulation from bone is not new – feedback from bone to pancreas and brain to control energy metabolism has been shown [16] but this is the first study that would point to integrins as part of a feedback loop.

Alternatively, integrins could play a role in the hypothalamus or pituitary itself; in communication in neuronal networks, differentiation of precursors into hormone-producing cells [17] or in actual hormone production and release. For example, the cell adhesion molecule E-cadherin, which plays a key role in epithelial mesenchymal transition, is involved in the organization and function of the pituitary somatotroph network and in the development of GH adenomas [18]. In addition, integrins are involved in the proliferation of pituitary folliculostellate cells [19]. A role for other cell adhesion molecules like integrins in hypothalamic and pituitary function would therefore be possible [20].

A further point of interest is that the reduction of growth in the mutant mice occurred mostly in the first month of life, and remained constant in the next 2 months, which the authors argued was not due to reduced food intake. IGF-1 concentration was also most severely affected at 1 month of age, and had almost normalized at 3 months of age. This growth and hormone pattern is reminiscent of that seen in constitutionally delayed growth or 'transient GH deficiency' in children, and may be a mouse model for this variant human growth pattern.

References

1. Ferrara N, Carver-Moore K, Chen H, Dowd M, Lu L, O'Shea KS, et al: Heterozygous embryonic lethality induced by targeted inactivation of the VEGF gene. Nature 1996;380:439–442.
2. Serini G, Valdembri D, Zanivan S, Morterra G, Burkhardt C, Caccavari F, et al: Class 3 semaphorins control vascular morphogenesis by inhibiting integrin function. Nature 2003;424:391–397.
3. Wang Y, Martin JF, Bai CB: Direct and indirect requirements of Shh/Gli signaling in early pituitary development. Dev Biol 2010;348:199–209.
4. Cassoni P, Marrocco T, Bussolati B, Allia E, Munaron L, Sapino A, et al: Oxytocin induces proliferation and migration in immortalized human dermal microvascular endothelial cells and human breast tumor-derived endothelial cells. Mol Cancer Res 2006;4:351–359.
5. Cattaneo MG, Chini B, Vicentini LM: Oxytocin stimulates migration and invasion in human endothelial cells. Br J Pharmacol 2008;153:728–736.
6. Fauquier T, Rizzoti K, Dattani M, Lovell-Badge R, Robinson IC: SOX2-expressing progenitor cells generate all of the major cell types in the adult mouse pituitary gland. Proc Natl Acad Sci USA 2008;105:2907–2912.
7. Treier M, O'Connell S, Gleiberman A, Price J, Szeto DP, Burgess R, et al: Hedgehog signaling is required for pituitary gland development. Development 2001;128:377–386.
8. Rizzoti K, Lovell-Badge R: Regenerative medicine: organ recital in a dish. Nature 2011;480:44–46.
9. Buslei R, Nolde M, Hofmann B, Meissner S, Eyupoglu IY, Siebzehnrubl F, et al: Common mutations of β-catenin in adamantinomatous craniopharyngiomas but not in other tumours originating from the sellar region. Acta Neuropathol 2005;109:589–597.
10. Hassanein AM, Glanz SM, Kessler HP, Eskin TA, Liu C: Beta-catenin is expressed aberrantly in tumors expressing shadow cells. Pilomatricoma, craniopharyngioma, and calcifying odontogenic cyst. Am J Clin Pathol 2003;120:732–736.
11. Andoniadou CL, Gaston-Massuet C, Reddy R, Schneider RP, Blasco MA, Le Tissier P, et al: Identification of novel pathways involved in the pathogenesis of human adamantinomatous craniopharyngioma. Acta Neuropathol 2012 (E-pub ahead of print).
12. Takuma N, Sheng HZ, Furuta Y, Ward JM, Sharma K, Hogan BL, et al: Formation of Rathke's pouch requires dual induction from the diencephalon. Development 1998;125:4835–4840.
13. Vallette-Kasic S, Brue T, Pulichino AM, Gueydan M, Barlier A, David M, et al: Congenital isolated adrenocorticotropin deficiency: an underestimated cause of neonatal death, explained by TPIT gene mutations. J Clin Endocrinol Metab 2005;90:1323–1331.
14. Bonnefont X, Lacampagne A, Sanchez-Hormigo A, Fino E, Creff A, Mathieu MN, et al: Revealing the large-scale network organization of growth hormone-secreting cells. Proc Natl Acad Sci USA 2005;102:16880–16885.
15. Jeong Y, Leskow FC, El-Jaick K, Roessler E, Muenke M, Yocum A, et al: Regulation of a remote Shh forebrain enhancer by the Six3 homeoprotein. Nat Genet 2008;40:1348–1353.
16. Karsenty G: Bone endocrine regulation of energy metabolism and male reproduction. C R Biol 2011;334:720–724.
17. Li L, Bennett SA, Wang L: Role of E-cadherin and other cell adhesion molecules in survival and differentiation of human pluripotent stem cells. Cell Adh Migr 2012;6:222–233.
18. Lekva T, Berg JP, Fougner SL, Olstad OK, Ueland T, Bollerslev J: Gene expression profiling identifies ESRP1 as a potential regulator of epithelial mesenchymal transition in somatotroph adenomas from a large cohort of patients with acromegaly. J Clin Endocrinol Metab 2012 (E-pub ahead of print).
19. Horiguchi K, Fujiwara K, Ilmiawati C, Kikuchi M, Tsukada T, Kouki T, et al: Caveolin 3-mediated integrin β_1 signaling is required for the proliferation of folliculostellate cells in rat anterior pituitary gland under the influence of extracellular matrix. J Endocrinol 2011;210:29–36.
20. Borghi N, Lowndes M, Maruthamuthu V, Gardel ML, Nelson WJ: Regulation of cell motile behavior by crosstalk between cadherin- and integrin-mediated adhesions. Proc Natl Acad Sci USA 2010;107:13324–13329.

    Evelien F. Gevers/Carles Gaston-Massuet/Mehul T. Dattani

Thyroid

Gabor Szinnai[a], Mireille Castanet[b], Aurore Carré[c] and Michel Polak[d]

[a]Paediatric Endocrinology, University Children's Hospital Basel, and Department of Biomedicine, University Basel, Basel, Switzerland
[b]Paediatric Endocrinology, Hôpital Charles Nicolle, Rouen, France
[c]UMR 8200 CNRS, Institut Gustave Roussy, Villejuif, France
[d]Paediatric Endocrinology, Gynecology and Diabetology, Hôpital Necker Enfants Malades, AP-HP, INSERM U845, Université Paris Descartes, Paris, France

In the last 12 months significant advances were achieved in important areas of thyroid research. Clinical outcome studies increased our knowledge on long-term effects of congenital hypothyroidism on fertility, maternal thyroid disorders during pregnancy on infant's cognitive development and anti-thyroid medication in children with autoimmune hyperthyroidism. Developmental research convincingly established the role of micro-RNAs for normal thyroid development and function, and elucidated new molecular mechanisms of thyroid hormone receptor-dependent pulmonary development. This year's highlight in thyroid genetics was the description of a new form of thyroid hormone resistance due to mutations in the thyroid hormone receptor-α subunit. This chapter aims at giving a representative overview of the key publications in thyroidology.

Clinical trials

Antenatal thyroid screening and childhood cognitive function

Lazarus JH, Bestwick JP, Channon S, Paradice R, Maina A, Rees R, Chiusano E, John R, Guaraldo V, George LM, Perona M, Dall'Amico D, Parkes AB, Joomun M, Wald NJ
Centre for Endocrine and Diabetes Sciences, Cardiff School of Medicine, Cardiff, UK
lazarus@cf.ac.uk
N Engl J Med 2012;366:493–501

Background: Thyroid hormone levels during pregnancy have been reported to be crucial for the cognitive function of the offspring.
Methods: The authors conducted a randomized trial in pregnant women at a gestation of 15 weeks 6 days, or less. The women provided blood samples for measurement of thyrotropin (TSH) and free thyroxine (free T_4) and were assigned either to a screening group (in which measurements were obtained immediately) or a control group (in which serum was stored and measurements were obtained shortly after delivery). Women with positive findings in the screening group (TSH levels above the 97.5th percentile, free T_4 levels below the 2.5th percentile, or both) were assigned to 150 µg levothyroxine per day. The primary outcome was IQ at 3 years of age in children of women with positive results, as measured in a blinded fashion by psychologists.
Results: The study was able to obtain a large group of 21,846 women with blood samples at a median gestational age of 12 weeks 3 days: 390 women in the screening group and 404 in the control group tested positive. The median gestational age at the start of levothyroxine treatment was 13 weeks 3 days. Children of women with positive results had mean IQ scores of 99.2 and 100.0 in the screening and control groups, respectively (difference 0.8; 95% confidence interval −1.1 to 2.6; p = 0.40). The proportions of children with an IQ <85 were 12.1% in the screening group and 14.1% in the control group (difference 2.1 percentage points; 95% CI −2.6 to 6.7; p = 0.39).
Conclusions: The authors concluded that antenatal screening (at a median gestational age of 12 weeks 3 days) and maternal treatment for hypothyroidism did not result in improved cognitive function in children at 3 years of age.

Mild maternal thyroid dysfunction at delivery of infants born ≤34 weeks and neurodevelopmental outcome at 5.5 years

Williams F, Watson J, Ogston S, Hume R, Willatts P, Visser T
Population Health Sciences, University of Dundee, Ninewells Hospital and Medical School Campus, Dundee, UK
f.l.r.williams@dundee.ac.uk
J Clin Endocrinol Metab 2012;97:1977–1985

Background: Many publications have demonstrated that mild maternal thyroid dysfunction during early pregnancy is associated with poor neurodevelopment in affected offspring. The authors did not find studies that focused on preterm infants. They wished to describe the relationship between mild maternal thyroid dysfunction at delivery of infants born ≤34 weeks of gestation and their neurodevelopment at 5.5 years of age.
Methods: The authors performed a follow-up study evaluating the association of delivery levels of maternal TSH, and free T_4 (FT_4) in 143 women with McCarthy Scale scores adjusted for 26 confounders of neurodevelopment in their 166 children.
Results: The authors observed after adjustment for confounders significant 3.2-, 2.1-, and 1.8-point decrements, respectively, in general cognitive index, verbal subscale, and the perceptual performance subscale for each milliunit per liter increment in maternal TSH. After adjustment, significant associations were found with maternal FT_4 for the general cognitive index, motor scale, and quantitative subscale; each picomole per liter decrease in FT_4 was associated with a significant increase of general cognitive index (+1.5 points), motor scale (+1.7 points), and quantitative subscale (+0.9 points), respectively.
Conclusions: The authors concluded that higher maternal levels of TSH at delivery of infants born preterm were associated with lower scores on the general cognitive index at 5.5 years of age.

Previous studies have suggested that maternal hypothyroxinemia during pregnancy can negatively affect cognitive function of the children. Two years ago a large-scale study demonstrated the consequences of low maternal T_4 on the offspring cognition and correlated the whole range of FT_4 during early pregnancy with cognition in early childhood [1].

Up to now there was a paucity of data providing evidence for beneficial outcome of infants of hypothyroxinemic mothers after iodine or T_4 supplementation in early gestation. Therefore, intervention studies with iodine or thyroxine supplementation were needed. Lazarus et al. realized a large-scale prospective controlled randomized study in comparing treatment versus observation in early gestation with puzzling results. The study did neither find a significant difference in child IQ at the age of 3 years when starting treatment at 13 weeks of gestation nor was the proportion of children with IQ <85 different in the screening group versus the control group. Was the time point of screening and treatment too late? Calvo et al. found that in early (5–12 GW) embryonic fluids FT_4 concentrations were at least one third of those in their euthyroid mothers. They concluded that the availability of FT_4 for embryonic and fetal tissues would decrease in hypothyroxinemic women and may result in adverse effects on the timely sequence of developmental events in the human fetus as early as the first trimester [2]. Could postnatal iodine deficiency be a confounding factor that may affect the results? (See Vanderpump et al. on iodine status of UK schoolgirls, below in this chapter.) Indeed, studies demonstrated that the IQ of schoolchildren in a developed country can be influenced by iodine intake [3]. For the moment, the Lazarus study does not provide new arguments for universal screening of maternal hypothyroidism, but further trials are ongoing (http://www.clinicaltrials.gov/ct/show/NCT00388297).

Differences between the published studies on neurodevelopment may be due to several factors: (1) definition of maternal hypothyroidism (elevated TSH, hypothyroxinemia or both?), (2) time point of thyroid status assessment during pregnancy, (3) age and tools of neurodevelopmental assessment of the child, (4) term versus preterm infants. In this context, Williams et al. confirmed the association between maternal TSH levels, as was shown earlier in term neonates [4], but also FT_4/T_4 and neurodevelopmental outcome in preterm infants.

Positive impact of long-term antithyroid drug treatment on the outcome of children with Graves' disease: national long-term cohort study

Leger J, Gelwane G, Kaguelidou F, Benmerad M, Alberti C
Assistance Publique-Hopitaux de Paris, Hôpital Robert-Debre, Service d'Endocrinologie Pediatrique, Centre de Reference des Maladies Endocriniennes Rares de la Croissance, INSERM Unite 676. Hôpital Robert-Debre, Paris France juliane.leger@rdb.aphp.fr
J Clin Endocrinol Metab 2012;97:110–119

Background: Drug-based therapy is usually the initial treatment for Graves' disease (GD) hyperthyroidism in children. The objective of the authors was to assess the effect of long-term carbimazole therapy on GD remission in children and its determinants.

Methods: The authors included 154 children newly diagnosed with GD between 1997 and 2002 in an observational prospective multicenter follow-up cohort study. The intention was to treat patients with three consecutive courses of carbimazole, each lasting 2 years. Definitive treatment was performed in cases of poor compliance with antithyroid drug (ATD) treatment, thyrotoxicosis relapse, or major adverse effects of ATD treatment. The authors used remission for at least 18 months after the completion of each course of ATD treatment as major outcome measure.

Results: The median duration of follow-up was 10.4 (9.0–12.1) years. Overall estimated remission rates (95% confidence interval) 18 months after the withdrawal of ATD treatment increased with time and were 20 (13–26), 37 (29–45), 45 (35–54), and 49 (40–57)% after 4, 6, 8, and 10 years of follow-up, respectively. An independent positive effect of less severe forms of hyperthyroidism at diagnosis (subhazard ratio of 1 for patients with FT_4 <35 pmol/l vs. 0.4 (0.20–0.80) for FT_4 ≥35 pmol/l; p = 0.01) and of the presence of other autoimmune conditions (subhazard ratio of 2.23 (1.19–4.18); p = 0.01) was documented on remission rate after medical treatment.

Conclusion: About half the patients achieved remission after carbimazole discontinuation, and there seems to be a plateau in the incidence of remission achieved after 8–10 years of ATD therapy.

This is a unique long-term follow-up study of a cohort of children affected by autoimmune hyperthyroidism. The first study on this cohort published in 2008 showed the following results which are worth mentioning [5]. The overall estimated relapse rate for hyperthyroidism was 59% (95% confidence interval 52–67%) at 1 year and 68% (95% confidence interval 60–76%) at 2 years after the end of treatment. Multivariate analysis showed that the risk of relapse was higher for patients of non-Caucasian origin (hazard ratio (HR) = 2.54, p < 0.001), with high serum thyroid-stimulating hormone receptor antibodies (TRAb) (HR = 1.21 by 10 U, p = 0.03) and FT_4 (HR = 1.18 by 10 pmol/l, p = 0.001) levels at diagnosis. Conversely, relapse risk decreased with increasing age at onset (HR = 0.74 per 5 years, p = 0.03) and duration of first course of ATD (HR = 0.57 per 12 months, p = 0.005). A prognostic score was constructed, allowing the identification of three different risk groups, with 2-year relapse rates of 46, 77, and 98%.

Interestingly, the presented study highlights the positive impact of lower initial severity of hyperthyroidism on remission in the long-term follow-up as observed in the short term. However, for unclear reasons, the multivariate analysis did not identify age at presentation, ethnicity and initial TRAb levels as related to remission rate in the long-term follow-up study.

The authors further suggest that children with autoimmune hyperthyroidism displaying good compliance without major adverse effects of antithyroid drugs may be offered continuous medical treatment up to 8–10 years before planning definitive treatment. Certainly this conclusion will be challenged by pediatric endocrinologists offering much earlier an ablative therapy for children with Graves' disease.

Is the incidence of congenital hypothyroidism really increasing? A 20-year retrospective population-based study in Quebec

Deladoey J, Ruel J, Giguere Y, Van Vliet G
Endocrinology Service and Research Center, Sainte-Justine Hospital and Department of Pediatrics, University of Montreal, Montreal, Que., Canada
johnny.deladoey@umontreal.ca
J Clin Endocrinol Metab 2011;96:2422–2429

Background: Changes in screening methods for congenital hypothyroidism (CH) may explain the reportedly increasing frequency of CH in the United States. In Quebec, the same initial TSH cutoff (15 mU/l) has been used for the last 20 years, but in 2001, the cutoff was decreased from 15 to 5 mU/l for the second test, which is requested when TSH is intermediate (15–30 mU/l) on the first.
Methods: The authors aimed (1) to assess the incidence of CH over the last 20 years in Quebec using a population-based retrospective study and (2) to compare the incidences of CH by etiology based on thyroid scintigraphy between 1990–2000 and 2001–2009.
Results: Of 1,660,857 screened newborns over 20 years, 620 had CH (incidence 1:2,679). Scintigraphy revealed dysgenesis (n = 389, 1:4,270), either due to ectopy (n = 290) or athyreosis (n = 99), goiter (n = 52, 1:31,940), normal-size gland in situ (n = 115, 1:14,442), and unknown morphology (n = 64, 1:25,950). 49 additional cases were identified with the new screening algorithm (i.e. 25 normal-size gland in situ, 12 unknown etiology, 10 ectopies, and 2 goiters). Consequently, the incidence of normal-size gland in situ or of unknown etiology more than doubled (1:22,222 to 1:9,836, p = 0.0015, and 1:43,824 to 1:17,143, p = 0.0018, respectively) but that of dysgenesis and goiter remained stable.
Conclusion: The authors demonstrated that the incidence of CH is influenced by minimal changes in TSH screening cutoffs. Decreasing the cutoffs resulted in identification of additional cases that have predominantly functional disorders (thyroid in situ).

The newborn screening program in Quebec requests a second specimen in babies who have borderline TSH elevation between 15 and 30 mU/l (whole blood) on the first test. Between 1990 and 2000, when the TSH cutoff on the second test was >15 mU/l, the overall incidence of CH was 1:2,898. Between 2001 and 2009, when the TSH cutoff on the second test was lowered to >5 mU/l, the incidence rose to 1:2,450. Lowering the cutoff from 15 to 5 mU/l led to the detection of 49 additional cases of congenital hypothyroidism. The investigators clearly established that the apparent increased incidence was in fact solely the result of the lowered TSH cutoff on the second test. Although the Quebec authors do not comment, one presumes that there were no significant changes in population demographics, as noted in the United States. The conclusion for the increased incidence in Quebec is in accordance with earlier reports [6, 7]. In addition, the majority of the additional cases detected with a lower TSH cutoff by these programs had a thyroid gland in situ. In their analysis of laboratory practices in US newborn screening programs, the authors concluded that 'while different laboratory methods and screening practices affected the incidence rates, additional, unknown factors contributed to the reported increased rate' [8]. The following questions are raised: What could be the exact cause of congenital hypothyroidism with thyroid in situ? Do mild cases of congenital hypothyroidism benefit from detection by newborn screening and early thyroid hormone treatment?

Hippocampal size and memory functioning in children and adolescents with congenital hypothyroidism

Wheeler SM, Willoughby KA, McAndrews MP, Rovet JF
The Hospital for Sick Children, Toronto, Ont., Canada
joanne.rovet@sickkids.ca
J Clin Endocrinol Metab 2011;96:E1427–1434

Background: Selective and persistent neurocognitive weaknesses may be seen in children affected by congenital hypothyroidism (CH) despite early diagnosis and treatment after newborn screening. One area of particular weakness is memory, especially on tasks known to be mediated by the hippocampus. The objective of the authors was to use magnetic resonance imaging to determine whether children and adolescents with CH have reduced hippocampal size and abnormal hippocampal growth patterns relative to peers and whether reduced hippocampal volumes in CH predict poor memory performance.

Methods: The authors included 35 CH patients and 44 controls aged 9–15 years in their study. All were assessed using standardized tests of intelligence and verbal and visual memory and received a magnetic resonance imaging scan. Parents completed a questionnaire of their everyday memory functioning (EMF). Right and left hippocampal volumes were measured by manual tracing.

Results: CH subjects scored significantly below controls on indices of verbal but not visual memory. EMF was also affected for some aspects more than for controls. CH subjects also had smaller hippocampal volumes, particularly on the left side. Unlike controls, who showed a positive relationship between age and hippocampal volumes, age was unrelated to hippocampal size in CH. Structure-function correlations revealed significant relationships between hippocampal volumes and EMF in controls and modest correlations between hippocampal volumes and memory test scores but not EMF in CH.

Conclusions: The authors concluded that compromised hippocampal development in CH may contribute to some of the memory weaknesses of the patients affected by CH.

The authors have a long-standing interest in neurocognitive function in patients with congenital hypothyroidism. With specific testing, subtle neuropsychological anomalies can be demonstrated in affected children who will appear as normal for the pediatrician. For those 'apparently normal' patients, the consequences for their daily life may be minor. However, the hippocampus is very much related to ageing and diseases of ageing such as neurodegenerative disorders [9]. Will patients with congenital hypothyroidism show a different ageing process than controls? One wonders whether we have really closed the 'developmental gap with early high dose levothyroxine treatment' as stated 16 years ago [10]. Is there still room for improvement, especially by trying to minimize the impact of the lack of thyroid hormone in utero?

Fecundity in young adults treated early for congenital hypothyroidism is related to the initial severity of the disease: a longitudinal population-based cohort study

Hassani Y, Larroque B, Dos Santos S, Ecosse E, Bouyer J, Leger J
Institut National de la Sante et de la Recherche Médicale (INSERM) (Y.H., J.B.), Centre for Research in Epidemiology and Population Health (CESP), UMR 1018, Reproduction and Child Development Team, Le Kremlin-Bicêtre, France; Clinical Epidemiology and Research Unit (B.L.), Hôpital Beaujon, Assistance Publique-Hôpitaux de Paris, Clichy, France; INSERM Unité Mixte de Recherche (UMR) S953 (B.L.), Epidemiological Research on Perinatal Health and Women's and Children's Health; Université Pierre et Marie Curie (B.L.), University Paris 06, Paris, France; Assistance Publique-Hôpitaux de Paris (S.D.S., E.E., J.L.), Hôpital Robert-Debré, Service d'Endocrinologie Pédiatrique, Centre de Reference des Maladies Endocriniennes Rares de la Croissance; INSERM UMR 676 (J.L.), and Paris Diderot University (J.L.), Sorbonne Paris Cite, Paris, France, and Paris-Sud University (J.B.), UMR 1018, Le Kremlin-Bicêtre, France
Juliane.leger@rdb.aphp.fr
J Clin Endocrinol Metab 2012;97:1897–1904

Background: Hypothyroidism, if untreated, is a source of impaired fecundity. Screening programs for CH have been running for only the last 30 years in most industrialized countries. Therefore, patients treated early for CH have yet to be evaluated in adulthood. The authors' objective was to assess the fecundity of young adults treated early for CH and its determinants.

Methods: Of 1,748 subjects diagnosed with CH in the first 10 years after the introduction of neonatal screening in France, 1,158 completed a questionnaire on fecundity at a mean age of 25.3 years. This self-administered questionnaire focused on first attempts to have a child and time to pregnancy. The control group was that used in an analogous study on subjects born between 1971 and 1985. Fecundability hazard ratios (HR) were adjusted for known fecundity confounders (age, smoking, and reproductive history).

Results: Globally, fecundability was similar for the CH and control group. However, women with athyreosis, with absence of bone maturation at the knee epiphyseal ossification centers, and a low serum-free T_4 concentration at diagnosis (<5 pmol/l), representing the most severe forms of CH, were associated with lower fecundity: HR = 0.68 (0.50–0.98) (p = 0.02), HR = 0.65 (0.45–0.94) (p = 0.02), and HR =

0.70 (0.50–0.97) (p = 0.03), respectively. However, fecundability was not associated with age at the start of treatment, initial levothyroxine dose, or the adequacy of hypothyroidism control.

Conclusion: Fecundity was lower in women suffering from the most severe form of the disease.

These data originate from a unique population-based, large-scale study of young adults affected by congenital hypothyroidism. The systematic study of this cohort in comparison with an appropriate control group provides important information on long-term health and socioeconomic status of adults with CH [11]. One could have postulated that patients with CH might have a lower fecundity than the control population. Counter-intuitively, the overall fecundity was comparable in CH patients with that in controls. Only the subgroup of the most affected women, suffering from athyreosis, had a lower fecundity, although fecundity was not associated with age at start of treatment, initial LT_4 dose, or control of hypothyroidism after 15 days of treatment. Given the observational nature of the study, the impact of in utero hypothyroidism on the hypothalamus-pituitary-ovary axis remains unclear.

Genetics: new findings in 'old' genes

Frequent TSH receptor genetic alterations with variable signaling impairment in a large series of children with nonautoimmune isolated hyperthyrotropinemia

Calebiro D, Gelmini G, Cordella D, Bonomi M, Winkler F, Biebermann H, de Marco A, Marelli F, Libri DV, Antonica F, Vigone MC, Cappa M, Mian C, Sartorio A, Beck-Peccoz P, Radetti G, Weber G, Persani L
Laboratorio di Ricerche Endocrino-Metaboliche, Università degli Studi di Milano, Milano, Italy
luca.persani@unimi.it
J Clin Endocrinol Metab 2012;97:E156–160

Background: Partial TSH resistance, characterized by isolated nonautoimmune hyperthyrotropinemia (NAHT) has been associated with heterozygous mutations in the TSH receptor gene (TSHR). The authors aimed to investigate the prevalence and clinical impact of TSHR alterations in a large series of pediatric patients with NAHT.

Methods: The authors performed a prospective multicenter study which included 153 unrelated patients with NAHT aged <18 years. Patients with thyroid dysgenesis or major associated congenital defects were excluded from the study.

Results: The frequency of heterozygous nonpolymorphic TSHR variations was 11.8%. The authors identified seven previously undescribed variations: a frameshift (p.Q33PfsX46), one intronic (g.IVS4+2A→G), and five novel missense mutations (p.P162L, p.Y466C, p.I583T, p.I607T, and p. R609Q). The missense variations variably affected TSHR membrane expression and G(s) and/or G(q/11) signaling. Several variations cosegregated with NAHT in the affected families. Parameters of thyroid function were similar between affected and unaffected family members.

Conclusions: The authors concluded that nonpolymorphic alterations in the TSHR gene were commonly associated with isolated NAHT in young patients. This study confirmed that partial TSH resistance is the most frequent inheritable cause of isolated NAHT. The authors provided further evidence that besides the well-known defects in G(s) signaling, TSHR genetic alternations found in NAHT may frequently impair the G(q/11) pathway.

A mutation in the thyroid hormone receptor-α gene

Bochukova E, Schoenmakers N, Agostini M, Schoenmakers E, Rajanayagam O, Keogh JM, Henning E, Reinemund J, Gevers E, Sarri M, Downes K, Offiah A, Albanese A, Halsall D, Schwabe JW, Bain M, Lindley K, Muntoni F, Khadem FV, Dattani M, Farooqi IS, Gurnell M, Chatterjee K
University of Cambridge Metabolic Research Laboratories and National Institute for Health Research Cambridge Biomedical Research Centre, Institute of Metabolic Science, Addenbrooke's Hospital, Cambridge, UK
N Engl J Med 2012;366:243–249

Background: Thyroid hormones exert their effects through α (TRα1) and 3 (TRβ1 and TRβ2) receptors. *Methods:* The authors describe a child with classic features of hypothyroidism (growth retardation, developmental retardation, skeletal dysplasia, and severe constipation) but only borderline-abnormal thyroid hormone levels. *Results:* Using whole-exome sequencing, they identified a de novo heterozygous nonsense mutation in a gene encoding thyroid hormone receptor-α (THRA) and generating a mutant protein that inhibits wild-type receptor action in a dominant negative manner. *Conclusions:* Their observations are consistent with defective human TRα-mediated thyroid hormone resistance and substantiate the concept of hormone action through distinct receptor subtypes in different target tissues.

During the last 12 months, no new gene with relevant role in the hypothalamus-pituitary-thyroid axis has been identified. However, new insights on the genetic basis of resistance syndromes in the thyroid axis have been published. The first paper focused on TSH resistance. It provides data on prevalence of heterozygous nonpolymorphic TSHR gene variations in a large pediatric cohort of patients with nonautoimmune hyperthyrotropinemia detected either by neonatal screening or by repeatedly increased TSH values during childhood. The prevalence of TSH resistance due to heterozygous TSHR mutations was 12%, which is higher than in other recent studies with comparable inclusion criteria, suggesting that in some settings heterozygous TSHR mutations are up to now the most frequent genetic cause of nonautoimmune hyperthyrotropinemia [12]. Important for clinical practice, only one third of patients were detected by neonatal screening and about half had no affected family members.

The second paper describes the use of whole-exome sequencing to identify a new and very severe form of thyroid hormone resistance due to the first described mutation in the thyroid hormone receptor-α (THRA) gene. In direct contrast to the more typical patients with thyroid hormone resistance due to THRB mutations, the clinical phenotype in this case was characterized by marked clinical hypothyroidism in the context of slightly decreased thyroxine and increased T_3 levels. The lack of elevation in thyroxine levels appears to be attributable to the persistence of normal central THRB signaling. There was differential responsiveness of target tissues to thyroxine treatment. Especially, the tissues highly expressing THRA (bone, heart, intestine) showed thyroid hormone resistance with no improvement of growth, chronic constipation and heart rate despite thyroxine treatment, consistent with the genetic findings.

Thyroid and lung: mechanism of the year

Thyroid hormone receptor repression is linked to type I pneumocyte-associated respiratory distress syndrome

Pei L, Leblanc M, Barish G, Atkins A, Nofsinger R, Whyte J, Gold D, He M, Kawamura K, Li HR, Downes M, Yu RT, Powell HC, Lingrel JB, Evans RM
Howard Hughes Medical Institute, Salk Institute for Biological Studies, La Jolla, CA, USA
evans@salk.edu
Nat Med 2011;17:1466–1472

Background: The lung epithelium mainly consists of type I pneumocytes, which mediate gas exchange, and type II pneumocytes, which produce surfactant proteins. Type II pneumocyte maturation is promoted by glucocorticoids through the glucocorticoid receptor and its cognate ligand and this mechanism underlies the use of glucocorticoid administration to treat infant respiratory distress syndrome. In contrast, the pathway controlling the formation of type I pneumocytes is poorly understood. The study aimed to investigate the role of the co-repressor SMRT (silencing mediator of retinoid and thyroid hormone receptors) for type I pneumocyte differentiation.

Methods: The authors generated SMRT knock-in mice (SMRTmRID) that specifically disrupted the interaction between SMRT and nuclear receptors.

Results: SMRTmRID mice died shortly after birth from a previously unidentified acute respiratory distress syndrome resulting from an abnormal terminal differentiation of the type I pneumocyte, while showing normal type II pneumocyte function. While unresponsive to glucocorticoids, treatment with antithyroid hormone drugs (propylthiouracil or methimazole) completely rescued SMRT-induced respiratory distress syndrome, suggesting an unrecognized and essential role for the thyroid hormone receptor in lung development. The authors further showed that the thyroid hormone receptor and SMRT controlled type I pneumocyte differentiation through Klf2, which, in turn, seemed to directly activate the type I pneumocyte gene program.

Conclusions: The thyroid hormone receptor was identified as a second nuclear receptor involved in lung development, specifically involved in type I pneumocyte differentiation. The authors suggested a possible new type of therapeutic option in the treatment of respiratory distress syndrome that is unresponsive to glucocorticoids.

The role of thyroid hormone receptors in different tissues and organs has been thought to be well characterized. The presented study suggests a new role of the nuclear thyroid hormone receptor during a critical time window of embryonic lung development by rescuing disordered terminal differentiation of type I pneumocytes in SMRTmRID mice by maternal treatment with PTU and MMI. In summary, the authors showed that association of SMRT and the thyroid hormone receptor are crucial for the development of type I pneumocytes and that thyroid hormone signaling is mediated by Klf2 in the lung. Future studies focusing on lung development in thyroid hormone receptor-deficient mice will be of great importance to further support the thyroid hormone receptor-dependent mechanism of the presented results in SMRTmRID mice.

New concerns linked to iodine deficiency

Low iodine content in the diets of hospitalized preterm infants

Belfort MB, Pearce EN, Braverman LE, He X, Brown RS
Division of Newborn Medicine, Hunnewell 438, Children's Hospital Boston, Boston, MA, USA
mandy.belfort@childrens.harvard.edu
J Clin Endocrinol Metab 2012;97:E632–636

Background: Iodine is the limiting substrate for thyroid hormone synthesis. Hypothyroidism due to iodine deficiency is a frequent cause of mental retardation worldwide. Preterm infants have a lower iodine store than term infants, rendering preterm infants particularly vulnerable to the effects of iodine deficiency. Currently it is unknown whether the dietary iodine intake meets the requirement for hospitalized preterm infants. The authors aimed to measure the iodine content of enteral and parenteral nutrition products commonly used for hospitalized preterm infants and estimate the daily iodine intake for a hypothetical 1-kg infant.

Methods: Mass spectrometry was used to measure the iodine concentration of a representative selection of (1) preterm infant formulas, (2) samples of pooled donor human milk with or without human milk fortifiers, (3) enteral supplements, and (4) a parenteral amino acid solution and a soy-based lipid emulsion. The daily iodine intake provided by diets based on 150 ml/kg body weight/day of formula, donor human milk with or without human milk fortifies, and parenteral nutrition was calculated.

Results: Preterm formula provided 16.4–28.5 µg/day of iodine, whereas unfortified donor human milk provided only 5.0–17.6 µg/day. The other enteral supplements contained almost no iodine, nor did a parenteral nutrition-based diet.

Conclusions: Typical enteral diets for hospitalized preterm infants, particularly those based on donor human milk, provide less than the recommended 30 µg/day of iodine, and parenteral nutrition provides almost no iodine. Additional iodine fortification should be considered.

Iodine status of UK schoolgirls: a cross-sectional survey

Vanderpump MP, Lazarus JH, Smyth PP, Laurberg P, Holder RL, Boelaert K, Franklyn JA
Department of Endocrinology, Royal Free Hampstead NHS Trust, London, UK
mark.vanderpump@nhs.net
Lancet 2011;377:2007–2012

Background: Iodine deficiency is the most common cause of preventable mental impairment worldwide. It is defined by WHO as mild if the population median urinary iodine excretion is 50–99 µg/l, moderate if 20–49 µg/l, and severe if <20 µg/l. No contemporary data were available for the UK. The authors aimed to assess iodine status of the UK population.
Methods: In a cross-sectional survey, the iodine status of girls at 14–15 years of age was investigated in nine different regions. Urinary iodine concentrations and tap water iodine concentrations were measured in summer and winter 2009. Ethnic origin, postal code, and a validated diet questionnaire assessing sources of iodine were recorded.
Results: From 810 participants, 737 urine samples and 664 questionnaires of dietary habits were available. Median urinary iodine excretion was 80.1 µg/l (IQR 56.9–109.0). Based on urinary iodine excretion and according to WHO definitions, mild iodine deficiency was present in 51% (n = 379) of participants, moderate deficiency in 16% (n = 120), and severe deficiency in 1% (n = 8). Prevalence of iodine deficiency differed in the nine analyzed geographical regions. Tap water iodine concentrations were low or undetectable and were not positively associated with urinary iodine concentrations. Multivariable general linear model analysis confirmed independent associations between low urinary iodine excretion and sampling in summer (p < 0.0001), geographical region (p < 0.0001), and low intake of milk (p = 0.03).
Conclusions: The data of this cross-sectional study suggest that the UK is iodine-deficient. The presented results have drawn attention to an urgent need for a comprehensive investigation of UK iodine status and implementation of evidence-based recommendations for iodine supplementation.

Two papers raised concerns about unexpected risk of iodine deficiency in the pediatric age group in developed countries. The first paper focused on preterm infant diet, as only few data were available on iodine content in enteral and parenteral nutrition of preterm babies. Belfort et al. examined the iodine content of infant formulas, human milk donor samples with or without fortifier, and parenteral nutrients used for preterm infant nutrition. Neither formulas nor human milk at a calculated fluid intake of 150 ml/kg/day provided the recommended minimal dose of 30 µg/kg iodine per day. Particularly donor human milk and parenteral solutions were poor in iodine. These results raise the concern of inadequate iodine supply to preterm infants, especially when receiving donor human milk. However, the study did not assess iodine status in the preterm infant group. Besides additional iodine fortification, a pragmatic way of improving human donor milk iodine content would be to promote systematic intake of the daily recommended dose of 150 µg iodine in all lactating women, however even that target may be insufficient in some lactating women [13].

The second paper by Vanderpump presents data from a cross-sectional study of iodine status of adolescents from the UK. According to the authors, the UK was thought to be iodine-sufficient, although no iodine food or salt iodination program exists. The study was initiated as the authors observed insufficient use of iodized salt and increasing number of pregnant women with iodine deficiency based on regional experiences in the context of lacking national data. The study results suggest that the UK is iodine-deficient, according to WHO definition of iodine deficiency. This surprising result is of 'potential major public health importance' as stated by the authors. An accompanying editorial reminded us that in many Western settings diet has long been 'accidentally' fortified due to the use of iodine in dairy cattle husbandry – but unfortunately those practices are now changing! Urgent systematic studies on iodine status in all age groups are needed together with plans for improving iodine uptake in the general population.

Deletion of the RNaseIII enzyme Dicer in thyroid follicular cells causes hypothyroidism with signs of neoplastic alterations

Rodriguez W, Jin L, Janssens V, Pierreux C, Hick AC, Urizar E, Costagliola S
Institut de Recherche Interdisciplinaire en Biologie Humaine et Moléculaire (I.R.I.B.H.M.), Faculté de Médecine,
Université Libre de Bruxelles (ULB), Brussels, Belgium
scostag@ulb.ac.be
PLoS One 2012;7:e29929

Background: Micro-RNAs (miRNAs) are small non-coding RNAs that regulate gene expression at mRNA posttranscriptional level. Functional maturation of most miRNAs requires processing of the primary transcript by Dicer, an RNaseIII-type enzyme. To date, the role of Dicer for normal miRNA processing and physiological organogenesis has been demonstrated by tissue-specific Dicer inactivation in several mouse models. The aim of this study was to investigate the role of Dicer for thyroid development and differentiation.
Methods: The authors generated mouse models in which Dicer expression has been inactivated at onset of thyroid development at the thyroid bud stage (embryonic day 8.5) and at the onset of thyroid functional and structural differentiation (embryonic day 14.5) in thyroid follicular cells.
Results: The early stages of thyroid organogenesis, preceding folliculogenesis, were unaffected by the loss of Dicer, presenting a normal bilobed thyroid gland in place. However, Dicer mutant mice were severely hypothyroid and died soon after weaning unless they were substituted with T_4. Tissue architecture was disturbed in Dicer knockout mice showing follicular disorganization and a strong downregulation of Nis expression. With increasing age, the thyroid tissue showed characteristics of neoplastic alterations as suggested by a marked proliferation of follicular cells and an ongoing dedifferentiation in the center of the thyroid gland, with a loss of Pax8, FoxE1, Nis and Tpo expression.
Conclusions: These data showed that loss of miRNA maturation due to Dicer inactivation results in severely disordered functional and structural thyroid differentiation.

The microRNA-processing enzyme Dicer is essential for thyroid function

Frezzetti D, Reale C, Cali G, Nitsch L, Fagman H, Nilsson O, Scarfo M, De Vita G, Di Lauro R
IRGS Biogem s.c.ar.l., Ariano Irpino, Italy and Dipartimento di Biologia e Patologia Cellulare e Moleculare, Università degli Studi di Napoli 'Federico II', Naples, Italy
rdilauro@unina.it
PLoS One 2011;6:e27648

Background: Dicer is a type III ribonuclease required for the biogenesis of microRNAs (miRNAs), a class of small non-coding RNAs. MiRNAs regulate gene expression at the posttranscriptional level.
Methods: A thyroid follicular cell (TFC)-specific Dicer conditional knockout mice was generated by the authors to investigate the functional role of Dicer and miRNAs for normal thyroid development and TFC function.
Results: The authors showed that thyroid organogenesis and early TFC differentiation were not affected by Dicer inactivation. However, severe hypothyroidism gradually developed after birth, leading to reduced body weight and shortened lifespan. Histological and molecular analyses of knockout mice revealed a dramatic loss of the thyroid gland follicular architecture associated with functional aberrations and downregulation of several TFC differentiation markers.
Conclusions: The presented data showed that an intact miRNAs processing machinery is essential for normal function of the thyroid, and indicate that deregulation of specific miRNAs could be involved in human thyroid dysfunctions.

With this 'double pack' of evidence for the role of miRNAs for thyroid function, a new mechanism of thyroid physiology has been convincingly established. Both groups used the same approach of thyrocyte-specific conditional Dicer inactivation to disrupt functional maturation of miRNAs from the onset of thyroid development on. Rodriguez et al. added a second mouse model with 'late' Dicer inactivation at onset of thyroid differentiation, providing identical results as 'early' inactivation.

While the central aspect of postnatal loss of tissue architecture and secretory function due to loss of gene expression of differentiation markers at 1 month of life is shown by both groups, further analyses are complementary: Frezetti et al. documented in detail the thyroid differentiation at embryonic day 15.5, while Rodriguez et al. showed a highly increased proliferation rate in 4-week-old mice in both of their knockout mice strains. In conclusion, as thyroid organogenesis and initial thyroid differentiation is normal in Dicer knockout mice, miRNAs seem to be mandatory for maintaining thyrocyte function and thyroid structure.

Thyroid stem cells: surely more to come

Efficient derivation of purified lung and thyroid progenitors from embryonic stem cells

Longmire TA, Ikonomou L, Hawkins F, Christodoulou C, Cao Y, Jean JC, Kwok LW, Mou H, Rajagopal J, Shen SS, Dowton AA, Serra M, Weiss DJ, Green MD, Snoeck HW, Ramirez MI, Kotton DN
Boston University Pulmonary Center, Boston University School of Medicine, Boston, MA, USA
dkotton@bu.edu

Cell Stem Cell 2012;10:398–411

Background: Nkx2-1 (NK2 homeobox 1, alternatively thyroid transcription factor 1) is a homeodomain-containing transcription factor expressed in lung, thyroid and brain. Two populations of Nkx2-1-expressing progenitor cells in the developing foregut endoderm give rise to the entire postnatal lung and thyroid epithelium. The aim of the study was to purify and characterize endodermal Nkx2-1-positive pneumocyte and thyrocyte precursors.
Methods: Embryonic stem cell culture and directed differentiation was performed by use of stage-specific selective inhibition and induction of key pathways.
Results: Efficient purification and directed differentiation of primordial lung and thyroid progenitors derived from mouse embryonic stem cells (ESCs) was realized in vitro by inhibition of TGF-β and BMP signaling, followed by combinatorial stimulation of BMP and FGF signaling. By use of an Nkx2-1(GFP) knock-in reporter, these progenitors were purified for expansion in culture. Transcriptome analyses revealed overlap of in ESC-derived Nkx2-1-positive cells with developing lung epithelium. Upon induction, they expressed a broad repertoire of markers indicative of lung and thyroid lineages.
Conclusions: The authors derived a pure population of Nkx2-1-expressing progenitors able to recapitulate the developmental milestones of lung/thyroid development.

Specific murine knockout models allowed dissecting the roles of different transcription factors and pathways for thyroid development during the last decade. However, up to now, knowledge on directed differentiation from pluripotent embryonic stem cells to specified thyrocyte progenitors was scarce. Longmire et al. were interested in the most proximal endodermal lineages, as thyroid and lung epithelia, and established in an elegant way a protocol of stepwise directed differentiation of embryonic stem cells to definitive endodermal progenitors (Foxa2+), lung/thyroid competent definitive endodermal progenitors (Foxa2+/Foxa3–), and Nkx2-1+ lung/thyroid progenitors, which finally expressed lung- or thyroid-specific differentiation markers. This technique overcomes the inability to access the very rare lung and thyroid progenitors within the developing endoderm and will allow studying early molecular events of thyroid specification and development.

Small-molecule MAPK inhibitors restore radioiodine incorporation in mouse thyroid cancers with conditional BRAF activation

Chakravarty D, Santos E, Ryder M, Knauf JA, Liao XH, West BL, Bollag G, Kolesnick R, Thin TH, Rosen N, Zanzonico P, Larson SM, Refetoff S, Ghossein R, Fagin JA
Human Oncology and Pathogenesis Program, Memorial Sloan-Kettering Cancer Center, New York, NY, USA
faginj@mskcc.org
J Clin Invest 2011;121:4700–4711

Background: Advanced human thyroid cancers, particularly those that are refractory to treatment with radioiodine (RAI), have a high prevalence of BRAF (v-raf murine sarcoma viral oncogene homolog B_1) mutations. The aim of the study was to evaluate the dependence of cancer biology BRAF expression.

Methods: The authors generated mice expressing the most commonly detected BRAF mutation in human papillary thyroid carcinomas (BRAF(V600E)) in thyroid follicular cells in a doxycycline-inducible (dox-inducible) manner.

Results: Dox induction of BRAF(V600E) induced highly penetrant and poorly differentiated thyroid tumors with abolished thyroid-specific gene expression and RAI incorporation. Discontinuation of dox extinguished BRAF(V600E) expression and re-established thyroid follicular architecture and normal thyroid histology. Treatment of mice with these thyroid cancers with small molecule inhibitors of either MEK or mutant BRAF reduced their proliferative index and partially restored thyroid-specific gene expression. Strikingly, treatment with the MAPK pathway inhibitors rendered the tumor cells susceptible to a therapeutic dose of RAI.

Conclusions: Thyroid tumors carrying BRAF(V600E) mutations are exquisitely dependent on the oncoprotein for viability. Genetic or pharmacological inhibition of its expression or activity is associated with tumor regression and restoration of RAI uptake in vivo in mice.

> BRAF mutations are associated with aggressive and radioiodine uptake-resistant thyroid carcinomas. The authors established a genetically reversible in vivo mouse model of BRAF mutation-dependent thyroid carcinogenesis to answer two questions: (1) How dependent are the dedifferentiated thyrocytes from ongoing BRAF mutation expression? (2) Is it possible by pharmacological means to inhibit the oncogenic potential of BRAF mutations? In analogy with reversible activation of oncogenes, such as MYC in hematopoietic cell lines, the authors demonstrated the high dependence of dedifferentiated thyroid follicular cells in vivo on the permanent effect of the oncogenic BRAF mutation for maintenance of the cancer phenotype [14]. Further, they were able to reverse biological consequences of oncogenic BRAF activation by two different MAPK-signaling pathway inhibitors. More precisely, as a consequence of sodium/iodide symporter (NIS) re-expression at the basolateral membrane, radioiodine uptake was restored to an extent that tumor cells were rendered susceptible to therapeutic doses of radioiodine. These promising results open new avenues for the treatment of human thyroid cancer.

Predictive factors of malignancy in pediatric thyroid nodules

Roy R, Kouniavsky G, Schneider E, Allendorf JD, Chabot JA, Logerfo P, Dackiw AP, Colombani P, Zeiger MA, Lee JA
Endocrine Surgery Section, The Johns Hopkins University School of Medicine, Baltimore, MD, USA
rashmiroymd@gmail.com
Surgery 2011;150:1228–1233

Background: According to the literature, thyroid nodules in children are more frequently malignant than in adult patients. The aim of the study was to identify clinical factors that may predict malignancy in pediatric thyroid nodules.

Methods: A retrospective analysis of 207 pediatric patients who underwent thyroidectomy for thyroid nodules was conducted over 15 years at two tertiary hospitals. Analyses examined predictive values of 16 clinicopathologic factors associated with cancer. Positive predictive values (PPVs) of fine-needle aspiration biopsy specimens (FNABs) were analyzed independently.

Results: Malignant thyroid histology was found in 41% of patients. Malignancy was more likely with family history of thyroid cancer (34.2 vs. 17.7%; p = 0.111), palpable lymphadenopathy (34.2 vs. 2.9%; p = 0.001), and hypoechoic nodules (52.2 vs. 19.2%; p = 0.016). Palpable lymphadenopathy indicated greater than 2-fold increased risk for malignancy (relative risk 2.18; 95% confidence interval 1.56–3.05). PPVs of FNAB results were 0.94 for malignancy, 0.63 for suspicious for malignancy, and 0.55 for indeterminate lesions. PPV for benign FNAB to be benign on final pathology was 0.71.

Conclusions: The authors concluded that malignancy was associated with family history of thyroid cancer and hypoechogenic lesions on ultrasonography; palpable lymphadenopathy had the greatest risk for malignancy. Further, a benign FNAB in children was not as accurate as in adults and the likelihood that an indeterminate nodule showed malignant histology was greater.

The 2009 revised American Association (ATA) guidelines for patients with thyroid nodules and differentiated thyroid cancer recommend that fine-needle aspiration biopsies should also be performed in children with thyroid nodules as in adults [15]. The aim of the study was first to identify clinical, radiological and pathological parameters which are associated with malignancy in the pediatric age group, and second to review the positive predictive value of fine-needle aspiration biopsies in their cohort. The study is of interest as it described a higher percentage of malignant thyroid nodules compared to earlier data, and found a relatively low positive predictive value of a benign fine-needle aspiration biopsy result in children. In summary, the authors conclude that the presence of the three identified clinical risk factors for malignancy should 'heighten suspicion for malignancy, even in the setting of a benign fine-needle aspiration biopsy, and certainly with an indeterminate biopsy'.

Chemotherapy and thyroid cancer risk: a report from the childhood cancer survivor study

Veiga LH, Bhatti P, Ronckers CM, Sigurdson AJ, Stovall M, Smith SA, Weathers R, Leisenring W, Mertens AC, Hammond S, Neglia JP, Meadows AT, Donaldson SS, Sklar CA, Friedman DL, Robison LL, Inskip PD
Radiation Epidemiology Branch, Division of Cancer Epidemiology and Genetics, National Cancer Institute, NIH, Department of Health and Human Services, Bethesda, MD, USA
veigal@mail.nih.gov
Cancer Epidemiol Biomarkers Prev 2012;21:92–101

Background: The thyroid gland is one of the most radiosensitive organs. Childhood cancer survivors treated with radiation are at elevated risk for thyroid cancer. However, the effect of chemotherapy alone and in combination with radiotherapy on thyroid cancer risk is unclear. The objective of this study was to evaluate the chemotherapy-related risk of thyroid cancer in childhood cancer survivors and the possible joint effects of chemotherapy and radiotherapy.

Methods: The Childhood Cancer Survival Study is the largest cohort study to date with detailed treatment-related information including 12,547 5-year survivors of childhood cancer diagnosed during 1970 through 1986. Chemotherapy and radiotherapy information was obtained from medical records, and radiation dose was estimated to the thyroid gland. Cumulative incidence and relative risks were calculated with lifetable methods and Poisson regression. Chemotherapy-related risks were analyzed separately in a radiation dose-dependent manner.

Results: Histologically confirmed thyroid cancer occurred in 119 patients. 30 years after the first childhood cancer treatment, the cumulative incidence of thyroid cancer was 1.3% (95% CI 1.0–1.6) for females and 0.6% (0.4–0.8) for males. Among patients with thyroid radiation doses of ≤20 Gy, treatment with alkylating agents was associated with a significant 2.4-fold increased risk of thyroid cancer (95% CI 1.3–4.5; p = 0.002). Chemotherapy risks decreased as radiation dose increased, with a significant decrease for patients treated with alkylating agents (p_{trend} = 0.03). No chemotherapy-related risk was evident for thyroid radiation doses more than 20 Gy.

Conclusions: Chemotherapy with alkylating agents increased thyroid cancer risk only if the radiation dose was <20 Gy.

Until now, most studies were unable to identify a significant association of chemotherapy and the risk of thyroid cancer as a second malignancy in childhood cancer survivors. New insights into thyroid cancer risk in this patient group come from the large Childhood Cancer Survival Study (CCSS). In a recent cohort analysis the authors observed a weak association of chemotherapy with thyroid cancer after adjustment for radiotherapy [16]. In the present study, they evaluated the possible joint effect of chemotherapy and radiation on thyroid cancer. They observed an increased risk for thyroid cancer in patients treated with alkalyting agents. However, this effect was only significant with a radiation dose <20 Gy, in accordance with the fact that high radiation doses result in cell killing, while in the lower radiation dose range cell-sparing predominates. Although lower than the effect of radiation, chemotherapeutic agents may increase the risk of thyroid cancer in pediatric cancer survivors.

Reviews of interest for the pediatric endocrinologist

The following three extensive guidelines and reviews focus on common thyroid diseases and provide the current state of knowledge for these clinical problems for the adult but also for the pediatric age group.

Guidelines of the American Thyroid Association for the diagnosis and management of thyroid disease during pregnancy and postpartum

Stagnaro-Green A, Abalovich M, Alexander E, Azizi F, Mestman J, Negro R, Nixon A, Pearce EN, Soldin OP, Sullivan S, Wiersinga W
Department of Medicine, George Washington University School of Medicine and Health Sciences, Washington, DC, USA
msdasg@gwumc.edu
Thyroid 2011;21:1081–1125

Hyperthyroidism and other causes of thyrotoxicosis: management guidelines of the American Thyroid Association and American Association of Clinical Endocrinologists

Bahn Chair RS, Burch HB, Cooper DS, Garber JR, Greenlee MC, Klein I, Laurberg P, McDougall IR, Montori VM, Rivkees SA, Ross DS, Sosa JA, Stan MN
Division of Endocrinology, Metabolism, and Nutrition, Mayo Clinic, Rochester, MN, USA
bahn.rebecca@mayo.edu
Thyroid 2011;21:593–646

Treatment of differentiated thyroid cancer in children: emphasis on surgical approach and radioactive iodine therapy

Rivkees SA, Mazzaferri EL, Verburg FA, Reiners C, Luster M, Breuer CK, Dinauer CA, Udelsman R
Department of Pediatrics, Yale Child Health Research Center, Yale University School of Medicine, New Haven, CT, USA
scott.rivkees@yale.edu
Endocr Rev 2011;32:798–826

References

1. Henrichs J, Bongers-Schokking JJ, Schenk JJ, et al: Maternal thyroid function during early pregnancy and cognitive functioning in early childhood: the generation R study. J Clin Endocrinol Metab 2010;95:4227–4234.
2. Calvo RM, Jauniaux E, Gulbis B, et al: Fetal tissues are exposed to biologically relevant free thyroxine concentrations during early phases of development. J Clin Endocrinol Metab 2002;87:1768–1777.
3. Santiago-Fernandez P, Torres-Barahona R, Muela-Martinez JA, et al: Intelligence quotient and iodine intake: a cross-sectional study in children. J Clin Endocrinol Metab 2004;89:3851–3857.

4. Haddow JE, Palomaki GE, Allan WC, et al: Maternal thyroid deficiency during pregnancy and subsequent neuropsychological development of the child. N Engl J Med 1999;341:549–555.
5. Kaguelidou F, Alberti C, Castanet M, Guitteny MA, Czernichow P, Leger J: Predictors of autoimmune hyperthyroidism relapse in children after discontinuation of antithyroid drug treatment. J Clin Endocrinol Metab 2008;93:3817–3826.
6. Mengreli C, Kanaka-Gantenbein C, Girginoudis P, et al: Screening for congenital hypothyroidism: the significance of threshold limit in false-negative results. J Clin Endocrinol Metab 2010;95:4283–4290.
7. Corbetta C, Weber G, Cortinovis F, et al: A 7-year experience with low blood TSH cutoff levels for neonatal screening reveals an unsuspected frequency of congenital hypothyroidism. Clin Endocrinol (Oxf) 2009;71:739–945.
8. Hertzberg V, Mei J, Therrell BL: Effect of laboratory practices on the incidence rate of congenital hypothyroidism. Pediatrics 2010;125(suppl 2):S48–53.
9. Li J, Pan P, Huang R, Shang H: A meta-analysis of voxel-based morphometry studies of white matter volume alterations in Alzheimer's disease. Neurosci Biobehav Rev 2012;36:757–763.
10. Dubuis JM, Glorieux J, Richer F, Deal CL, Dussault JH, Van Vliet G: Outcome of severe congenital hypothyroidism: closing the developmental gap with early high-dose levothyroxine treatment. J Clin Endocrinol Metab 1996;81:222–227.
11. Leger J, Ecosse E, Roussey M, Lanoe JL, Larroque B: Subtle health impairment and socioeducational attainment in young adult patients with congenital hypothyroidism diagnosed by neonatal screening: a longitudinal population-based cohort study. J Clin Endocrinol Metab 2011;96:1771–1782.
12. Narumi S, Muroya K, Abe Y, et al: TSHR mutations as a cause of congenital hypothyroidism in Japan: a population-based genetic epidemiology study. J Clin Endocrinol Metab 2009;94:1317–1323.
13. Mulrine HM, Skeaff SA, Ferguson EL, Gray AR, Valeix P: Breast-milk iodine concentration declines over the first 6 months' postpartum in iodine-deficient women. Am J Clin Nutr 2010;92:849–856.
14. Felsher DW, Bishop JM: Reversible tumorigenesis by MYC in hematopoietic lineages. Mol Cell 1999;4:199–207.
15. Cooper DS, Doherty GM, Haugen BR, et al: Revised American Thyroid Association management guidelines for patients with thyroid nodules and differentiated thyroid cancer. Thyroid 2009;19:1167–1214.
16. Bhatti P, Veiga LH, Ronckers CM, et al: Risk of second primary thyroid cancer after radiotherapy for a childhood cancer in a large cohort study: an update from the childhood cancer survivor study. Radiat Res 2010;174:741–752.

Growth and Growth Factors

Stefano Cianfarani

Molecular Endocrinology Unit, Bambino Gesù Children's Hospital, Department of Systems Medicine, 'Tor Vergata' University, Rome, Italy

Whereas in previous years many studies were focused on new potential indications for GH therapy, in the last 12 months, the attention of researchers has been focusing on possible long-term adverse effects of such treatment. Two preliminary reports from the SAGhE European study, which represents the first effort to assess long-term safety in children receiving GH, have been published generating concern and controversy as they apparently lead to opposite conclusions. The publication of the final and comprehensive results of this study is needed before drawing any conclusions. Another interesting novelty is the evidence for a role of IGF-II in postnatal metabolism. IGF-II has always been associated with brain and pancreas development in fetus and cancer growth in postnatal life, now it seems to be living a second life as a metabolic regulator. Finally, in basic science research, the attention has been focusing on the interplay between GH receptor signaling in specific organs and whole-body glucose metabolism. Although the results have been obtained in animal models carrying selective gene deletions, potential implications for a better understanding of physiological factors regulating glucose homeostasis and for therapeutic fallout can be envisaged.

New Concerns

Meta-analysis and dose-response meta-regression: circulating insulin-like growth factor I (IGF-I) and mortality

Burgers AM, Biermasz NR, Schoones JW, Pereira AM, Renehan AG, Zwahlen M, Egger M, Dekkers OM
Departments of Endocrinology and Metabolism, Leiden University Medical Center, Leiden, The Netherlands
o.m.dekkers@lumc.nl
J Clin Endocrinol Metab 2011;96:2912–2920

Background: Epidemiological studies have shown that circulating IGF-I concentrations are positively associated with cancer risk and inversely with risk of cardiovascular disease. The aim of this study was to perform a meta-analysis and meta-regression of population-based reports to quantify the robustness of these relationships.
Methods: The search was performed in PubMed, EMBASE, Web of Science, and Cochrane Library from 1985 to September 2010 to identify the population-based cohort studies and (nested) case-control studies reporting on the relation between circulating IGF-I and mortality.
Results: Twelve studies, with 14,906 participants, were selected. All-cause mortality was significantly increased in subjects with low as well as high IGF-I, with a hazard ratio (HR) of 1.27 (95% CI 1.08–1.49) and HR of 1.18 (95% CI 1.04–1.34), respectively. Dose-response meta-regression showed a U-shaped relation of IGF-I and all-cause mortality (p = 0.003). The predicted HR for the increase in mortality comparing the 10th with the 50th percentile was 1.56 (95% CI 1.31–1.86); the predicted HR comparing the 90th with the 50th percentile was 1.29 (95% CI 1.06–1.58). Four studies also reported the association of IGFBP-3 levels with all-cause mortality. This meta-analysis showed a higher mortality for subjects in the lowest category of IGFBP-3 compared with the middle category with a HR of 1.40 (95% CI 1.17–1.68).
Conclusions: IGF-I and IGFBP-3 are associated with mortality. Both low and high IGF-I concentrations are associated with increased cancer and cardiovascular disease mortality, whereas only low IGFBP-3 is associated with increased mortality.

The IGFs are increasingly recognized to be important growth factors in many tumor types and virtually all human cancer cells express IGF receptors and produce IGFs, IGFBPs, and IGFBP proteases. Type I IGF receptor is actively involved in the control of cell growth and differentiation, and mutations of IGF-I receptor result in a tumorigenic or mitogenic effect of IGF-I [1]. Preliminary short-term clinical trials aimed at testing the efficacy of anti-IGF-IR monoclonal antibodies in patients with sarcomas have shown promising results [2, 3]. In the 1990s, a series of papers based on data from prospective cohorts showed that circulating IGF-I levels were positively correlated with the risk of many types of cancers, including colorectal, breast and prostate cancer, whereas circulating IGFBP-3 concentrations were inversely correlated with the risk of these cancers. These observations were consistent with the mitogenic and anti-apoptotic effects of IGF-I and the proapoptotic effects of IGFBP-3. A recent review summarizes the evidence from epidemiological studies that support the association between raised circulating levels of IGF-I and the risk of certain cancers [4]. We used to think of high IGF1 as a risk factor for cancer and low IGF1 – for cardiovascular morbidity. The current study reveals, for the first time, a U-shaped curve relating IGF-I levels to both cancer and cardiovascular disease mortality. According to this model, low as well as high IGF-I concentrations would be associated with increased mortality risk. Transferring this finding to clinical practice, the goal of GH replacement therapy should be to maintain the IGF-I levels around the average. However, we should be cautious in interpreting these results as they could be affected by different IGF-I and IGFBP-3 assays, by confounding factors such as nutritional status, and by genetic background which alone may account for up to 40% of the variability of IGF-I concentrations.

Long-term mortality after recombinant growth hormone treatment for isolated growth hormone deficiency or childhood short stature: preliminary report of the French SAGhE study

Carel JC, Ecosse E, Landier F, Meguellati-Hakkas D, Kaguelidou F, Rey G, Coste J
Pediatric Endocrinology and Diabetology, Hôpital Robert-Debré, Paris, France
jean-claude.carel@inserm.fr
J Clin Endocrinol Metab 2012;97:416–425

Background: Few independent studies have addressed the issue of long-term safety of GH therapy in childhood. The aim of this study, which represents the first report from the SAGhE (Safety and Appropriateness of Growth hormone treatments in Europe) project, was to determine the long-term mortality of patients treated with recombinant GH in childhood in France.

Methods: This was a population-based cohort study. 6,928 children with idiopathic isolated GH deficiency (n = 5,162), neurosecretory dysfunction (n = 534), idiopathic short stature (n = 871), or born short for gestational age (n = 335) who started treatment between 1985 and 1996 were enrolled in the study. Follow-up data on vital status were available in September 2009 for 94.7% of the patients.

Results: All-cause mortality was increased in treated subjects (standardized mortality ratio (SMR) 1.33, 95% confidence interval (CI) 1.08–1.64). The use of GH doses >50 µg/kg/day was associated with increased mortality rates (SMR 2.94, 95% CI 1.22–7.07, hazard ratio 2.79, 95% CI 1.14–6.82). Whereas all type cancer-related mortality was not increased, bone tumor-related mortality resulted in being significantly increased (SMR 5.00, 95% CI 1.01–14.63). Data analysis also showed an increase in mortality due to cardiovascular disease (SMR 3.07, 95% CI 1.40–5.83) and cerebrovascular events (SMR 6.66, 95% CI 1.79–17.05).

Conclusions: Subjects treated with GH during childhood showed increased mortality rate which was associated with the use of higher GH doses. Bone tumors and cerebrovascular diseases resulted to be the main causes of death. These results highlight the need for further studies on long-term morbidity and mortality after GH treatment in childhood.

Long-term mortality and causes of death in isolated GHD, ISS, and SGA patients treated with recombinant growth hormone during childhood in Belgium, the Netherlands, and Sweden: preliminary report of three countries participating in the EU SAGhE study

Sävendahl L, Maes M, Albertsson-Wikland K, Borgström B, Carel JC, Henrard S, Speybroeck N, Thomas M, Zandwijken G, Hokken-Koelega AC
Division of Pediatric Endocrinology, Karolinska University Hospital Q2:08, Stockholm, Sweden
lars.savendahl@ki.se
J Clin Endocrinol Metab 2012;97:E213–217

Background: The preliminary data from SAGhE (Safety and Appropriateness of Growth hormone treatments in Europe) consortium, released from the French Unit, have shown an increased mortality rate in adults treated with GH during childhood. The aim of this second paper from SAGhE consortium was to report the preliminary data on long-term mortality in the same diagnostic groups of the French study, in Belgium, the Netherlands, and Sweden.

Methods: Data were retrieved from national registries of GH-treated patients and vital status from National Population Registries. Causes of death were retrieved from a National Cause of Death Register (Sweden), Federal and Regional Death Registries (Belgium), or individual patient records (the Netherlands). Patients with isolated GH deficiency or idiopathic short stature or born small for gestational age, being started on recombinant GH treatment during childhood between 1985 and 1997, irrespective of treatment duration, and who had attained 18 years of age by the end of year 2009 (the Netherlands) or the end of year 2010 (Belgium and Sweden) were included. Vital status was available for approximately 98% of these 2,543 patients, corresponding to 46,556 person-years of observation. The standardized mortality ratios were not calculated.

Results: 21 deaths were identified, the majority being caused by accidents and suicides (76%). Not a single case of death caused by cancer or cardiovascular or cerebrovascular diseases was observed.

Conclusions: These results, strikingly in contrast with the French data, highlight the need of exercising extreme caution in drawing conclusions based on preliminary data from a single country and the importance to wait for the final results of the whole EU SAGhE consortium.

After many years of the industry dominance as gatekeepers of GH therapy, we now have two reports generated by public funding. Both Carel's and Sävendahl's reports stem from the same EU SAGhE project which was started in 2009 in eight countries (France, Sweden, Belgium, the Netherlands, Switzerland, Germany, United Kingdom and Italy). The French study began 3 years before the European consortium and that is the reason why they could finish data collection and analysis earlier than the other countries. Sweden, Belgium and the Netherlands, taking advantage of the existence of national registries of GH-treated patients, could achieve the endpoint of mortality rates well in advance the end of the project which is scheduled for November 2012. The fact that these two preliminary reports show opposite results in the long-term mortality of subjects treated with GH during childhood is both interesting and puzzling. Whereas the French data raise concern on the risk of cancer and cerebrovascular diseases, in the other three countries not a single case of death from cancer or cerebrovascular disease was observed. It is hard to prove whether differences in genetics, environment, or, more simply, confounding factors might account for this discrepancy. This kind of study is certainly worthwhile and these two preliminary reports stress the importance to replicate these surveys in different contexts. An editorial by Rosenfeld et al. [5] underscores the need of a joint effort involving all the stakeholders (physicians, regulatory agencies, pharmaceutical companies, patients and their families), to invest resources and expertise in setting up an international task force aimed at addressing the still controversial issue of long-term GH safety.

New Paradigms

Insulin-like growth factor 2/H19 methylation at birth and risk of overweight and obesity in children

Perkins E, Murphy SK, Murtha AP, Schildkraut J, Jirtle RL, Demark-Wahnefried W, Forman MR, Kurtzberg J, Overcash F, Huang Z, Hoyo C
Department of Community and Family Medicine, Duke University, Durham, NC, USA
cathrine.hoyo@duke.edu
J Pediatr 2012;161:31–39

Background: Childhood obesity may be the expression of an early adaptive response which can be driven by epigenetic mechanisms driving the expression of genes involved in energy balance, ultimately leading to overweight and obesity. Higher circulating insulin-like growth factor 2 (IGF2) protein levels have been associated with obesity. The aim of this study was to determine whether altered methylation in differentially methylated regions (DMRs) regulating IGF2 expression at birth, is associated with the risk of overweight or obesity in early childhood.

Methods: Methylation analyses were performed in cord blood leukocytes of 204 newborns by using pyrosequencing. Anthropometric and feeding data were collected at age 1 year. Methylation differences were compared between children >85th percentile and children ≤85th percentile of weight-for-age at 1 year by adjusting for postnatal caloric intake, maternal cigarette smoking, and race/ethnicity.

Results: The methylation percentages at the H19 imprint center DMR was higher in infants with weight >85th percentile (62.7%; 95% CI 59.9–65.5%) than in infants with weight ≤85th percentile (59.3%; 95% CI 58.2–60.3%; p = 0.02).

Conclusions: The finding that children who were overweight or obese at age 1 year had higher methylation percentages at the H19 DMR at birth suggests that IGF2 methylation status may play a key role in the development of overweight or obesity in early childhood, and may represent a useful marker of obesity risk.

Epigenetic mechanisms are commonly associated with gene silencing, genomic imprinting and transcriptional regulation of tissue-specific gene expression during cellular differentiation. In humans, evidence that epigenetic changes predispose the organism to type 2 diabetes stems among others from studies on individuals who were prenatally exposed to famine during the Dutch Hunger Winter of 1944–45 that showed a higher risk for obesity and obesity-related chronic disease [6]. These individuals were at higher risk for cardiovascular and metabolic diseases in adulthood [7], and periconceptional exposure to famine was associated with lower methylation of the IGF-II gene six decades later [8]. In the present study, for the first time, an association between IGF2 methylation and risk of obesity has been observed in early childhood. Interestingly, the authors report that breastfeeding modified the magnitude of IGF2 methylation, thus suggesting an interplay between prenatal environment (nutrient transfer from mother to fetus) and early postnatal feeding behavior which could stabilize or change the epigenetic patterns acquired in utero. Although cause-and-effect could not be established in this epidemiological study, these results warrant further investigations aimed at clarifying the role of IGF2 epigenetic changes in obesity and its metabolic consequences. Methylation patterns may represent early markers of long-term metabolic risk, offering the possibility to identify high-risk individuals thus driving early targeted interventions.

Associations between paternally transmitted fetal IGF2 variants and maternal circulating glucose concentrations in pregnancy

Petry CJ, Seear RV, Wingate DL, Manico L, Acerini CL, Ong K, Hughes IA, Dunger DB
Department of Paediatrics, University of Cambridge, Cambridge, UK
cjp1002@cam.ac.uk
Diabetes 2011;60:3090–3096

Background: Genomic variation in the fetal genome, in particular in fetal growth genes, could affect maternal metabolism in pregnancy and alter the mother's risk of developing gestational diabetes mellitus. The aim of this study was to determine whether polymorphisms in the paternally transmitted fetal IGF2 gene was associated with maternal glucose concentrations in the third trimester of pregnancy.

Methods: A total of 17 single nucleotide polymorphisms (SNPs) in the IGF2 gene region were genotyped in 1,160 mother/partner/offspring trios from the prospective Cambridge Baby Growth Study (n = 845 trios) and the retrospective Cambridge Wellbeing Study (n = 315 trios) (3,480 samples in total). Associations were tested between the inferred parent-of-origin fetal alleles, Z scores of maternal glucose concentrations 60 min after an oral glucose load performed at weeks 27–29 of pregnancy, and offspring birth weights.

Results: Paternally transmitted fetal rs6578987, rs680, rs10770125, and rs7924316 alleles were associated with increased maternal glucose concentrations in the third trimester of pregnancy and placental IGF-II contents at birth (p = 0.03). In contrast, no association was observed between maternally transmitted fetal IGF2 genotypes and maternal glucose concentrations.

Conclusions: The association between polymorphic variation in a paternally transmitted fetal gene, namely, IGF2, and maternal glucose concentrations in pregnancy is described for the first time. These findings support the hypothesis that variations in fetal imprinted genes regulate the maternal availability of nutrients.

Pregnant mice carrying pups with targeted disruption of 13 kb genetic region, including the imprinted H19 gene and IGF2 control element, show increased circulating glucose concentrations in late pregnancy [9]. This finding prompted the authors to test the hypothesis that functional variation in the

                                                    Stefano Cianfarani

fetal IGF2 gene alters maternal glucose concentrations in human pregnancy. The results of the present study demonstrate that specific polymorphisms in paternally imprinted fetal IGF2 are associated with increased maternal glucose concentrations in pregnancy and could thus affect the risk of gestational diabetes in the mother. These data are consistent with SRS and BWS imprinting findings and with Haig's parental conflict hypothesis, which suggests that paternally expressed fetal imprinted genes will tend to increase fetal growth, whereas maternally expressed genes will tend to restrain it [10]. These effects are probably achieved through modifications in fetal and placental nutritional demand and supply, and alterations in maternal glucose concentrations. However, no association between any of the IGF2 fetal variants and offspring birth weight was observed. The authors speculate that probably the effect sizes on maternal glucose concentrations were too small to make a detectable difference in birth weight. Important limitations of this study are the lack of paternity testing and the unavailability of maternal BMI in the vast majority of the study cohort. Nevertheless, this report represents a major breakthrough in prenatal programming for adult health and disease research, showing that mother-fetus interaction is bidirectional, the developing host influencing maternal metabolism according to paternally transmitted genetic information.

Higher levels of IGF-I and adrenal androgens at age 8 years are associated with earlier age at menarche in girls

Thankamony A, Ong K, Ahmed ML, Ness AR, Holly JM, Dunger DB
University Department of Paediatrics, University of Cambridge, Addenbrooke's Hospital, Cambridge, UK
dbd25@cam.ac.uk
J Clin Endocrinol Metab 2012;97:E786–790

Background: Earlier age at menarche has been associated with low birth weight, rapid weight gain during infancy, and childhood obesity. A role of intrauterine programming has been suggested but the endocrine mechanisms underlying these associations are still unclear. The aim of this study was to relate hormone levels at age 8 years with the timing of menarche.
Methods: A total of 329 girls from the Avon Longitudinal Study of Parents and Children (ALSPAC) prospective study provided blood samples at mean age 8.1 years (range 8.0–8.5) for hormone measurements, and were followed longitudinally to establish age at menarche. Age at menarche was reported by questionnaire and categorized as before 12.0, 12.0–13.0, or later than 13 years.
Results: Earlier menarche was associated with greater body weight, height, and body mass index at age 8 years. Among the endocrine variables, after adjustment for body mass index and height only IGF-I, androstenedione, and DHEAS remained significantly associated with earlier menarche.
Conclusions: These findings support direct roles of IGF-I and adrenal androgens on the regulation of pubertal maturation.

This study confirms earlier evidence that body size closely relates to the timing of pubertal development; girls with greater weight, height, BMI and waist circumference undergoing earlier puberty. This finding is consistent with a direct role of childhood obesity on the secular trends in pubertal timing previously suggested by the same research team [11]. An original finding is that IGF-I levels are an independent predictor of early menarche, suggesting a direct role of IGF-I in controlling pubertal timing in humans [12]. IGF-I may, in fact, act at multiple sites such as hypothalamus, pituitary, and ovaries to modulate the reproductive system [13]. The association between the concentrations of adrenal androgens and the timing of menarche is less surprising since adrenarche is a well-known preliminary stage heralding the onset of puberty. Low birth weight and rapid weight gain in infancy are associated with increased levels of IGF-I and adrenal androgens, suggesting that these hormones may mediate the effects exerted by intrauterine and early postnatal programming on childhood growth and pubertal development.

Three-year efficacy and safety of LB03002, a once-weekly sustained-release growth hormone (GH) preparation, in prepubertal children with GH deficiency (GHD)

Péter F, Bidlingmaier M, Savoy C, Ji HJ, Saenger PH
Department of Pediatrics, Albert Einstein College of Medicine, Bronx, NY, USA
PHSaenger@aol.com
J Clin Endocrinol Metab 2012;97:400–407

Background: The availability of a GH depot preparation might considerably improve the management of children on GH therapy. LB03002 is a novel once-weekly sustained-release formulation of recombinant human GH (rhGH) that could potentially offer patients and caregivers a suitable alternative to daily subcutaneous injections. The aim of this study was to explore the optimal LB03002 dose to stimulate long-term longitudinal growth and to establish the long-term safety profile of the compound.

Methods: GH-naive prepubertal GH-deficient children were randomized to four groups who received: (1) 0.2 mg/kg/week LB03002 for 12 months, followed by 0.5 mg/kg/week for another 24 months (n = 13); (2) 0.5 mg/kg/week LB03002 for 36 months (n = 13); (3) 0.7 mg/kg/week LB03002 for 12 months, followed by 0.5 mg/kg/week for another 24 months (n = 13), or (4) conventional therapy with daily GH 0.03 mg/kg/day for 24 months, switched to 0.5 mg/kg/week LB03002 for 12 months (n = 12). Height measurements were taken at baseline and after 6, 12, 24, and 36 months, and height and height velocity were calculated.

Results: During the first 12 months of treatment, catch-up growth was observed in all treatment groups, with a dose-dependent pattern of response in the three LB03002 groups. Whereas patients treated with the lower dose of LB03002 showed a reduced growth response in comparison with those receiving daily GH injections, the growth responses for the 0.5 and 0.7 mg/kg/week LB03002 groups were comparable to the daily GH group during the first year. There were no significant differences in height SD score gain between any groups at 24 and 36 months. Bone maturation and IGF-I levels did not differ for any LB03002 dose compared with daily GH. No significant change in mean fasting glucose and glycosylated hemoglobin concentrations was observed in any treatment group at any time.

Conclusions: LB03002 treatment of prepubertal GHD children for up to 3 years resulted in an efficacy and safety profile that did not differ from that of conventional daily GH regimen. 0.5 mg/kg/week appeared to be the optimal dose for long-term treatment.

Long-term GH therapy in children is currently based on daily subcutaneous injections, which makes it cumbersome for patients and their caregivers, leading to a reduced adherence to treatment and potentially affecting the long-term growth response. Pharmaceutical research in this field has been focusing on the development of GH depot preparations to be given once or twice weekly. A previous depot GH preparation tested over a period of 1 year did not provide satisfactory results in comparison with the conventional daily therapy [14]. LB03002 is a novel once-weekly sustained-release formulation of recombinant human GH (rhGH), manufactured using the yeast *Saccharomyces cerevisiae* as the expression system, contained in sodium hyaluronate microparticles, which are suspended in medium-chain triglycerides before injection. This is the first study reporting on the efficacy and safety of LB03002 administered once per week over a period of 3 years. These preliminary data look promising, showing a growth response and safety profile comparable to conventional daily therapy. However, this study was designed as a dose-finding study, and thus, the overall number of treated patients was small, and follow-up limited to 36 months. Therefore, data on adult height and longer safety assessment are needed before drawing any conclusions.

Beneficial effects of growth hormone treatment on cognition in children with Prader-Willi syndrome: a randomized controlled trial and longitudinal study

Siemensma EP, Tummers-de Lind van Wijngaarden RF, Festen DA, Troeman ZC, van Alfen-van der Velden AA, Otten BJ, Rotteveel J, Odink RJ, Bindels-de Heus GC, van Leeuwen M, Haring DA, Oostdijk W, Bocca G, Mieke Houdijk EC, van Trotsenburg AS, Hoorweg-Nijman JJ, van Wieringen H, Vreuls RC, Jira PE, Schroor EJ, van Pinxteren-Nagler E, Pilon JW, Lunshof LB, Hokken-Koelega AC
Dutch Growth Research Foundation/Erasmus MC Rotterdam, Rotterdam, The Netherlands
e.siemensma@kindengroei.nl
J Clin Endocrinol Metab 2012 (E-pub ahead of print)

Background: Data on GH effect on mental development are few and conflicting. GH therapy has been suggested to improve mental development in conditions associated with mild or severe cognitive impairment such as children born small for gestational age or with Down syndrome. Short-term GH treatment significantly improved mental and motor development in infants with Prader-Willi syndrome (PWS), compared with randomized controls. The aim of this study was to investigate the effect of GH treatment on cognitive functioning in children with PWS followed over a period of 4 years.

Methods: 50 prepubertal children with PWS aged 3.5–14 years were studied in a randomized controlled GH trial. Cognitive functioning was measured biennially by short forms of the WPPSI-R or WISC-R, depending on age. Total IQ (TIQ) score was estimated based on two subtest scores.

Results: Whereas in GH-treated children mean SD scores of all subtests and mean TIQ score remained similar compared to baseline, in untreated controls mean subtest SD scores and mean TIQ score decreased with time. This decline was significant for the Similarities and Vocabulary subtests. After 4 years of GH treatment, mean SD scores on the Similarities and Block design subtests were significantly higher than at baseline.

Conclusions: GH treatment prevents deterioration of certain cognitive skills in children with PWS and improves abstract reasoning and visuospatial skills during 4 years of GH treatment. Children with a more severe mental impairment at baseline had more benefit from GH treatment.

The issue of a potential beneficial effect of GH therapy on mental development is under debate as the available data are conflicting [15]. The authors previously reported an improvement of mental and motor performance in infants with PWS undergoing 12 months of GH therapy [16]. In this study they show that children with PWS undergo a spontaneous deterioration of cognitive skills, which can be partially prevented by GH treatment. Another interesting finding was that children with a maternal uniparental disomy had a significantly lower score on the Block design subtest but a better response during GH treatment than children with a mutation, suggesting that the more is the mental impairment at baseline, the more is the benefit induced by GH treatment. It is noteworthy that these effects of GH therapy were independent of IGF-I circulating levels, suggesting either a paracrine/autocrine IGF-I action or a direct GH effect on the brain [17]. If these results will be confirmed by other trials in larger cohorts of patients, the goals of GH treatment in children with PWS will comprise not only the normalization of height and the improvement of body composition, but also the prevention of mental deterioration. However, these findings and conclusions should be taken with caution. The average age of children with PWS treated with GH was 7.4 years and, although the authors quote a review reporting an effect of GH on adult brain, it seems unlikely that the GH action on a mature brain may be so relevant to have an impact on function. The other explanation provided for explaining the improved cognitive skills during GH treatment was the improvement of sleep apnea in children with PWS induced by therapy. A significant positive effect of GH on sleep apnea has never been proved. On the contrary, GH therapy has been related to tonsillar and adenoid hypertrophy and consequent worsening of obstructive apnea [18].

Three-year growth hormone treatment in short children with X-linked hypophosphatemic rickets: effects on linear growth and body disproportion

Živičnjak M, Schnabel D, Staude H, Even G, Marx M, Beetz R, Holder M, Billing H, Fischer DC, Rabl W, Schumacher M, Hiort O, Haffner D, Nephrologie HRSGotAfPEaGfP
Department of Pediatric Kidney, Liver, and Metabolic Diseases, Hannover Medical School, Hannover, Germany
zivicnjak.miroslav@mh-hannover.de
J Clin Endocrinol Metab 2011;96:E2097–2105

Background: Despite adequate replacement therapy, children with X-linked hypophosphatemic rickets (XLH) fail to achieve a normal adult height. They show progressive disproportional stunting characterized by reduced leg growth associated with normal trunk growth. Preliminary studies showed that GH therapy increases height velocity in short XLH patients during short-term trials. However, GH was also suggested to worse preexisting body disproportions. The aim of this study was to determine the effects of 3 years of GH treatment on stature and body proportions in short children with XLH.

Methods: The study design was a 3-year randomized controlled open-label GH study in short prepubertal children with XLH (n = 16) on phosphate and calcitriol treatment. 76 XLH patients on conservative treatment represented the control group. Changes in SD scores (SDS) of stature and linear body segments were the main outcome measures.

Results: Growth of XLH patients at time of enrollment was severely impaired (–3.3 SDS), leg length (–3.8 SDS) being particularly affected by disease, whereas sitting height (–1.7 SDS) was preserved. GH therapy was effective in inducing a sustained increase in linear growth (stature +1.1 SDS; sitting height +1.3 SDS; leg length +0.8 SDS; arm length +1.1 SDS; each p < 0.05 vs. baseline). However, mean height SDS at the end of the 3-year trial did not significantly differ between treated and control group. Sitting height index remained stable in both the GH-treated patients and in study controls but increased further in the XLH-reference population. During the 3-year observation period, bone age tended to increase faster in GH-treated patients compared with controls.

Conclusions: Three-year GH treatment in short children with XLH resulted partly effective in improving linear growth without progression of body disproportion.

GH therapy has been proposed in various conditions associated with short stature even when GH secretion is not impaired. If proved beneficial XLH might represent a further indication for a pharmacologic rather than replacement treatment, with all the precautions discussed above about GH and IGF-1 potential untoward effects in the long run. Children with XLH, though undergoing specific therapy with large doses of oral phosphate and calcitriol, fail to achieve normal adult height and show progressive disproportional stunting mainly due to a continuously diminished leg growth during the prepubertal growth period [19]. Previous reports have shown that GH treatment increases growth velocity mildly and has a small effect on adult height in short XLH patients [20, 21], although some studies indicated that GH might aggravate the preexisting body disproportion in XLH patients [22]. The results of these preliminary reports looked promising though only few patients were enrolled in nonrandomized trials. The present study conducted over a period of 3 years on a relatively large cohort of XLH patients still offers conflicting results showing an acceleration of growth, with no detrimental effect on body proportions, but at the same time, an acceleration of bone maturation in GH-treated subjects. At the end of the treatment period, no significant difference in height between GH-treated and untreated children was observed. Let us wait until the completion of growth in these patients before we prescribe GH for unproven indications. Most of all, no long-term results also means no evidence for safety.

Light stimuli control neuronal migration by altering of insulin-like growth factor 1 (IGF-1) signaling

Li Y, Komuro Y, Fahrion JK, Hu T, Ohno N, Fenner KB, Wooton J, Raoult E, Galas L, Vaudry D, Komuro H
Department of Neurosciences, Lerner Research Institute, The Cleveland Clinic Foundation, Cleveland, OH, USA
komuroh@ccf.org
Proc Natl Acad Sci USA 2012;109:2630–2635

Background: Environmental cues, such as temperature and light, intervene in brain development by controlling neuronal proliferation and migration. The aim of this study was to determine the role of light stimuli in neuronal cell migration.
Methods: Newborn mice were exposed to a standard light-dark cycle and the migration of cerebellar granule cells in the external granular layer (EGL) was determined at postnatal day 10. Serum and cerebellum IGF-I levels were assessed by ELISA. Microexplant cultures of postnatal day 3 (P3) mouse cerebella were used to test the effect of IGF-I on cell migration. The activity of IGF-1 receptors was specifically inhibited by the use of picropodophyllin (PPP).
Results: Granule cells migrated faster during light cycles and more slowly during dark cycles in early postnatal mouse cerebella. Cerebellar and serum IGF-1 levels of P10 mice depended on light stimuli: IGF-1 levels being high during light cycles, when granule cells migrated faster, and low during dark cycles, when granule cells migrated more slowly. The addition of IGF-I to the culture medium of mouse cerebella stimulated migration in a dose-dependent manner by enhancing PI3K- and PKC-related signaling pathways through the activation of IGF-1 receptors. The inhibition of IGF-1 receptors decelerated granule cell migration during light cycles (high IGF-1 levels) but did not alter migration during dark cycles (low IGF-1 levels).
Conclusions: These results suggest that during early postnatal development, light stimuli control granule cell migration by altering the activity of IGF-1 receptors through modification of cerebellar IGF-1 levels.

The mechanisms underlying the link between environmental stimuli and brain development are largely unknown. This study for the first time elegantly demonstrates that cerebellum development, particularly the migration of cerebellar granule cells in early postnatal life, s regulated by light stimuli. Even more interestingly, light acts through modulation of local (cerebellar) IGF-I levels; thus IGF-I representing the final mediator of light effects on early cerebellum maturation. Circulating IGF-1 crosses the blood-brain barrier easily [23], but is also synthesized in the developing cerebellum [24]. The potential clinical implications of these findings are the following: (1) our ancestors raised their infants in the open, while we hide them in semi-dark rooms. Alterations in the exposure of human babies to light stimuli may affect granule cell migration and may have long-lasting consequences on brain development and function later in life, because the cell density and dendrite length of granule cells are significantly reduced at an adult age in the cerebellum of mice exposed to altered light stimuli during early postnatal development. (2) IGF-I, a well-known neurotrophic factor, plays a key role in mediating the light-induced brain maturation and may represent a molecule effective in restoring normal development of cerebellum in babies at high risk of cerebellar damage.

Noonan syndrome-causing SHP2 mutants inhibit insulin-like growth factor 1 release via growth hormone-induced ERK hyperactivation, which contributes to short stature

De Rocca Serra-Nédélec A, Edouard T, Tréguer K, Tajan M, Araki T, Dance M, Mus M, Montagner A, Tauber M, Salles JP, Valet P, Neel BG, Raynal P, Yart A
Institut National de la Santé et de la Recherche Médicale U1048 and Université Paul Sabatier, Institut des Maladies Métaboliques et Cardiovasculaires, Toulouse, France
armelle.yart@inserm.fr
Proc Natl Acad Sci USA 2012;109:4257–4262

Background: Noonan syndrome (NS), a genetic disease clinically characterized by heart defects, facial dysmorphism and short stature. Half of the patients with NS carry activating mutations of the tyrosine phosphatase SHP2 (PTPN11) but the mechanism through which SHP2 induces growth retardation is still undefined. The aim of this study was to explore how SHP2 mutations may alter GH response.

Methods: A mouse model of NS expressing the D61G mutant of SHP2 and different cellular approaches were used.

Results: Early postnatal growth retardation in mutant mice was associated with reduced IGF-I and IGFBP-3 circulating levels. The experiments in cell lines revealed a negative effect of SHP2 on GH-induced IGF-I production whereas a positive effect of SHP2 on GH-evoked ERK1/2 phosphorylation was observed. Furthermore, SHP2 cooperated in GH-induced RAS activation by dephosphorylation of the adaptor Grb2-associated binder-1 (GAB1) on its RAS GTPase-activating protein (RASGAP) binding sites. NS mutant mice showed increased ERK1/2 phosphorylation upon GH treatment. Finally, treatment with a specific inhibitor of ERK1/2 restored a normal GH-induced IGF-I production and partially rescued growth retardation.

Conclusions: SHP2 mutants show inhibition of GH-induced IGF-1 release through RAS/ERK1/2 hyperactivation, a mechanism that could ultimately lead to growth failure. These findings open avenue for potential treatments based on the modulation of RAS/ERK1/2 in NS caused by PTPN11 mutations.

Clinical data show that children with NS carrying PTPN11 (SHP2) mutations display reduced IGF-I levels [25]. The SHP2 mutant mice used in this study showed similar growth phenotype, characterized by early onset of growth retardation and reduction of both IGF-I and IGFBP-3 levels. Interestingly, whereas liver-selective *IGF1* gene disruption, determining a 75% reduction of circulating IGF-I, was not associated with growth failure [26], the 40% reduction of IGF-I concentrations in NS mice was accompanied by severe growth retardation, suggesting a concomitant impairment of local IGF-I autocrine/paracrine actions, particularly in bone and cartilage. The merit of this study was to elucidate the mechanism underlying the association of SHP2 mutation and growth failure. The authors identified in the dysregulation of RAS/ERK1/2 activation the critical checkpoint affecting IGF-I secretion, eventually leading to growth failure. The finding of the negative influence of mutated SHP2 on GH-induced IGF-I production may have potential clinical implications. GH treatment has been shown to stimulate growth in children with NS [27] but long-term efficacy results are modest. The results of this study clearly show that subjects with SHP2 mutations have partial GH insensitivity which may account for the moderate response to therapy. In the light of these data, short children with NS might need a higher GH dose, IGF-I therapy or a MEK inhibitor which has already been shown to improve growth and alleviate cardiac and craniofacial defects in animal models of NS [28].

Skeletal muscle mitochondrial function is associated with longitudinal growth velocity in children and adolescents

McCormack SE, McCarthy MA, Farilla L, Hrovat MI, Systrom DM, Grinspoon SK, Fleischman A
Program in Nutritional Metabolism and Neuroendocrine Unit, Massachusetts General Hospital and Harvard Medical School, Boston, MA, USA
afleischman@partners.org
J Clin Endocrinol Metab 2011;96:E1612–1618

Background: Mitochondrial diseases are associated with the impairment of growth suggesting that mitochondrial function, providing energy and substrates, may play a key role in longitudinal growth. The aim of this study was to determine the relationship between mitochondrial function and linear growth in healthy children and adolescents.

Methods: 29 children aged 8–15 years were enrolled in this prospective longitudinal study. Fasting laboratory studies and an estimate of mitochondrial function (as assessed by the time to recovery of phosphocreatine (PCr) concentration after submaximal quadriceps extension/flexion exercise using ^{31}P magnetic resonance spectroscopy) were obtained at baseline and annually for 2 years.

Results: Data were complete at the 1 year time point for 23 subjects. More rapid skeletal muscle oxidative phosphorylation, as suggested by a shorter time to PCr recovery after submaximal exercise, was significantly associated with growth velocity in the subsequent year. This result was significant in the first year. In multivariate modeling, baseline mitochondrial function remained significantly and independently associated with growth, controlling for age, gender, pubertal stage, body mass index Z-score, height Z-score, sex steroid levels and IGF-I concentrations.

Conclusions: A novel association between mitochondrial function, expressed by time to recovery of PCr concentration after submaximal exercise, and linear growth in childhood and adolescence is shown.

The growth process requires both energy and substrate to fulfill physiological demands. Consistent with the pivotal role played by mitochondria in energy metabolism during growth is the observation that mitochondrial diseases are often associated with growth impairment. This study for the first time shows an association between linear growth and mitochondrial function as investigated by an indirect and noninvasive method based on ^{31}P magnetic resonance spectroscopy. This association might be explained by a GH-dependent regulation of mitochondrial function [29]. However, there are many potential biases affecting the interpretation of these results. The small size and the heterogeneity of the study cohort, including both prepubertal and pubertal children of whom two thirds were overweight, calls for caution in drawing conclusions. Moreover, association does not necessarily mean causation. Nevertheless, the originality of the results and their potential physiological and clinical fallout warrant further large-scale studies to elucidate the extent of the interplay between muscle energy production and growth plate growth and maturation during childhood and adolescence.

Important for clinical practice

Incidence of diabetes mellitus and evolution of glucose parameters in growth hormone-deficient subjects during growth hormone replacement therapy: a long-term observational study

Luger A, Mattsson AF, Koltowska-Häggström M, Thunander M, Góth M, Verhelst J, Abs R
Clinical Division of Endocrinology and Metabolism, Medical University of Vienna, Vienna, Austria
anton.luger@meduniwien.ac.at

Diabetes Care 2012;35:57–62

Background: Growth hormone (GH) exerts anti-insulin effects in liver and muscle and GH therapy has been associated with the risk of developing insulin resistance and diabetes. The aim of the current study was to determine the incidence of diabetes during GH replacement therapy (GHRT) in adult patients. In addition, results of a longitudinal study analyzing yearly fasting plasma glucose and HbA_{1c} concentrations in a subgroup of patients over an observation period of 6 years are reported.
Methods: KIMS database was the data source. Only patients with severe adult-onset GH deficiency and naive to GH treatment were selected. A total of 5,143 GH-deficient patients (mean age ± SD, 49 ± 13 years) were analyzed. Mean observation time was 3.9 years. Total number of patient-years was 20.106. Observed number of cases-to-expected number of cases (O/E) ratios of patients diagnosed with diabetes were calculated, and stratified for age and sex. The expected number of cases was calculated using normal population-based age- and sex-specific reference incidence rates from Sweden and three additional European regions, plus one US region.
Results: 523 patients (10.2%) developed diabetes after a median period of 1.7 years. Patients who developed diabetes were significantly older, had higher BMI, waist circumference, waist-to-hip ratio, and triglyceride concentrations, and had significantly higher systolic and diastolic blood pressure and significantly lower HDL cholesterol concentrations than those who did not develop diabetes. Overall diabetes incidence was 2.6 per 100 patient-years, significantly higher than the expected according to the Swedish reference, the overall O/E ratio was 6.0 (95% CI 5.5–6.6), as well as to the four other populations references, the O/E ratios ranging from 2.11 (1.86–2.39) to 5.22 (4.76–5.72). In the subgroup of patients with available yearly fasting glucose and HbA_{1c} data over a period of 5 years, plasma glucose concentrations increased from 84.4 ± 0.9 to 89.5 ± 0.8 mg/dl (0.70 mg/dl/year) and HbA_{1c} increased from 4.74 ± 0.04 to 5.09 ± 0.13% (0.036%/year).
Conclusions: Diabetes incidence appears to be increased in GH-deficient patients receiving GHRT, thus strongly suggesting that patients on GHRT, particularly those with an adverse baseline risk profile, should be carefully followed regarding parameters of glucose metabolism.

Although this study reports data from a large database of adult patients (KIMS), the results are relevant for clinical practice raising concern on the safety of GH replacement therapy, and should drive the attitude of pediatric endocrinologists as well. Indeed the finding of increased incidence of diabetes in adult patients undergoing GH replacement therapy strengthen the results of previous studies reporting a similar increase in metabolic risk in both adults and children treated with GH [30–32]. These data should prompt the clinicians who treat subjects with GH to monitor glucose homeostasis especially in those patients with predisposing factors (i.e. familial history for type 2 diabetes, high BMI and waist circumference, etc.). As in the case of the potential cancer risk associated with long-term GH therapy, it may be argued that the metabolic risk may be intrinsically related to the disease (GH deficiency) rather than to treatment, and that, ideally, only a randomized controlled trial might clarify the real impact of GH therapy on the development of diabetes. However, realistically speaking, it is extremely unlikely that a study involving an ideal age-, sex- and risk factor-matched GH-deficient group not receiving GHRT in a prospective controlled trial will ever be performed. Regulatory authorities in several countries have recently questioned the beneficial effect of GH in adult GHD. This paper adds another point to the hesitant. Alternatively, we may be giving GH in a wrong fashion; after all, normal secretion of GH is pulsatile.

A novel missense mutation in the SH2 domain of the STAT5B gene results in a transcriptionally inactive STAT5B associated with severe IGF-I deficiency, immune dysfunction, and lack of pulmonary disease

Scaglia PA, Martínez AS, Feigerlová E, Bezrodnik L, Gaillard MI, Di Giovanni D, Ballerini MG, Jasper HG, Heinrich JJ, Fang P, Domené HM, Rosenfeld RG, Hwa V
Department of Pediatrics, CDRC 2250, Oregon Health and Science University, Portland, OR, USA
hwav@ohsu.edu
J Clin Endocrinol Metab 2012;97:E830–839

Background: Signal transducer and activator of transcription 5b (STAT5B) deficiency accounts for rare forms of GH insensitivity (GHI) characterized by IGF-I deficiency (IGFD), and severe immune dysregulation manifesting as progressive worsening of pulmonary function. The aim of this study was to report the phenotype of a patient with a novel mutation of STAT5B.

Patient: A girl from Argentina developed severe generalized seborrheic dermatitis at the age of 1 year. Autoimmune thyroiditis was diagnosed at 4.5 years, and she was started on L-T$_4$ therapy. In later years, she developed severe varicella with cutaneous infection and *Streptococcus pyogenes* septicemia. Impairment of pulmonary function was not observed throughout childhood or adolescence. She concomitantly exhibited severe growth failure, achieving an adult height of 124.7 cm. Endocrine evaluations (normal provocative GH tests, low serum IGF-I, –3.7 SDS, and IGF-binding protein-3, –4.5 SDS) were consistent with primary IGF-I deficiency.

Results: Sequencing of the *STAT5B* gene revealed a T→C transition in exon 16, corresponding to the second nucleotide of codon 646 (c.1937T3C), which changed phenylalanine (Phe, F) to serine (Ser, S) (p.Phe646Ser; p.F646S). In reconstitution studies, GH-induced phosphorylation of the STAT5B p.F646S variant was observed but was consistently less than that detected with wild-type STAT5B. Similar observations were made when treated with IFN-γ. These findings suggested that STAT5B p.F646S had retained the ability to associate with critical pY motifs on the GHR and IFN-γ receptors.

Conclusion: A novel homozygous *STAT5B* missense mutation, located within the critical SH2 domain, was identified in a patient with profound postnatal growth failure due to IGF deficiency but who lacked the severe chronic pulmonary disease and immunodeficiency observed in the patient carrying the first described *STAT5B* missense mutation in SH2 domain.

This case report describes the clinical features of a novel homozygous missense mutation in the *STAT5B* gene. This is the ninth case of STAT5B deficiency. Functional studies and clinical presentation of this novel mutation were compared with p.A630P missense mutation previously identified in the same critical SH2 domain. Unlike the previously described missense mutation however, this new mutation was associated with a residual capacity of *STAT5B* to be phosphorylated in response to GH and IFN-γ, although could not drive transcription. Another striking difference between the 2 patients was the absence of pulmonary symptoms in the new case, despite a diagnosed T-cell lymphopenia and other immune irregularities. The mechanism underlying the relative immune competency in this and all previous patients relates to the overlap in STAT signaling between GH and several cytokines and interferon. This case confirms the critical importance of the SH2 domain for mediating the GH-induced regulation of *IGF1* expression. Moreover, this patient shows a new genotype-phenotype association among the STAT5B mutations, mainly characterized by the severe growth failure, which is typical of patients carrying other types of STAT5B mutations, but spared pulmonary function.

Food for thought

Targeted loss of GHR signaling in mouse skeletal muscle protects against high-fat diet-induced metabolic deterioration

Vijayakumar A, Wu Y, Sun H, Li X, Jeddy Z, Liu C, Schwartz GJ, Yakar S, LeRoith D
Division of Endocrinology, Diabetes, and Bone Diseases, the Department of Medicine, Mount Sinai School of Medicine, New York, NY, USA
derek.leroith@mssm.edu
Diabetes 2012;61:94–103

Background: It is difficult to distinguish the metabolic actions directly exerted by growth hormone (GH) in tissues from those mediated by IGF-I and/or insulin. The aim of this study was to identify the direct metabolic effects of GH in the muscle using mice with selective postnatal inactivation of growth hormone receptor (GHR) gene in skeletal muscle.

Methods: Specific GHR inactivation in muscle was achieved using the Cre/loxP system (mGHRKO model). Body composition analysis was performed using the EchoMRI 3-in-1 NMR system. Total triglycerides (TG) were extracted from the liver and gastrocnemius using the chloroform-methanol method. Metabolic cage studies were performed in unrestrained mice fed a high-fat (60% fat) diet (HFD) for 12–14 weeks. The metabolic state of the mGHRKO mice was characterized under lean and obese states.

Results: High-fat diet feeding in the mGHRKO mice was associated with reduced adiposity, improved insulin sensitivity, lower systemic inflammation, decreased muscle and hepatic triglyceride content, and greater energy expenditure compared with control mice. The obese mGHRKO mice also had an increased respiratory exchange ratio, suggesting increased carbohydrate utilization. Muscles of obese mGHRKO mice had decreased *socs2* and muscles of both lean and obese mGHRKO mice showed a higher interleukin-15 and lower myostatin expression relative to controls.

Conclusions: These data suggest a role for muscle GHR signaling in mediating whole-body insulin resistance in obesity either by altering substrate utilization or by modifying energy expenditure.

As most GH actions are mediated by IGF-I via endocrine, paracrine and autocrine actions, it is difficult to dissect pure GH actions from those actually mediated by IGF-I. The selective postnatal knockout of muscle GHR has enabled the authors to elucidate the role of skeletal muscle GHR signaling in regulating metabolism. The inactivation of muscle GHR has revealed a novel role of muscle GHR signaling in facilitating cross-talk between muscle and other metabolic tissues such as liver and adipose tissue, probably via the regulation of secreted myokines, such as myostatin. However, these results are in contrast with that of Mavalli et al. [33] showing in a similar model of selective muscle inactivation of GHR increased body weight, body adiposity, and circulating TG levels and worsened insulin sensitivity. The discrepancies between the two studies may arise from the different genetic background of the mice used or from the different timing of GHR inactivation. Therefore, different animal models of muscle GHR inactivation yield different opposite results, suggesting that the genetic, endocrine and metabolic mechanisms involved in the interplay between muscle GHR signaling and metabolism are complex and still largely unknown. We knew that GHD and GHIS are associated with muscle weakness and adiposity; here may lay the mechanism.

Growth hormone receptor regulates β-cell hyperplasia and glucose-stimulated insulin secretion in obese mice

Wu Y, Liu C, Sun H, Vijayakumar A, Giglou PR, Qiao R, Oppenheimer J, Yakar S, LeRoith D
Endocrinology/Diabetes and Bone Disease, The Mount Sinai School of Medicine, New York, NY, USA
shoshana.yakar@mssm.edu
J Clin Invest 2011;121:2422–2426

Background: β cells express the GH receptor and GH stimulates insulin gene expression, biosynthesis, and release in β cells of rodents and humans. However, it is unclear whether these effects are directly exerted by GH or are mediated by IGF-I or by changes in body composition. The aim of this study was to determine the role of GHR in determining β-cell mass and function during normal and pathophysiological conditions.

Methods: Specific *Ghr* inactivation in β cells was achieved using the Cre/loxP system to generate β-cell-specific GHRKO mice.

Results: βGHRKO mice fed a standard chow diet showed impaired glucose-stimulated insulin secretion but had no changes in islet size or insulin content. When challenged with a high-fat diet (HFD), βGHRKO mice exhibited impaired β-cell hyperplasia and a β-cell secretory defect, with deterioration of glucose homeostasis. Obese βGHRKO mice exhibited decreased β-cell proliferation.

Conclusions: Deletion of GHR specifically in pancreatic islet β cells was associated with a lack of compensatory hyperplasia in response to HFD-induced obesity, thus suggesting that GH receptor plays critical roles in glucose-stimulated insulin secretion and β-cell compensation in response to a high-fat diet.

This is another paper reporting the structural and functional consequences of targeted loss of GHR, in this case specifically in the pancreatic β cell. The objective was to clarify the role, if any, of GH and its receptor in regulating β-cell proliferation and function in mice either fed a standard chow diet or a high-fat diet. Previous studies yielded conflicting results showing that loss of GHR in β cells was followed by reduced β-cell mass, impaired glucose tolerance, and increased insulin sensitivity. However, these animals displayed compromised growth and significant changes in body adiposity, thus questioning a direct causal effect of GHR ablation [34]. Furthermore, the ablation of STAT5A/B had negligible effects on β-cell mass or function under normal conditions, but in obese mice was associated with hyperglycemia and glucose intolerance [35]. These results are consistent with a metabolic role played by GHR during obesogenic conditions, GHR ablation negatively influencing glucose-stimulated insulin secretion and β-cell compensation in response to a high-fat diet. These targeted knockout studies are valuable in identifying the direct actions exerted by specific molecules, in this case GHR. However, physiology is far more complex involving a network of interactions among multiple players influencing each other. Therefore, it would be simplistic and potentially misleading trying to speculate that GHR may mediate potential protective effects on β cells in conditions of overfeeding.

References

1. Blakesley VA, Kalebic T, Helman LJ, Stannard B, Faria TN, Roberts CT, et al: Tumorigenic and mitogenic capacities are reduced in transfected fibroblasts expressing mutant insulin-like growth factor (IGF)-I receptors. The role of tyrosine residues 1250, 1251, and 1316 in the carboxy-terminus of the IGF-I receptor. Endocrinology 1996;137:410–417.
2. Olmos D, Postel-Vinay S, Molife LR, Okuno SH, Schuetze SM, Paccagnella ML, et al: Safety, pharmacokinetics, and preliminary activity of the anti-IGF-1R antibody figitumumab (CP-751,871) in patients with sarcoma and Ewing's sarcoma: a phase 1 expansion cohort study. Lancet Oncol 2010;11:129–135.
3. Toretsky JA, Gorlick R: IGF-1R targeted treatment of sarcoma. Lancet Oncol 2010;11:105–106.
4. Clayton PE, Banerjee I, Murray PG, Renehan AG: Growth hormone, the insulin-like growth factor axis, insulin and cancer risk. Nat Rev Endocrinol 2011;7:11–24.
5. Rosenfeld RG, Cohen P, Robison LL, Bercu BB, Clayton P, Hoffman AR, et al: Long-term surveillance of growth hormone therapy. J Clin Endocrinol Metab 2012;97:68–72.
6. Roseboom T, de Rooij S, Painter R: The Dutch famine and its long-term consequences for adult health. Early Hum Dev 2006;82:485–491.
7. Lumey L, Stein A, Kahn H, van der Pal-de Bruin K, Blauw G, Zybert P, et al: Cohort profile: the Dutch Hunger Winter families study. Int J Epidemiol 2007;36:1196–1204.
8. Heijmans B, Tobi E, Stein A, Putter H, Blauw G, Susser E, et al: Persistent epigenetic differences associated with prenatal exposure to famine in humans. Proc Natl Acad Sci USA 2008;105:17046–17049.
9. Petry CJ, Evans ML, Wingate DL, Ong KK, Reik W, Constância M, et al: Raised late pregnancy glucose concentrations in mice carrying pups with targeted disruption of H19δ13. Diabetes 2010;59:282–286.
10. Haig D: Genetic conflicts in human pregnancy. Q Rev Biol 1993;68:495–532.
11. Ong KK, Ahmed ML, Dunger DB: Lessons from large population studies on timing and tempo of puberty (secular trends and relation to body size): the European trend. Mol Cell Endocrinol 2006;254/255:8–12.

12. Zhao J, Xiong DH, Guo Y, Yang TL, Recker RR, Deng HW: Polymorphism in the insulin-like growth factor 1 gene is associated with age at menarche in Caucasian females. Hum Reprod 2007;22:1789–1794.
13. Daftary SS, Gore AC: IGF-1 in the brain as a regulator of reproductive neuroendocrine function. Exp Biol Med (Maywood) 2005;230:292–306.
14. Reiter EO, Attie KM, Moshang T, Silverman BL, Kemp SF, Neuwirth RB, et al: A multicenter study of the efficacy and safety of sustained release GH in the treatment of naive pediatric patients with GH deficiency. J Clin Endocrinol Metab 2001;86:4700–4706.
15. Scheepens A, Möderscheim TA, Gluckman PD: The role of growth hormone in neural development. Horm Res 2005;64(suppl 3):66–72.
16. De Lind van Wijngaarden RF, Siemensma EP, Festen DA, Otten BJ, van Mil EG, Rotteveel J, et al: Efficacy and safety of long-term continuous growth hormone treatment in children with Prader-Willi syndrome. J Clin Endocrinol Metab 2009;94:4205–4215.
17. Lobie PE, García-Aragón J, Lincoln DT, Barnard R, Wilcox JN, Waters MJ: Localization and ontogeny of growth hormone receptor gene expression in the central nervous system. Brain Res Dev Brain Res 1993;74:225–233.
18. Tauber M, Diene G, Molinas C, Hébert M: Review of 64 cases of death in children with Prader-Willi syndrome. Am J Med Genet A 2008;146:881–887.
19. Zivičnjak M, Schnabel D, Billing H, Staude H, Filler G, Querfeld U, et al: Age-related stature and linear body segments in children with X-linked hypophosphatemic rickets. Pediatr Nephrol 2011;26:223–231.
20. Saggese G, Baroncelli GI, Bertelloni S, Perri G: Long-term growth hormone treatment in children with renal hypophosphatemic rickets: effects on growth, mineral metabolism, and bone density. J Pediatr 1995;127:395–402.
21. Baroncelli GI, Bertelloni S, Ceccarelli C, Saggese G: Effect of growth hormone treatment on final height, phosphate metabolism, and bone mineral density in children with X-linked hypophosphatemic rickets. J Pediatr 2001;138:236–243.
22. Haffner D, Nissel R, Wühl E, Mehls O: Effects of growth hormone treatment on body proportions and final height among small children with X-linked hypophosphatemic rickets. Pediatrics 2004;113:e593–596.
23. Reinhardt RR, Bondy CA: Insulin-like growth factors cross the blood-brain barrier. Endocrinology 1994;135:1753–1761.
24. Bartlett WP, Li XS, Williams M, Benkovic S: Localization of insulin-like growth factor-1 mRNA in murine central nervous system during postnatal development. Dev Biol 1991;147:239–250.
25. Binder G, Neuer K, Ranke MB, Wittekindt NE: PTPN11 mutations are associated with mild growth hormone resistance in individuals with Noonan syndrome. J Clin Endocrinol Metab 2005;90:5377–5381.
26. Yakar S, Liu JL, Stannard B, Butler A, Accili D, Sauer B, et al: Normal growth and development in the absence of hepatic insulin-like growth factor I. Proc Natl Acad Sci USA 1999;96:7324–7329.
27. Romano AA, Dana K, Bakker B, Davis DA, Hunold JJ, Jacobs J, et al: Growth response, near-adult height, and patterns of growth and puberty in patients with Noonan syndrome treated with growth hormone. J Clin Endocrinol Metab 2009;94:2338–2344.
28. Wu X, Simpson J, Hong JH, Kim KH, Thavarajah NK, Backx PH, et al: MEK-ERK pathway modulation ameliorates disease phenotypes in a mouse model of Noonan syndrome associated with the Raf1(L613V) mutation. J Clin Invest 2011;121:1009–1025.
29. Makimura H, Stanley TL, Sun N, Hrovat MI, Systrom DM, Grinspoon SK: The association of growth hormone parameters with skeletal muscle phosphocreatine recovery in adult men. J Clin Endocrinol Metab 2011;96:817–823.
30. Cutfield WS, Wilton P, Bennmarker H, Albertsson-Wikland K, Chatelain P, Ranke MB, et al: Incidence of diabetes mellitus and impaired glucose tolerance in children and adolescents receiving growth-hormone treatment. Lancet 2000;355:610–613.
31. Attanasio AF, Jung H, Mo D, Chanson P, Bouillon R, Ho KK, et al: Prevalence and incidence of diabetes mellitus in adult patients on growth hormone replacement for growth hormone deficiency: a surveillance database analysis. J Clin Endocrinol Metab 2011;96:2255–2261.
32. Child CJ, Zimmermann AG, Scott RS, Cutler GB, Battelino T, Blum WF, et al: Prevalence and incidence of diabetes mellitus in GH-treated children and adolescents: analysis from the GeNeSIS observational research program. J Clin Endocrinol Metab 2011;96:E1025–1034.
33. Mavalli MD, DiGirolamo DJ, Fan Y, Riddle RC, Campbell KS, van Groen T, et al: Distinct growth hormone receptor signaling modes regulate skeletal muscle development and insulin sensitivity in mice. J Clin Invest 2010;120:4007–4020.
34. Liu JL, Coschigano KT, Robertson K, Lipsett M, Guo Y, Kopchick JJ, et al: Disruption of growth hormone receptor gene causes diminished pancreatic islet size and increased insulin sensitivity in mice. Am J Physiol Endocrinol Metab 2004;287:E405–413.
35. Jackerott M, Møldrup A, Thams P, Galsgaard ED, Knudsen J, Lee YC, et al: STAT5 activity in pancreatic β-cells influences the severity of diabetes in animal models of type 1 and 2 diabetes. Diabetes 2006;55:2705–2712.

Bone, Growth Plate and Mineral Metabolism

Outi Mäkitie[a] and Ola Nilsson[b]

[a]Pediatric Endocrinology and Metabolic Bone Diseases, Children's Hospital, Helsinki University Central Hospital and University of Helsinki, Helsinki, Finland
[b]Center for Molecular Medicine and Pediatric Endocrinology Unit, Department of Women's and Children's Health, Karolinska Institutet and Karolinska University Hospital, Stockholm, Sweden and Program in Developmental Endocrinology and Genetics, Eunice Kennedy Shriver National Institute of Child Health and Human Development, Bethesda, MD, USA

It is a challenge to select only a handful of papers from the abundance of high-quality new literature on skeletal physiology and pathology. Last year's chapter described the expanding role of the skeleton in whole-body homeostasis [1]; the present knowledge has been thoroughly covered in a review article by Karsenty and Feron [2]. This year's selected papers discuss new mechanisms in osteoblast and osteoclast communication and their functional regulation. New therapies, such as enzyme-replacement therapy for life-threatening hypophosphatasia and a novel tyrosine kinase inhibitor for achondroplasia, although in their early phases, provide new hope for these debilitating illnesses. The whole-exome sequencing approach has uncovered the genetic background of 'idiopathic' infantile hypercalcemia and acrodysostosis. These discoveries open exciting avenues for further research and are likely to expand our knowledge on not only the pathology behind the disorders but also on the physiological processes in mineral and skeletal homeostasis. Such development can be seen in hereditary vitamin D-resistant rickets caused by unfunctioning vitamin D receptor. The lively discussion on vitamin D target levels – still poorly defined for the pediatric age group – continues. But in the midst of these debates it is good to be reminded about the importance of accurate means to measure serum 25-OH-vitamin D: if the results are unreliable, the target levels are of little value.

Mechanism of the year
Acrodysostosis is Albright's close relative

Recurrent *PRKAR1A* mutation in acrodysostosis with hormone resistance

Linglart A, Menguy C, Couvineau A, Auzan C, Gunes Y, Cancel M, Motte E, Pinto G, Chanson P, Bougneres P, Clauser E, Silve C
INSERM Unité 986, Hôpital St. Vincent de Paul, Paris, France
N Engl J Med 2011;364:2218–2226

Background: The skeletal features of acrodysostosis resemble the Albright's hereditary osteodystrophy in patients with pseudohypoparathyroidism type 1a, but defects in the α-stimulatory subunit of the G-protein (GNAS) are not present in patients with acrodysostosis.
Methods: The authors used candidate-gene approach to test the hypothesis that a gene defect elsewhere in the cyclic AMP (cAMP)-dependent protein kinase A signaling pathway downstream of GNAS might be involved.
Results: Three unrelated patients with acrodysostosis and resistance to multiple hormones were studied. The authors found a heterozygous germline mutation p.R368X in the gene encoding PRKAR1A, the cAMP-dependent regulatory subunit of protein kinase A in all 3 patients. Functional studies showed that the mutated subunit impaired the protein kinase A response to stimulation by cAMP.
Conclusion: Acrodysostosis with hormone resistance is caused by *PRKAR1A* mutation and decreased protein kinase A sensitivity to cAMP. This explains hormone resistance and skeletal similarities with patients with pseudohypoparathyroidism type 1a.

Exome sequencing identifies *PDE4D* mutations as another cause of acrodysostosis

Michot C, Le Goff C, Goldenberg A, Abhyankar A, Klein C, Kinning E, Guerrot AM, Flahaut P, Duncombe A, Baujat G, Lyonnet S, Thalassinos C, Nitschke P, Casanova JL, Le Merrer M, Munnich A, Cormier-Daire V
INSERM U781, Département de Génétique, Université Paris Descartes, Sorbonne Paris Cite, Hôpital Necker Enfants Malades, Paris, France
Am J Hum Genet 2012;90:740–745

Background: Acrodysostosis is a rare autosomal-dominant condition with facial dysostosis, severe brachydactyly, and short stature. Moderate intellectual disability may also be present. Recently, a recurrent mutation in *PRKAR1A* has been identified in 3 individuals with acrodysostosis and resistance to multiple hormones.
Methods: The authors looked for *PRKAR1* mutations in 10 unrelated patients with acrodysostosis, and performed exome sequencing in mutation-negative patients.
Results: De novo *PRKAR1A* mutations were identified in 5 out of the 10 individuals. Four patients had p.Arg368* and 1 had p.Tyr373His. Exome sequencing identified heterozygous mutations in the phosphodiesterase 4D (*PDE4D*) gene as another cause for acrodysostosis. *PDE4D* encodes a class IV cAMP-specific phosphodiesterase that regulates cAMP concentration. Altogether, 4 out of 10 patients harbored heterozygous de novo *PDE4D* mutations (p.Pro225Thr, p.Phe226Ser, p.Ser190Ala and p.Thr587Pro). The 4 individuals with *PDE4D* mutations shared common clinical features, namely characteristic midface and nasal hypoplasia and moderate intellectual disability, but no hormone resistance. However, resistance to PTH and TSH was consistently observed in the 5 cases with *PRKAR1A* mutations.
Conclusion: The findings further support the key role of the cAMP signaling pathway in skeletogenesis.

Exome sequencing identifies *PDE4D* mutations in acrodysostosis

Lee H, Graham JM Jr, Rimoin DL, Lachman RS, Krejci P, Tompson SW, Nelson SF, Krakow D, Cohn DH
Department of Human Genetics, University of California-Los Angeles, CA, USA
Am J Hum Genet 2012;90:746–751

Background: Acrodysostosis is a dominantly-inherited, multisystem disorder with skeletal, endocrine, and neurological abnormalities.
Methods: The authors performed exome sequencing on 5 genetically independent cases with acrodysostosis to identify the underlying genetic cause.
Results: Three different heterozygous missense mutations in *PDE4D*, encoding cAMP-specific phosphodiesterase 4D, were found in 3 of the cases. Two additional cases were heterozygous for de novo missense mutations in *PRKAR1A*, which encodes the cAMP-dependent regulatory subunit of protein kinase A.
Conclusion: These findings demonstrate that acrodysostosis is genetically heterogeneous and underscore the exquisite sensitivity of many tissues to alterations in cAMP homeostasis.

These three papers elucidate the genetic defects underlying acrodysostosis, a rare autosomal dominant skeletal dysplasia. The condition has some similarity with pseudohypoparathyroidism 1A, especially when hormone resistance is present. Several hormones activate G-protein-coupled receptors, which then activate G-protein and adenylyl cyclase, generating intracellular cAMP. In turn, cAMP activates protein kinase A, resulting in the phosphorylation of specific proteins that mediate the effects of these hormones. In pseudohypoparathyroidism type 1a defective α-stimulatory subunit of the G-protein (GNAS) fails to activate the signaling cascade. These three papers show that defects within the same signaling pathway but downstream of GNAS underlie acrodysostosis (fig. 1). The main clinical features of acrodysostosis include facial dysostosis with nasal hypoplasia, severe brachydactyly, and short stature. Moderate intellectual disability may be present. Some patients have resistance to multiple hormones, including PTH, TSH, growth hormone-releasing hormone, and gonadotropins. Altogether, four different *PRKAR1A* mutations were identified in 10 of the reported 18 patients with acrodysostosis; one of the mutations was recurrent and all mutations were located in exon 11. As in other skeletal dysplasias, these are gain-of-function mutations as they decrease protein kinase A sensitivity to cAMP. Seven patients were found to have different heterozygous de novo mutations in the *PDE4D* gene. Phenotype-genotype correlation suggested that patients with *PRKAR1A* mutations were

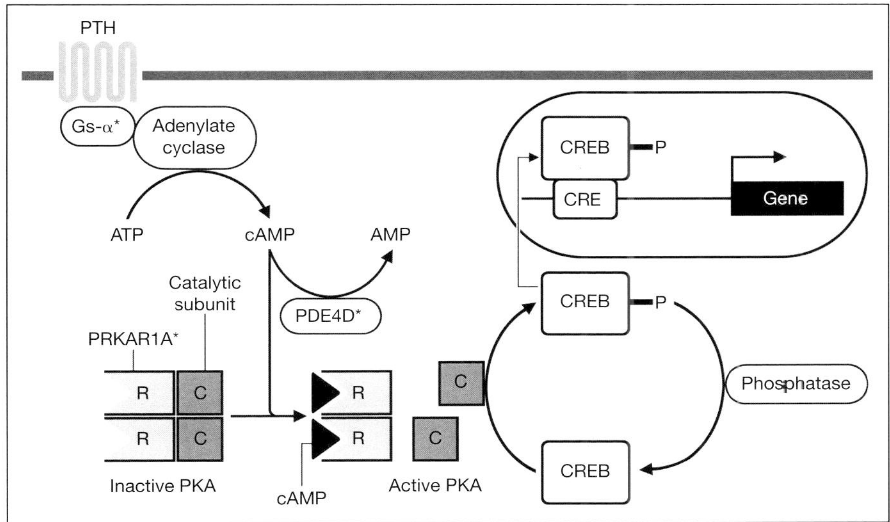

Fig. 1. Ligand binding activates Gs-α and stimulates cAMP synthesis. PRKAR1A binds cAMP, leading to dissociation and activation of PKA and the subsequent phosphorylation of cAMP response element binding (CREB), nuclear translocation, and expression of target genes. PDE4D activity modulates cAMP levels. The asterisks indicate mutated genes in Albright hereditary osteodystrophy (*GNAS*) and in acrodysostosis (*PDE4D* or *PRKAR1A*).

more likely to have short stature and hormone resistance while patents with *PDE4D* gene mutations had the characteristic facial dysostosis and intellectual disability, usually normal stature and no hormone resistance. There was however phenotypic overlap, which is not surprising considering that the defects involve the same signaling cascade. These three reports provide intriguing new information regarding the cAMP-mediated signaling in disorders within pediatric endocrinology.

New mechanisms
All the good in one molecule?

Osteoprotection by semaphorin 3A

Hayashi M, Nakashima T, Taniguchi M, Kodama T, Kumanogoh A, Takayanagi H
Department of Cell Signaling, Graduate School of Medical and Dental Sciences, Tokyo Medical and Dental University, Tokyo, Japan

Nature 2012;485:69–74

Background: Skeletal homeostasis requires in addition to hormones also local factors that regulate bone-forming osteoblasts and bone-resorbing osteoclasts. Osteoprotegerin protects bone by inhibiting osteoclastic bone resorption, but no factor has yet been identified that could locally regulate both osteoclasts and osteoblasts.

Methods: The authors used osteoblasts from mice that lacked osteoprotegerin to identify other factors involved in the regulation of bone homeostasis locally. The function of the identified semaphorin 3A (Sema3A) was then characterized in various animal models and cell assays.

Results: Sema3A was found to exert an osteoprotective effect by both suppressing osteoclastic bone resorption and increasing osteoblastic bone formation. The binding of Sema3A to neuropilin-1 (Nrp1) inhibited RANKL-induced osteoclast differentiation. In addition, Sema3A and Nrp1 binding stimulated osteoblast and inhibited adipocyte differentiation through the canonical Wnt/β-catenin signaling pathway. The *Sema3a–/–* mice displayed osteopenic phenotype; a similar phenotype was shown in mice with a disrupted Sema3A-binding site in Nrp1. Intravenous Sema3A administration in mice increased bone volume and expedited bone regeneration.

Conclusion: The authors conclude that Sema3A inhibits osteoclast differentiation and promotes osteoblastic bone formation and is thus a promising new therapeutic agent in bone and joint diseases.

Bone formation is linked to bone resorption through coupling factors, and skeletal homeostasis requires a balance between these two processes. The differentiation of bone-resorbing osteoclasts is regulated by cells expressing the key osteoclast differentiation factor, RANKL. Osteoblastic cells counterbalance the function of RANKL by producing a soluble decoy receptor for RANKL, osteoprotegerin (Opg). The authors used osteoblast cultures from Opg-deficient mice and show that another factor, Sema3A – a signaling protein involved in the regulation of axonal growth, is a potent direct inhibitor of osteoclastogenesis. Sema3A inhibits the differentiation of osteoclast precursor cells into osteoclasts, thus preventing excessive bone degradation. However, it also promotes osteoblastic bone formation: newly formed osteoblasts secreted Sema3A to augment and coordinate their own differentiation and bone-forming activity. The activity of Sema3A is initiated by its binding to a cell-surface receptor neuropilin-1. Mice deficient of Sema3A and mice with a defective neuropilin-1 receptor, unable to bind Sema3A, both show an osteoporotic phenotype, which is due to enhanced bone degradation and reduced bone formation. The authors went on to investigate whether an intravenous injection of Sema3A could prevent bone loss in a mouse model of menopause. Remarkably, the Sema3A injection inhibited bone degradation and promoted bone formation. Such a potential therapeutic agent would be superior to any presently available medication for the treatment of osteoporosis. The authors optimistically state that Sema3A represents the long sought soluble molecule with the capacity to bring both osteoblasts and osteoclasts into a condition that favors bone mineral increase. The findings are indeed promising and will hopefully lead to the development of a combined antiresorptive and bone-increasing agent capable of promoting bone regeneration.

New mechanisms
Moving from D to E in skeletal alphabets

Vitamin E decreases bone mass by stimulating osteoclast fusion

Fujita K, Iwasaki M, Ochi H, Fukuda T, Ma C, Miyamoto T, Takitani K, Negishi-Koga T, Sunamura S, Kodama T, Takayanagi H, Tamai H, Kato S, Arai H, Shinomiya K, Itoh H, Okawa A, Takeda S
Department of Orthopedic Surgery, Tokyo Medical and Dental University, Tokyo, Japan
Nat Med 2012;18:589–594

Background: Bone homeostasis requires a balance between osteoblastic bone formation and osteoclastic bone resorption. Osteoclasts are multinucleated cells that are formed by mononuclear preosteoclast fusion. It is known that vitamin D plays a pivotal role in maintaining skeletal integrity. However, the role of vitamin E in bone remodeling is unknown.

Methods: The authors used mice deficient in α-tocopherol transfer protein (Ttpa(–/–) mice), a mouse model of genetic vitamin E deficiency, as well as cell-based assays to study the role of vitamin E in bone metabolism.

Results: The Ttpa(–/–) mice had high bone mass as a result of a decrease in bone resorption. Cell-based assays indicated that α-tocopherol stimulated osteoclast fusion, independent of its antioxidant capacity. This was mediated by induction of the expression of dendritic-cell-specific transmembrane protein (DC-STAMP), which is an essential molecule for osteoclast fusion and encoded by *Tm7sf4*. Indeed, the bone abnormality seen in Ttpa(–/–) mice was rescued by a *Tm7sf4* transgene. Moreover, wild-type mice or rats fed an α-tocopherol-supplemented diet, which contains a comparable amount of α-tocopherol to common human supplements, lost bone mass.

Conclusion: These results show that serum vitamin E is a determinant of bone mass by regulating osteoclast fusion.

With all the noise about vitamin D and bone, vitamin E seems to have been forgotten; when first identified, its deficiency was believed to cause rickets. In this study the authors apply mouse models to elucidate the mechanisms through which vitamin E might influence skeletal homeostasis. Vitamin E, a lipid-soluble antioxidant, is believed to be protective against arteriosclerotic change and the aging process and is one of the most widely used supplements. Vitamin E is a mixture of tocopherols and tocotrienols. After intestinal absorption it is transported to the liver, where α-tocopherol transfer protein (α-TTP) selectively transfers α-tocopherol into lipoproteins. Consequently, α-tocopherol is the predominant isoform of vitamin E in the body. Mice deficient of α-TTP (*Ttpa*–/– mice) had, compared to wild-type mice, higher bone mass in both vertebrae and long bones as a consequence of lower bone resorption and unaltered bone formation. The skeletal phenotype was reversed by supplemental α-tocopherol. α-Tocopherol stimulated osteoclast differentiation while osteoblast differentiation remained unaltered. Vitamin E affected the later stage of osteoclast differentiation and stimulated osteoclast fusion, resulting in increased osteoclast size, nuclear number and bone-resorbing capacity per osteoclast. Finally, the authors fed the mice with α-tocopherol with doses comparable to those present in vitamin E supplements. This induced a 20% decrease in bone mass with concomitant increase in bone resorption and osteoclast size after 8 weeks, suggesting that excessive use of vitamin E may be deleterious for bone. Human studies on vitamin E and bone health have been limited and show conflicting results. A recent paper by Hamidi et al. [3] evaluated the effects of vitamin E on bone turnover markers among US postmenopausal women. The vitamin E users had significantly higher levels of α-tocopherol while levels of δ-tocopherol, another vitamin E isomer mostly obtained from dietary sources, were lower. This constellation associated with lower levels of bone formation and unaltered bone resorption marker status, suggesting uncoupling of bone formation and resorption. Based on these studies it seems that while E may have beneficial anti-inflammatory and antioxidant properties (poorly documented), it may also mediate adverse skeletal effects with increased bone loss and/or diminished bone formation.

New mechanisms
TSH, the osteoblast-stimulating hormone

Thyroid-stimulating hormone induces a Wnt-dependent, feed-forward loop for osteoblastogenesis in embryonic stem cell cultures

Baliram R, Latif R, Berkowitz J, Frid S, Colaianni G, Sun L, Zaidi M, Davies TF
Thyroid Research Laboratory, Mount Sinai School of Medicine, and James J Peters VA Medical Center, New York, NY, USA
Proc Natl Acad Sci U S A 2011;108:16277–16282

Background: The thyroid-stimulating hormone (TSH) can bypass the thyroid to exert a direct protective effect on the skeleton. Thus in hyperthyroidism a low TSH level, in addition to high thyroid hormone level, may contribute to bone loss. Mouse genetic, cell-based, and clinical studies have previously established that TSH inhibits osteoclastic bone resorption. However, the direct influence of TSH on the osteoblast has remained unclear.

Methods: The authors used a model system developed from murine embryonic stem cells, induced to form mature mineralizing osteoblasts, and measured TSH-induced changes in osteoblastic markers.

Results: TSH stimulated osteoblast differentiation primarily through the activation of protein kinase Cδ and the upregulation of the noncanonical Wnt components frizzled and Wnt5a. Their findings suggested that a TSH-induced, fast-forward short loop in bone marrow permits Wnt5a production, which enhances osteoblast differentiation and also stimulates osteoprotegerin secretion to attenuate bone resorption by neighboring osteoclasts.

Conclusion: The authors conclude that TSH promotes osteoblast differentiation and that this osteoblastogenic effect of TSH is mediated by the noncanonical Wnt pathway and that protein kinase Cδ is a downstream mediator of TSH action. This loop uncouples bone formation from bone resorption with a net increase in bone mass.

Previous studies have established that TSH receptors are expressed in bone cells and that absent TSH receptor signaling causes high-turnover bone loss [4, 5]. TSH inhibits bone resorption directly by acting on osteoclastic TSH receptors. However, TSH also seems to stimulate bone formation through a direct action on the osteoblast. The authors used embryonic stem cells to further characterize the effects of TSH on osteoblasts. Osteoblastic differentiation of the embryonic stem cells was significantly enhanced in the presence of TSH and activation of the TSH receptor. TSH also potently stimulated the production of osteoprotegerin, an inhibitor of osteoclastic bone resorption. These actions of TSH were primarily exerted through the noncanonical Wnt pathway. Based on these observations, the authors hypothesize that not only low thyroid hormone levels but also high TSH in children with congenital hypothyroidism might have an effect on skeletal development. It remains to be elucidated in future studies whether these observations in embryonic stem cells can be translated to clinical practice.

New paradigms
The multi-tasking osteocyte

Demonstration of osteocytic perilacunar/canalicular remodeling in mice during lactation

Qing H, Ardeshirpour L, Pajevic PD, Dusevich V, Jahn K, Kato S, Wysolmerski J, Bonewald LF
School of Dentistry, University of Missouri-Kansas City, Kansas City, MO, USA
J Bone Miner Res 2012;27:1018–1029

Background: Lactation is associated with a significant decline in bone mineral density (BMD) both in humans and mice. Osteoclasts are thought to be solely responsible for the removal of bone matrix. The authors hypothesized that osteocytes might also play a role in mobilizing bone mineral during lactation.

Methods: Various mouse models were used to study the effects of lactation, weaning and unloading on gene expression profiles, BMD, bone microstructure and scanning electron microscopy findings.

Results: Gene array analysis of osteocytes from lactating animals revealed an elevation of genes known to associate with osteoclastic bone resorption including tartrate-resistant acid phosphatase (TRAP) and cathepsin K that returned to virgin levels upon weaning. Infusion of PTHrP, known to be elevated during lactation, induced TRAP activity and cathepsin K expression in osteocytes concurrent with osteocytic remodeling. Conversely, animals lacking the PTH type 1 receptor in osteocytes failed to express TRAP or cathepsin K or to remodel their osteocyte perilacunar matrix during lactation.

Conclusion: The findings show that osteocytes remove mineralized matrix through molecular mechanisms similar to those utilized by osteoclasts. Osteocytes thus have an active role in the regulation of calcium homeostasis during lactation.

In humans, lactation associates with a 5–8% decline in maternal BMD and may occasionally lead to severe symptomatic postpartum osteoporosis with vertebral fractures [6]. Previous studies have suggested that this is not only caused by increased osteoclast activity but other mechanisms may play a role. The authors here elegantly show that osteocytes can remove mineral from their surroundings and subsequently replace it in a cyclical fashion. This so-called osteocytic osteolysis seems to be a part of normal adaptation of bone and calcium metabolism to the demands of reproduction. This study provides more evidence for the significant role of the osteocyte in bone health and disease. Osteocytes are the most abundant cells in the bone tissue. They orchestrate skeletal remodeling by regulating osteoblasts and osteoclasts on the bone surface, participate in phosphate homeostasis, and mediate the effects of mechanical forces on the skeleton. And as shown here, they also participate in calcium homeostasis. A truly good all-around player in the bone!

miR-34s inhibit osteoblast proliferation and differentiation in the mouse by targeting SATB2

Wei J, Shi Y, Zheng L, Zhou B, Inose H, Wang J, Guo XE, Grosschedl R, Karsenty G
Department of Genetics and Development, College of Physicians and Surgeons, Columbia University, New York, NY, USA

J Cell Biol 2012;197:509–521

Background: It has been suggested that microRNAs (miRNAs) may be involved in the regulation of osteoblast proliferation and/or differentiation but this has not been shown in vivo.

Methods: The authors used osteoblast cell lines to screen for microRNAs whose expression increases during osteoblast differentiation. The function of the miRNAs was studied in various osteoblast-specific gain- and loss-of-function mouse models.

Results: The authors identified members of the miR-34 family as regulators of osteoblast proliferation and differentiation. Further in-vivo experiments revealed that miR-34b and -34c affected skeletogenesis during embryonic development, as well as bone mass accrual after birth, through two complementary cellular and molecular mechanisms. First, they inhibited osteoblast proliferation by suppressing cyclin D1, CDK4, and CDK6 accumulation. Second, they inhibited terminal differentiation of osteoblasts, at least in part through the inhibition of SATB2, a nuclear matrix protein that is a critical determinant of osteoblast differentiation. Genetic evidence obtained in the mouse confirmed the importance of SATB2 regulation by miR-34b/c.

Conclusion: These results are the first to identify a family of microRNAs involved in bone formation in vivo and to identify a specific genetic pathway by which these microRNAs regulate osteoblast differentiation.

MicroRNAs (miRNAs) are small noncoding RNAs that downregulate expression of their target genes by either mRNA degradation or translational inhibition. They thus provide a novel dimension to post-transcriptional control by directly inhibiting mRNA translation. This mode of action implies that regulation of mRNA and/or protein levels can proceed faster than transcriptional mechanisms. Consequently, miRNAs mediate rapid fine tuning of gene expression. Previous studies have suggested that miRNAs are involved in osteoblast maturation [7]. However, in-vivo data have been lacking. In this study the authors screened for miRNAs whose expression significantly increased during osteoblast differentiation. Of the several potential miRNAs, they selected miR-34b and miR-34c for further studies since, in addition to increased expression during osteoblastogenesis, their expression was restricted mainly to osteoblasts. Mice overexpressing miR-34c in the osteoblasts had low bone mass with decreased osteoblast number and bone formation rate, while osteoclast activity was unchanged. In contrast, osteoblast-specific ablation of miR-34b and -34c resulted in significant increase in bone mass and osteoblast number. The authors identified specific targets for miR-34-mediated regulation. One of these was SATB2, which is a transcription factor belonging to the family of special AT-rich binding proteins and involved in craniofacial patterning and osteoblast differentiation [8]. This work shows that miRNAs have an important role in the regulation of bone formation. In fact, it is likely that miRNAs contribute to every phase of skeletogenesis, from embryonic bone development to maintenance of adult bone homeostasis by regulating the growth, differentiation and activity of the involved cells; the current knowledge has been elegantly reviewed by Lian et al. [9]. However, the role of miRNAs in pathologic human skeletal disorders such as osteoporosis and osteoarthritis remains largely unknown.

Denosumab treatment for fibrous dysplasia

Boyce A, Chong W, Yao J, Gafni R, Kelly M, Chamberlain C, Bassim C, Cherman N, Ellsworth M, Kasa-Vubu J, Farley F, Molinolo A, Bhattacharyya N, Collins M
Skeletal Clinical Studies Unit, Craniofacial and Skeletal Diseases Branch, National Institute of Dental and Craniofacial Research, NIH, and National Institute of Child Health and Development, NIH
J Bone Miner Res 2012;27:1462–1470

Background: Fibrous dysplasia (FD) is caused by somatic activating mutations in the cAMP-regulating protein, Gs-α. These lead to replacement of normal bone by proliferative osteogenic precursors, resulting in bone deformity, fractures, and pain. RANKL, a cell surface protein involved in osteoclastogenesis, is overexpressed in FD. This prompted the authors to use denosumab, a humanized monoclonal antibody to RANKL, in the treatment of FD.
Methods: The authors present a 9-year-old boy with severe FD and a rapidly expanding femoral lesion. Immunohistochemical staining on a pretreatment bone biopsy showed marked RANKL expression. The patient was started on monthly denosumab, with an initial starting dose of 1- and 0.25-mg/kg dose escalations every 3 months.
Results: Over 7 months of treatment the patient showed marked reduction in pain, bone turnover markers, and tumor growth rate. Denosumab did not affect healing of a femoral fracture that occurred while on denosumab treatment. After treatment onset the patient developed hypophosphatemia and secondary hyperparathyroidism, and needed supplementation with phosphorus, calcium and calcitriol. Bone turnover markers showed rapid and sustained suppression. However, with discontinuation of denosumab there was a rapid and dramatic rebound of bone turnover markers, with the resorption maker CTX (reflecting osteoclast activity) exceeding pretreatment levels, and severe hypercalcemia.
Conclusion: Denosumab led to dramatic reduction of FD expansion and bone pain. However, the medication was associated with clinically significant disturbances in mineral metabolism both while on treatment and after discontinuation. Denosumab treatment of FD warrants further study to confirm efficacy and safety.

Fibrous dysplasia (FD) is a relatively common skeletal disorder in which normal bone is replaced by fibro-osseous tissue, leading to fracture, functional impairment, deformity and pain. FD may be isolated or occur in association with cutaneous hyperpigmentation and hyperfunctioning endocrinopathies. FD in combination with one or more extraskeletal manifestations is termed McCune-Albright syndrome (MAS). The treatment of endocrinopathies in MAS may be challenging. However, the often widely spread and expanding polyostotic skeletal lesions may cause even greater challenges, as in the patient reported here. Bisphosphonates have been used in the treatment of childhood-onset FD but especially in the polyostotic forms the efficacy is often questionable and is limited to relief of FD-related pain [10]. Against this background, denosumab, a fully-humanized monoclonal RANKL antibody, is a tempting therapeutic alternative. RANKL is expressed by osteogenic cells and plays a key role in osteoclastogenesis. By binding to its receptor on osteoclast progenitor membranes, RANKL promotes osteoclast differentiation and leads to increased bone resorption. RANKL inhibition via denosumab has recently been shown to be effective in the treatment of giant cell granulomas of bone, which like FD are derived from bone marrow stromal cells [11]. The treatment response in this patient was very promising as there was a marked reduction in the size of FD lesions, bone turnover markers and in bone pain. However, there were significant disturbances in mineral homeostasis after treatment cessation. Two months after the last infusion the patient developed severe symptomatic hypercalcemia (S-Ca 4.5 mmol/l); bone turnover markers were extremely elevated. With hydration, intravenous pamidronate and calcitonin the disturbances slowly normalized within 5 months. This apparently first case description of denosumab treatment in the pediatric age group suggests that this new medication may be efficacious in the treatment of severe polyostotic FD. At the same time it calls for caution when considering denosumab in children: the withdrawal effects may be unpredictable and exceptionally severe.

A novel tyrosine kinase inhibitor restores chondrocyte differentiation and promotes bone growth in a gain-of-function Fgfr3 mouse model

Jonquoy A, Mugniery E, Benoist-Lasselin C, Kaci N, Le Corre L, Barbault F, Girard AL, Le Merrer Y, Busca P, Schibler L, Munnich A, Legeai-Mallet L
INSERM U781, Université Paris Descartes-Hôpital Necker-Enfants Malades, Paris, France
Hum Mol Genet 2012;21:841–851

Background: Novel tyrosine kinase inhibitors are small molecular weight inhibitors of tyrosine phosphorylation that specifically inhibit the activity of tyrosine kinases, e.g. epidermal growth factor receptor (EGFR), fibroblast growth factor receptors (FGFRs), and the insulin receptor. Members of this new class of pharmaceuticals have shown to be useful in the treatment of a variety of malignancies. The specific inhibition of subclasses of receptors raises the hope that specific treatments for other conditions caused by increased tyrosine phosphorylation may be within reach. Along this line, the authors tested the hypothesis that a novel tyrosine kinase inhibitor targeting the increased intracellular signaling of FGFR3 may normalize the growth and growth plate histology of mice with an activating mutation in the FGFR3, the 'achondroplasia mice'.

Methods: The authors used an ex-vivo culture model of femurs from Fgfr3(Y367C/+) dwarf and wild-type mice to study the effect of a novel tyrosine kinase inhibitor, A31, selected for its inhibitory effect on FGFR3 signaling.

Results: In their model system, A31 was able to normalize growth plate morphology, chondrocyte differentiation, proliferation, cell cycle regulator expression, as well as growth of cultured achondroplasia-mice femurs.

Conclusion: The findings suggest that specific tyrosine kinase inhibitors that target FGFR3 may provide an efficacious treatment of FGFR3-related chondrodysplasias.

In order to find a treatment for achondroplasia, several strategies aimed at reducing the excessive activity of FGFR3 have been proposed, including strategies to inhibit FGFR3 tyrosine kinase activity, to promote its degradation, or to antagonize its downstream signaling [12, 13]. In this article the authors show proof-of-concept for an appealing approach; inhibition of FGFR3 tyrosine kinase activity using a small molecular FGFR3 tyrosine kinase inhibitor. The authors find that growth and histology of ex-vivo cultured achondroplasia-mice femurs can be normalized by exposure to this specific inhibitor. This is an in-vitro finding and it is very possible that this finding may not be possible to replicate in vivo due to lack of efficient kinase inhibition or unacceptable side effects from other tyrosine kinases. Nevertheless, the finding that it is possible to reverse the effects of a constitutively active FGF receptor in cultured femurs makes it plausible that an inhibitor that is sufficiently specific to reverse the bone phenotype in vivo could be developed. Tyrosine kinase inhibition may thus be the most promising strategy currently being pursued in the quest for a specific treatment for achondroplasia, the most common form of skeletal dysplasia in humans.

Ablation of the proapoptotic protein Bax protects mice from glucocorticoid-induced bone growth impairment

Zaman F, Chrysis D, Huntjens K, Fadeel B, Sävendahl L
Pediatric Endocrinology Unit, Department of Women's and Children's Health, Astrid Lindgren Children's Hospital, Karolinska Institutet, Stockholm, Sweden
Farasat.Zaman@ki.se
PLoS One 2012;7:e33168

Background: Glucocorticoid (GC)-induced growth suppression is a common adverse effect during treatment of inflammatory disorders and malignancies. Several approaches, including growth hormone and IGF1 treatment, have been used to mitigate this unwanted side effect of GC treatment. In this experimental study, the authors use a different approach, targeting the proapoptotic gene Bax to test the hypothesis that Bax deficiency will prevent GC-induced apoptosis of growth plate chondrocytes and thereby prevent GC-induced growth impairment.
Methods: The authors used a combination of in-vitro and in-vivo studies including mice with targeted deletion of Bax to test their hypothesis.
Results: Dexamethasone activated Bax in chondrocytes by inducing a conformational change, resulting in its translocation to the mitochondria, and thus activating the intrinsic apoptotic pathway. Conversely, silencing of Bax blocked dexamethasone-induced apoptosis. Finally and most importantly, Bax-deficient female mice exhibited a near-normal growth rate, and were protected against glucocorticoid-induced bone growth impairment.
Conclusion: The findings suggest that the proapoptotic protein Bax is an important mediator of the growth-inhibiting effects of GC treatment in growth plate chondrocytes. Targeting of Bax may therefore be a possible strategy to circumvent the negative effect of GC treatment on longitudinal bone growth.

Glucocorticoids continue to be a widely used anti-inflammatory agent. In children, long-term use causes severe skeletal side effects, including growth retardation through multiple mechanisms including direct inhibition of growth plate chondrocyte proliferation, increased apoptosis, and likely also indirectly via effects on the GH/IGF-1 axis. Preventive measures targeting GC-induced apoptosis of growth plate chondrocytes appear particularly appealing since apoptosis may deplete the pool of resting and/or proliferative chondrocytes and, if so, would negatively affect the potential for future catch-up growth. The authors show that the growth-inhibiting effect of dexamethasone is prevented in Bax-deficient mice. The study does not address the effect of Bax deficiency on the desired, anti-inflammatory effects of GC treatment. If, in fact, Bax targeting does reverse some of the negative effects of GC treatment in humans without abolishing the anti-inflammatory effects, Bax targeting, presumably by small molecules or peptides, might turn out to be an attractive therapeutic approach to a common problem in children with chronic autoimmune conditions requiring long-term GC treatment. However, as we know, it is a long way from a knockout mouse to the growing child.

Role of fibroblast growth factor 21 (FGF21) in undernutrition-related attenuation of growth in mice

Kubicky RA, Wu S, Kharitonenkov A, De Luca F
St. Christopher's Hospital for Children, Philadelphia, PA, USA
francesco.deluca@drexelmed.edu
Endocrinology 2012;153:2287–2295

Background: Insufficient caloric intake is known to inhibit skeletal growth, but the underlying hormonal/ molecular mechanisms are not fully understood. Short-term caloric restriction is associated with reduced hepatic GH sensitivity as well as increased serum levels of FGF21. The authors explore the hypothesis that increased FGF21 activity during caloric restriction may result in reduced GH sensitivity and thereby contribute to the decrease in growth rate that occurs during food restriction.

Methods: The authors created FGF21 knockout mice (*fgf21* KO). These mice were subjected to 4 weeks of food restriction and the effect of FGF21 deficiency on growth inhibition and liver GH sensitivity was assessed.

Results: After the period of food restriction, *fgf21* KO mice exhibited greater body and tibial growth than wild-type (wt) littermates. Daily injections of recombinant human FGF21 in food-restricted *fgf21* KO mice prevented these differences. GH binding and GH receptor expression were reduced in the liver and in the growth plate of food-restricted wt mice (compared to wt mice fed ad libitum), whereas they were similar between food-restricted and ad libitum fed KO mice. In addition, a single injection of GH induced greater liver signal transducer and activator of transcription 5 phosphorylation and IGF-I mRNA in food-restricted KO mice than in wt mice. Lastly, in the tibial growth plate of food-restricted wt mice, FGF21 mRNA and protein expression was greater than that of wt mice fed ad libitum.

Conclusion: The findings suggest that inhibition of growth plate chondrogenesis and longitudinal bone growth during periods of low caloric intake is, in part, due to increased FGF21 activity and that this effect is due to antagonistic effect of FGF21 on GH action in the liver. In addition, the findings of FGF21 expression in growth plate cartilage and its upregulation during food restriction may suggest that FGF21 not only acts to regulate growth in an endocrine manner, but also may act locally to modulate growth.

FGF21 has extensively been reviewed in the *Yearbook* series and by others as a metabolic hormone with glucagon-like effects that is secreted from the liver in response to extended fasting [14]. FGF21 also acts in an autocrine fashion in several tissues, including adipose. The growth inhibition of food restriction is generally assumed to be mediated via the GH-IGF-I axis. In most mammals, fasting is associated with reduced IGF-I levels and reduced GH sensitivity in the liver. However, little is known of the molecular mechanism of this phenomenon. In this article, the authors show evidence that the upregulation of FGF21 expression during malnutrition may induce GH insensitivity in the liver. In addition, the finding of increased expression of FGF21 in growth plate cartilage suggests that FGF21 may also inhibit growth directly at the growth plate through the growth-inhibiting capacity of FGF receptors 1 and 3, expressed on proliferative and hypertrophic growth plate chondrocytes. These are interesting findings that provide a mechanistic explanation to the growth retardation that occurs during fasting or food restriction and may explain a common clinical problem in pediatrics.

SOCS2 is the critical regulator of GH action in murine growth plate chondrogenesis

Pass C, Macrae VE, Huesa C, Ahmed SF, Farquharson C
Bone Biology Group, Division of Developmental Biology, The Roslin Institute and Royal (Dick) School of Veterinary Studies, The University of Edinburgh, Roslin, Midlothian, and Bone & Endocrine Research Group, Royal Hospital for Sick Children, Glasgow, UK
J Bone Miner Res 2012;27:1055–1066

Background: GH acts locally on the growth plate to promote bone growth. Suppressor of cytokine signalling-2 (SOCS2) is a negative regulator of GH signaling and bone growth via inhibition of the JAK/STAT pathway. Consequently, SOCS2 targeting in mice (SOCS2–/–) results in increased longitudinal bone growth. The authors have previously demonstrated that this effect is due to loss of SOCS2 inhibition of GH signaling. In this follow-up study the authors clarify the mechanisms for the SOCS2-mediated inhibition of GH signaling in the growth plate.

Methods: The authors used wild-type and SOCS2–/– mice and a combination of in-vitro and in-situ models to study the role of SOCS2-mediated inhibition.

Results: In SOCS 2–/– mice longitudinal bone growth rates, growth plate widths and chondrocyte proliferation are increased. The authors clarified the molecular mechanism for this finding as they showed that SOCS2, in contrast to SOCS1 and SOCS3 expression, was increased in cultured chondrocytes following GH challenge and that GH stimulated chondrocyte STATs-1, -3 and -5 phosphorylation in SOCS2–/– but not in SOCS2 overexpressing cells. In addition, GH exposure of fetal metatarsal organ cultures stimulated growth of SOCS2–/– but not wild-type bones. The stimulatory effect of GH on SOCS2–/– metatarsal growth was blocked by a PI3K inhibitor, suggesting that this effect of GH is mediated through increased IGF1.

Conclusions: SOCS2 is crucial in modulating the local effects of GH on chondrocyte STAT activation, chondrocyte proliferation, and bone growth.

GH exerts most of its growth-promoting effect through IGF1, but it also stimulates growth by a direct action at the growth plate. In contrast to IGF1, the direct action of GH is frequently nonsignificant when assessed by in-vitro models of growth plate chondrogenesis, i.e. cultured chondrocytes or growth plate or whole-bone organ cultures. Interestingly, cultured metatarsal bones from SOCS2-deficient mice respond to GH with a solid increase in growth rate. However, as the authors show, this local effect of GH is mediated mostly through local production of IGF1, thus supporting the hypothesis that most of the growth-promoting effects of GH are mediated by IGF1.

Mutations in *CYP24A1* and idiopathic infantile hypercalcemia

Schlingmann KP, Kaufmann M, Weber S, Irwin A, Goos C, John U, Misselwitz J, Klaus G, Kuwertz-Broking E, Fehrenbach H, Wingen AM, Guran T, Hoenderop JG, Bindels RJ, Prosser DE, Jones G, Konrad M
University Children's Hospital, Münster, Germany
N Engl J Med 2011;365:410–421

Background: In Britain in the 1950s there was increased incidence of idiopathic infantile hypercalcemia during a period of high vitamin D supplementation in fortified milk products. The authors investigated the molecular basis of idiopathic infantile hypercalcemia, which is characterized by severe hypercalcemia, failure to thrive, vomiting, dehydration, and nephrocalcinosis.

Methods: A candidate-gene approach was applied in a cohort of familial cases of idiopathic infantile hypercalcemia with suspected autosomal recessive inheritance. Identified mutations were evaluated with the use of a mammalian expression system.

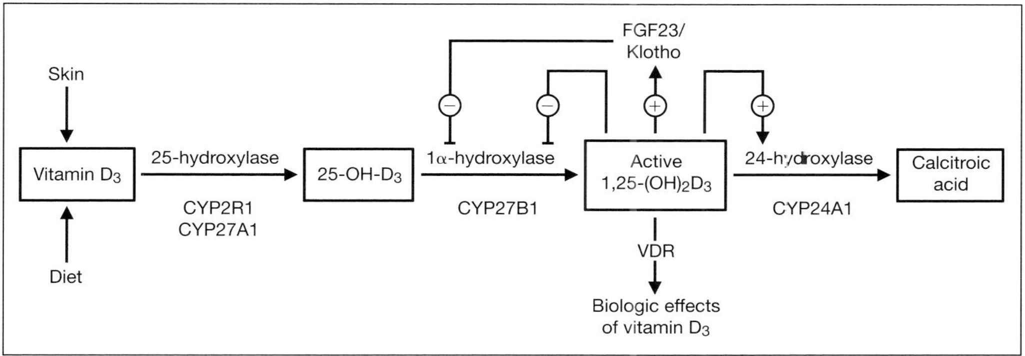

Fig. 2. Vitamin D undergoes 25-hydroxylation in the liver and 1α-hydroxylation in the kidney, resulting in the formation of active 1,25-dihydroxyvitamin D_3 (1,25-OH_2D_3), which binds to the vitamin D receptor (VDR). The 1,25-OH_2D_3 is catabolized by CYP24A1 to water-soluble calcitroic acid. The enzymatic activities of CYP27B1 and CYP24A1 are tightly controlled by the levels of 1,25-OH_2D_3, serum calcium, and parathyroid hormone. In addition, 1,25-OH_2D_3 exerts negative feedback on CYP27B1 through fibroblast growth factor 23 (FGF23) and Klotho.

Results: Sequence analysis of *CYP24A1*, which encodes 25-hydroxyvitamin D 24-hydroxylase, the key enzyme of 1,25-dihydroxyvitamin D degradation, revealed recessive mutations in 6 affected children. Subsequently, *CYP24A1* mutations were identified in a cohort of infants who developed severe hypercalcemia after bolus prophylaxis with vitamin D. Functional characterization revealed a complete loss of function in all *CYP24A1* mutations.

Conclusion: The *CYP24A1* mutations explain the increased sensitivity to vitamin D in patients with idiopathic infantile hypercalcemia and are a genetic risk factor for hypercalcemia during vitamin D prophylaxis in otherwise healthy infants.

The authors studied a cohort of 6 patients from four families with idiopathic infantile hypercalcemia – an enigmatic condition so far. The inheritance pattern suggested an autosomal recessive condition. A second cohort consisted of 4 patients with suspected vitamin D intoxication in whom severe hypercalcemia developed after bolus prophylaxis with vitamin D. The authors looked for mutations in four candidate genes that encode key enzymes involved in vitamin D metabolism: *CYP24A1, CYP27B1, FGF23 and KL* (encoding Klotho) (fig. 2). In both cohorts, loss-of-function mutations in the *CYP24A1* gene were identified. These abolished the enzyme's capacity to degrade 1,25-dihydroxyvitamin D into 24,25-dihydroxyvitamin D, thereby rendering the subjects susceptible to vitamin D toxicity. The study by Dauber et al. [15] took another approach with a patient with severe infantile hypercalcemia. The patient presented at the age of 10 months with hypercalcemia, suppressed PTH, hypercalciuria, nephrocalcinosis and normal 25-OH and 1,25-OH_2 vitamin D levels. Whole-exome sequencing of the patient's DNA identified a homozygous 3-bp in-frame deletion in the *CYP24A1* gene. In accordance with this, the serum levels of 24,25-dihydroxyvitamin D were undetectable. Streeten et al. [16] described hypercalcemia in an adult patient with a homozygous loss-of-function mutation in the same gene. Interestingly, in the report by Dauber et al. [15] the patient's mother, a heterozygous mutation carrier, had nephrolithiasis. This may suggest hypercalciuria and presence of a carrier phenotype. These reports together provide solid evidence for the causative role of *CYP24A1* mutations in idiopathic hypercalcemia. However, several questions remain unanswered: What is the natural course of hypercalcemia as some probands became asymptomatic with time while others only developed symptoms at adult age? What is the mechanism behind hypercalcemia? Probably what counts is the intracellular 1,25-dihydroxyvitamin D concentration, as the measured circulating 1,25-dihydroxyvitamin D levels tended to be normal. And finally, do the heterozygous mutation carriers have normal calcium homeostasis? In any case, this study opens a new view to infantile hypercalcemia.

Enzyme-replacement therapy in life-threatening hypophosphatasia

Whyte MP, Greenberg CR, Salman NJ, Bober MB, McAlister WH, Wenkert D, Van Sickle BJ, Simmons JH, Edgar TS, Bauer ML, Hamdan MA, Bishop N, Lutz RE, McGinn M, Craig S, Moore JN, Taylor JW, Cleveland RH, Cranley WR, Lim R, Thacher TD, Mayhew JE, Downs M, Millan JL, Skrinar AM, Crine P, Landy H
Center for Metabolic Bone Disease and Molecular Research, Shriners Hospital for Children, St. Louis, MO, USA
mwhyte@shrinenet.org
N Engl J Med 2012;366:904–913

Background: Hypophosphatasia results from mutations in the *TNSALP* gene encoding the tissue-nonspecific isozyme of alkaline phosphatase. Consequent accumulation of inorganic pyrophosphate leads to rickets or osteomalacia. Severely affected infants often die from respiratory insufficiency or have persistent bone disease. ENB-0040, a bone-targeted recombinant human TNSALP, prevents the manifestations of hypophosphatasia in Tnsalp knockout mice.

Methods: The authors carried out a multinational, open-label study of treatment with ENB-0040 in infants and young children with life-threatening or debilitating perinatal or infantile hypophosphatasia. The primary objective was the healing of rickets, as assessed radiographically. Motor and cognitive development, respiratory function, and safety were evaluated, as well as the pharmacokinetics and pharmacodynamics of ENB-0040.

Results: Of the 11 patients recruited, 10 completed 6 months of therapy and 9 completed 1 year. At 6 months the authors observed healing of rickets and improvement in developmental milestones and pulmonary function. Plasma levels of inorganic pyrophosphate and pyridoxal 5'-phosphate diminished. Increases in serum parathyroid hormone accompanied skeletal healing, often necessitating dietary calcium supplementation. There was no evidence of hypocalcemia, ectopic calcification, or serious adverse events.

Conclusion: ENB-0040, an enzyme-replacement therapy, significantly improved radiographic abnormalities and pulmonary and physical function in infants and young children with life-threatening hypophosphatasia.

Hypophosphatasia is characterized by defective skeletal mineralization. It ranges in severity from neonatally lethal forms with almost entirely absent mineralization to late-onset mild forms with minor skeletal or dental problems. Attempts to normalize mineralization with intravenous infusions of plasma enriched in soluble alkaline phosphatase have been unsuccessful. The present study reports preliminary results of an open-label study with an investigational recombinant enzyme-replacement therapy in 11 patients with life-threatening perinatal or infantile hypophosphatasia. All patients were younger than 3 years of age at study onset. The study preparation was given as one initial intravenous infusion followed by subcutaneous injections three times per week. Ten of the 11 patients completed the 6-month study period and continued treatment in the study extension. The enzyme-replacement therapy resulted in a significant improvement of radiological signs, showing improved mineralization, bone growth and normalization of bone shape. This was translated to improved respiratory function, mobility and well-being. Side effects were scarce and the treatment was overall well tolerated. The paper carefully documents the major biochemical, radiographic and clinical outcome measures in the study cohort. The findings are extremely important and interesting and provide hope for children with this life-threatening disease. This study, however, has to be seen as a preliminary short-term pilot study and more studies and long-term follow-up data are needed to confirm the positive results. Further studies will hopefully provide more solid ground for optimism. The unavoidable question in the near future will be where to draw the line when deciding about the therapy target group – a much larger patient population suffers from milder forms of hypophosphatasia and although not life-threatening, the disease is severely incapacitating. Will this new treatment be available to them too?

Long-term higher urinary calcium excretion within the normal physiologic range predicts impaired bone status of the proximal radius in healthy children with higher potential renal acid load

Shi L, Libuda L, Schonau E, Frassetto L, Remer T
Research Institute of Child Nutrition, Rheinische Friedrich-Wilhelms University Bonn, Dortmund, Germany
shi@fke-do.de
Bone 2012;50:1026–1031

Background: Reduced bone mineral density (BMD) has been observed in children with idiopathic hypercalciuria. The authors evaluated whether higher urinary calcium excretion within the normal physiologic range influenced bone characteristics in healthy children.
Methods: Urinary calcium excretion was quantified in 603 24-hour urine samples from 154 healthy children and adolescents, and parallel 3-day weighed dietary records were analyzed repeatedly during the 4 years preceding evaluation of proximal forearm bone status by peripheral quantitative computed tomography (pQCT). Urinary potential renal acid load (uPRAL) was determined according to urine ionogram by subtracting measured quantitatively important mineral cations from nonbicarbonate anions.
Results: Urinary calcium excretion was significantly associated with volumetric BMD (p = 0.04), almost significantly with cortical bone mineral content (BMC) (p = 0.05), but not with bone cross-sectional area (CSA), or strength-strain index. When the analyses were stratified by uPRAL, calcium excretion was negatively associated with volumetric BMD (p = 0.007), cortical BMC (p = 0.001), and cortical CSA (p = 0.004) in those children with higher uPRALs, but not in those with low uPRALs (p > 0.3).
Conclusion: Long-term higher calciuria within the physiological range predicts reduced diaphyseal bone mass and bone density particularly in children with long-term unfavorable higher dietary acid load, i.e. with lower fruit and vegetable intake.

While several studies have explored the influence of calcium intake on skeletal characteristics, this study takes a look at the output, namely urinary calcium excretion. This is impacted by the intake, but not solely by calcium intake but also by salt and protein intake and dietary acid load. Genetic factors also play a role. This meticulously performed longitudinal study in 6- to 18-year-old children evaluated the impact of urinary calcium excretion, within the normal physiologic range, on bone health. Those with supranormal urinary calcium excretion (exceeding 4 mg or 0.1 mmol/kg body weight) were excluded. Dietary intakes during the 4 preceding years were collected, parallel to 24-hour urine samples, to determine the degree of calcium excretion. The skeletal characteristics were determined by pQCT of the nondominant forearm. The authors observed significant differences in urinary potential renal acid load (uPRAL) but this alone did not associate with any of the pQCT-derived bone parameters. In contrast, urinary calcium excretion was a significant determinant of volumetric bone density especially when diet acid load was high: calcium excretion demonstrated significant negative associations with cortical bone mineral content, cortical cross-sectional area and cortical volumetric BMD in subjects belonging to the highest tertile of uPRAL. Urine calcium excretion was most significantly determined by sodium and nitrogen excretion, dietary acid load and by growth velocity, and less so by dietary calcium intake. Furthermore, there was no positive association between calcium intake and diaphyseal bone status, challenging the idea that increased dietary calcium consumption has consistent beneficial effects on bone health. The present study shows that several other factors need to be considered in order to optimize bone health during childhood and adolescence. The diet-independent urinary calcium excretion is important for bone health even when within the physiologic range. A long-term reduction in dietary acid load may have a positive overall effect on bone health. This can be obtained by high fruit and vegetable intake, which provides alkaline salts to compensate for the high acid load from protein-rich Western diet. It seems that this study, as so many others in various areas of medicine, comes to the same conclusion – more fruits and vegetables for all of us!

25-Hydroxyvitamin D assay variations and impact on clinical decision-making

Barake M, Daher RT, Salti I, Cortas NK, Al-Shaar L, Habib RH, Fuleihan Gel H
Division of Endocrinology, Department of Internal Medicine, American University of Beirut-Medical Center, Riad El Solh, Beirut, Lebanon
J Clin Endocrinol Metab 2012;97:835–843

Background: Several new automated 25-hydroxyvitamin D (25-OHD) assays are available. These methods often show variability in results.

Methods: The authors measured 25-OHD levels in 494 patients using two different methods, Immunodiagnostic Systems RIA (IDS-RIA) and DiaSorin Liaison assays. Sources of variability between the assays were investigated in 83 samples that were retested in the US reference laboratory, and by reviewing the performance reports issued by the International Vitamin D External Quality Assessment Scheme, DEQAS.

Results: The Liaison method gave significantly lower values than IDS-RIA. The mean bias was −5 ng/ml (range −38.1 to +18.7 ng/ml, p < 0.001); the absolute difference was independent of 25-OHD value. Interassay variability was also detected in values obtained in the reference laboratory and in DEQAS reports. The values impacted clinical decision-making regarding vitamin D treatment. Using 20 ng/ml as the target 25-OHD level, 52% required treatment when tested by Liaison and 36% when tested by IDS-RIA (p < 0.001). Using 30 ng/ml as the desirable level, the proportions were 79 and 64%, respectively (p < 0.001). The two assays agreed in only 41–68% of the subjects.

Conclusion: The 25-OHD assays have a significant impact on the results, patient classification, and treatment recommendations. Such variability should not be ignored when determining and applying vitamin D guidelines. Universal assay standardization is urgently needed.

Approximately 1 billion people worldwide are suspected to have vitamin D deficiency or insufficiency. Vitamin D deficiency has been associated with not only musculoskeletal health but also with cancer, cardiovascular disease, diabetes, and autoimmune disorders. Serum 25-OH-vitamin D (25-OHD) is widely used as a marker for vitamin D status and to guide replacement needs. Controversy exists regarding the optimal target level of serum 25-OHD. Recent recommendations include a target >20 ng/ml (50 nmol/l) by the Institute of Medicine [17] or 30 ng/ml (75 nmol/l) by the International Osteoporosis Foundation [18] and The Endocrine Society 2011 Clinical Practice Guidelines [19]. In children, 50 nmol/l is generally regarded as the lower limit for vitamin D sufficiency [20]. However, these guidelines are of little value if the methodology whereby we determine 25-OHD status is not valid. In this paper the researches quantified the sources of variability in 25-OHD measurements that occurred during a shift in assays from a traditional RIA to a more rapid automated assay. In IDS-RIA the 25-OHD concentration is inversely proportional to the bound radioactivity whereas DiaSorin Liaison uses chemiluminescent immunoassay. In the cohort of 494 patients the two methods gave consistently different results with an interassay CV of 20.6 ± 14.2%; the IDS-RIA values were on average 5 ng/ml (12.5 nmol/l) higher (range −38.1 to +18.7 ng/ml, or −95.2 to +46.7 nmol/l). These differences had a significant influence on clinical decision-making (fig. 3). Clinicians should be aware of this variability and stay alert about not only the results but the methodology behind the measured 25-OHD values. With a huge fraction of children anywhere having vitamin D insufficiency, do we really need to measure 25-OHD on every child? And even more so when the assay is only partly reliable. D is a vitamin; it needs to be added in the diet or taken as a supplement.

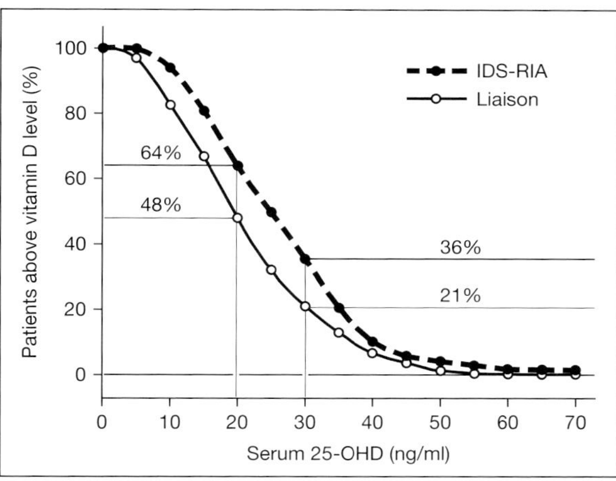

Fig. 3. Proportion of subjects by serum 25-OHD level in the study cohort using the DiaSorin Liaison and the IDS-RIA assays. S-25-OHD 20 ng/ml corresponds to 50 nmol/l and 30 ng/ml to 75 nmol/l.

Concepts revised
What is vitamin D really needed for?

Calcium absorption, kinetics, bone density, and bone structure in patients with hereditary vitamin D-resistant rickets

Tiosano D, Hadad S, Chen Z, Nemirovsky A, Gepstein V, Militianu D, Weisman Y, Abrams SA
Division of Pediatric Endocrinology, Meyer Children's Hospital, Rambam Health Care Campus, Haifa, Israel
d_tiosano@rambam.health.gov.il

J Clin Endocrinol Metab 2011;96:3701–3709

Background: Hereditary 1,25-dihydroxyvitamin D-resistant rickets (HVDRR), caused by mutations in the vitamin D receptor gene, results in severe hypocalcemia and rickets and in childhood requires treatment with high-dose calcium supplements. Surprisingly, calcium metabolism recovers postpubertally. This study evaluated the role of vitamin D receptor in intestinal fractional calcium absorption (FCA), bone calcium accretion, bone mineral density (BMD), and bone structure from infancy to adulthood.
Methods: The authors investigated 17 HVDRR patients aged 1.5–37 year. FCA and bone calcium accretion were determined by stable calcium isotopes; BMD was assessed by dual-energy x-ray absorptiometry and bone structure by high-resolution magnetic resonance imaging.
Results: FCA in patients aged 1.5–17 years was significantly lower than in age-matched controls (p < 0.00004), whereas in patients aged 18–26 years, it was higher than in controls (p < 0.001). In patients older than 29 years FCA was comparable to controls. Patients aged 18–26 years had higher bone calcium accretion than controls (p < 0.02) while bone calcium accretion in patients under 18 and over 29 years of age did not differ from controls. Femoral-neck BMD Z-score was −2.38 ± 0.3 in patients under 18 years and 0.28 ± 0.87 in postpubertal patients (p < 0.0001). High-resolution magnetic resonance imaging showed similar bone structure and bone parameters in HVDRR patients and controls.
Conclusion: These findings in HVDRR patients suggest that calcium absorption is highly vitamin D-dependent from infancy until the end of puberty, after which other mechanisms, independent of vitamin D, are substantially involved in calcium absorption.

Monogenic human disorders provide unique models to study physiology. Here the authors have carefully evaluated a relatively large cohort of patients with a rare recessive disorder in which loss-of-function mutations in the vitamin D receptor (VDR) gene render the receptor unresponsive to 1,25-(OH)$_2$D. Vitamin D resistance results in severe rickets, hypocalcemia, hypophosphatemia, elevated PTH and 1,25-(OH)$_2$D, and in alopecia. During infancy and childhood of these patients, extremely high doses of calcium are needed to control hypocalcemia and rickets. However, calcium requirements spontaneously normalize after puberty. This can be explained by lower calcium demand after cessation of growth and by activation of VDR-independent mechanisms of calcium absorption postpubertally. Intestinal calcium absorption and bone calcium accretion, studied with stable calcium isotopes, showed unique profiles. Postpubertally, intestinal calcium absorption increased to levels exceeding those in the controls. Studies in VDR knockout mice have shown that during pregnancy and lactation VDR-independent intestinal calcium absorption and skeletal mineralization are upregulated; this may be mediated by placental lactogen and prolactin. The present study shows that such mechanisms are activated also at the end of puberty, suggesting that sex hormones may stimulate intestinal calcium transport. The findings raise several questions that can be only partly answered based on the available data. Firstly, what are the VDR-independent intestinal mechanisms for calcium absorption and how are they regulated by various hormones and at different stages of growth and puberty. Interestingly, the gastric mucosa in male and female adult rats has a substantial aromatase activity [21] and if present also in humans, suggests a role for estrogen in this process. Secondly, it is intriguing that skeletal characteristics in these individuals with complete 1,25-(OH)$_2$D resistance showed no difference from healthy controls in young adulthood. The question arises, what indeed is the role of vitamin D in the skeletal development and homeostasis? And lastly, what is the overall health outcome of these individuals who are deprived from all the nonskeletal benefits of vitamin D because of a receptor problem? There is much more to be learnt.

Reviews
Bones – connecting people

The contribution of bone to whole-organism physiology

Karsenty G, Ferron M
Department of Genetics and Development, College of Physicians and Surgeons, Columbia University, New York, NY, USA
gk2172@columbia.edu
Nature 2012;481:314–320

Background: The mouse genetic revolution has shown repeatedly that most organs have more functions than expected. To uncover these, there is a need for a whole-organism study of physiology.
Methods: This paper reviews the current knowledge on the interactions between bone and other organ systems.
Results: Moving from molecular and cellular approach to whole-organism studies in the evaluation of skeletal physiology has broadened our understanding of the various skeletal functions and revealed important connections between bone and other organs such as the brain, pancreas and gut.
Conclusions: A whole-organism approach is needed to understand the physiological role of the skeleton. This approach is likely to shed new light on the pathogenesis of degenerative diseases affecting multiple organs.

Recent years have significantly broadened our view about skeletal functions. Some of these new discoveries were highlighted in last year's *Yearbook* [1]. The key molecule mediating signals from the skeleton to other organs is osteocalcin, an osteoblast-specific molecule, which has a function in the regulation of whole-body glucose homeostasis and energy expenditure [22, 23]. Furthermore, osteocalcin regulates male fertility [24]. In this review the authors summarize the details of these and other connections as they are presently understood. However, the authors conclude that if so much has been learned in such a short time about the physiology of one organ, it is likely that several other aspects will be discovered with similar whole-organism approach in the near future. This approach is based on the ideas that firstly, no body function is determined by one organ alone, and second, different organs exert opposite influences on the same function to regulate it tightly and maintain homeostasis. Furthermore, the cardinal rule of endocrinology applies to most systems: a regulated organ talks back to another regulating one to limit its influence. Interestingly, the bone seems to play a key role in the communication and networking with other organs.

References

1. Mäkitie O, Nilsson O: Bone, growth plate and mineral metabolism; in Carel J-C, Hochberg Z (eds): Yearbook of Pediatric Endocrinology 2011. Basel, Karger, 2011, pp 63–80.
2. Karsenty G, Ferron M: The contribution of bone to whole-organism physiology. Nature 2012;481:314–320.
3. Hamidi MS, Corey PN, Cheung AM: Effects of vitamin E on bone turnover markers among US postmenopausal women. J Bone Miner Res 2012;27:1368–1380.
4. Abe E, Marians RC, Yu W, Wu XB, Ando T, Li Y, et al: TSH is a negative regulator of skeletal remodeling. Cell 2003;115:151–162.
5. Iida K, Hino Y, Ohara T, Chihara K: A case of myxedema coma caused by isolated thyrotropin-stimulating hormone deficiency and Hashimoto's thyroiditis. Endocr J 2011;58:143–148.
6. Segal E, Hochberg I, Weisman Y, Ish-Shalom S: Severe postpartum osteoporosis with increased PTHrP during lactation in a patient after total thyroidectomy and parathyroidectomy. Osteoporos Int 2011;22:2907–2911.
7. Zhang Y, Xie RL, Croce CM, Stein JL, Lian JB, van Wijnen AJ, et al: A program of microRNAs controls osteogenic lineage progression by targeting transcription factor Runx2. Proc Natl Acad Sci USA 2011;108:9863–9868.
8. Dobreva G, Chahrour M, Dautzenberg M, Chirivella L, Kanzler B, Farinas I, et al: SATB2 is a multifunctional determinant of craniofacial patterning and osteoblast differentiation. Cell 2006;125:971–986.
9. Lian JB, Stein GS, van Wijnen AJ, Stein JL, Hassan MQ, Gaur T, et al: MicroRNA control of bone formation and homeostasis. Nat Rev Endocrinol 2012;8:212–227.
10. Plotkin H, Rauch F, Zeitlin L, Munns C, Travers R, Glorieux FH: Effect of pamidronate treatment in children with polyostotic fibrous dysplasia of bone. J Clin Endocrinol Metab 2003;88:4569–4575.
11. Thomas D, Henshaw R, Skubitz K, Chawla S, Staddon A, Blay JY, et al: Denosumab in patients with giant-cell tumour of bone: an open-label, phase 2 study. Lancet Oncol 2010;11:275–80.
12. Yasoda A, Komatsu Y, Chusho H, Miyazawa T, Ozasa A, Miura M, et al: Overexpression of CNP in chondrocytes rescues achondroplasia through a MAPK-dependent pathway. Nat Med 2004;10:80–86.
13. Laederich MB, Horton WA: FGFR3 targeting strategies for achondroplasia. Expert Rev Mol Med 2012;14:e11.
14. Potthoff MJ, Kliewer SA, Mangelsdorf DJ: Endocrine fibroblast growth factors 15/19 and 21: from feast to famine. Genes Dev 2012;26:312–324.
15. Dauber A, Nguyen TT, Sochett E, Cole DE, Horst R, Abrams SA, et al: Genetic defect in CYP24A1, the vitamin D 24-hydroxylase gene, in a patient with severe infantile hypercalcemia. J Clin Endocrinol Metab 2012;97:E268–274.
16. Streeten AE, Zarbalian K, Damcott CM: CYP24A1 mutations in idiopathic infantile hypercalcemia. N Engl J Med 2011;365:1741–1742.
17. Ross AC, Manson JE, Abrams SA, Aloia JF, Brannon PM, Clinton SK, et al: The 2011 report on dietary reference intakes for calcium and vitamin D from the Institute of Medicine: what clinicians need to know. J Clin Endocrinol Metab 2011;96:53–58.
18. Dawson-Hughes B, Mithal A, Bonjour JP, Boonen S, Burckhardt P, Fuleihan GE, et al: IOF position statement: vitamin D recommendations for older adults. Osteoporos Int 2010;21:1151–1154.
19. Holick MF, Binkley NC, Bischoff-Ferrari HA, Gordon CM, Hanley DA, Heaney RP, et al: Evaluation, treatment, and prevention of vitamin D deficiency: an Endocrine Society clinical practice guideline. J Clin Endocrinol Metab 2011;96:1911–1930.
20. Misra M, Pacaud D, Petryk A, Collett-Solberg PF, Kappy M: Vitamin D deficiency in children and its management: review of current knowledge and recommendations. Pediatrics 2008;122:398–417.
21. Ueyama T, Shirasawa N, Numazawa M, Yamada K, Shelangouski M, Ito T, et al: Gastric parietal cells: potent endocrine role in secreting estrogen as a possible regulator of gastro-hepatic axis. Endocrinology 2002;143:3162–3170.
22. Lee NK, Sowa H, Hinoi E, Ferron M, Ahn JD, Confavreux C, et al: Endocrine regulation of energy metabolism by the skeleton. Cell 2007;130:456–469.
23. Ferron M, Wei J, Yoshizawa T, Del Fattore A, DePinho RA, Teti A, et al: Insulin signaling in osteoblasts integrates bone remodeling and energy metabolism. Cell 2010;142:296–308.
24. Oury F, Sumara G, Sumara O, Ferron M, Chang H, Smith CE, et al: Endocrine regulation of male fertility by the skeleton. Cell 2011;144:796–809.

Reproductive Endocrinology

Lena Sahlin and Olle Söder

Paediatric Endocrinology Unit, Department of Women's and Children's Health, Astrid Lindgren Children's Hospital, Karolinska Institutet and Karolinska University Hospital, Stockholm, Sweden

This chapter has a selection of papers published during the last year dealing with many important aspects of reproductive endocrinology. They include endocrine treatments, gender differences in brain imaging, care for children with gender dysphoria, genetic studies in disorders of sexual development and reproductive disorders, puberty, markers of gonadal function and many others. The chapter aims at presenting a mix of experimental and clinical papers advancing the field of reproductive endocrinology with implications for a better understanding of human physiology and better care for children with endocrine disorders. The present selection of papers obviously represents our own bias but we hope you find them interesting to read and helpful for your daily professional activity. There is limited space for everything to be covered within the frame of this chapter but there are also additional publications dealing with subjects related to reproductive endocrinology in other chapters of this *Yearbook*.

New treatments

Aromatase inhibitors in pediatrics

Wit JM, Hero M, Nunez SB
Department of Pediatrics, J6S, Leiden University Medical Center, Leiden, The Netherlands
j.m.wit@lumc.nl
Nat Rev Endocrinol 2012;8:135–147

Background: The enzyme CYP19 aromatase catalyzes the rate-limiting step in the conversion of androgens to estrogens in many tissues. Translational studies have revealed a major role for this enzyme in epiphyseal plate closure, which has promoted interest in the use of inhibitors of aromatase to improve longitudinal growth and adult height of children. The relatively novel selective aromatase inhibitors letrozole and anastrozole have been reported to be used off-label in pediatrics for several medical conditions.
Methods: This paper reviews the reported use of aromatase inhibitors in pediatric practice. Their use in the following medical conditions in children is presented: hyperestrogenism, such as aromatase excess syndrome, Peutz-Jeghers syndrome, McCune-Albright syndrome and functional follicular ovarian cysts; hyperandrogenism, e.g. testotoxicosis (also known as familial male-limited precocious puberty), congenital adrenal hyperplasia; pubertal gynecomastia, and short stature and/or pubertal delay in boys.
Results: Reported data suggest that aromatase inhibitors are probably effective in the treatment of patients with aromatase excess syndrome or testotoxicosis, partially effective in Peutz-Jeghers and McCune-Albright syndrome, but probably ineffective in gynecomastia. Insufficient data are available in patients with congenital adrenal hyperplasia or functional ovarian cysts.
Conclusions: Aromatase inhibitors appear effective in increasing adult height of boys with short stature and/or pubertal delay but safety concerns, including vertebral deformities, a decrease in serum HDL cholesterol levels and increase of erythrocytosis, are reasons for caution.

Aromatase inhibitors seem to have a role in the treatment of certain rare endocrine disorders in children but these patients should be handled by specialists with an ambition to add an accumulating experience to increase the evidence base. Additional studies with long-lasting follow-up are required to understand better the efficacy and safety of these drugs in pediatric endocrinology. At the present stage of knowledge, common use of these potent drugs to improve longitudinal growth of boys is not recommended.

Effect of oxandrolone and timing of pubertal induction on final height in Turner's syndrome: randomized, double-blind, placebo-controlled trial

Gault EJ, Perry RJ, Cole TJ, Casey S, Paterson WF, Hindmarsh PC, Betts P, Dunger DB, Donaldson MD
University of Glasgow Department of Child Health, Royal Hospital for Sick Children, Glasgow, UK
BMJ 2011;342:d1980

Background: The nonaromatizable androgen oxandrolone has been used as an adjuvant to stimulate longitudinal growth in children including those with Turner's syndrome. This clinical study examines the effect of oxandrolone and the timing of pubertal induction on final height in girls with Turner's syndrome receiving a standard dose of growth hormone.

Methods: A randomized, double-blind, placebo-controlled trial was performed in the settings of 36 pediatric endocrinology departments in UK hospitals. Girls with Turner's syndrome aged 7–13 years at recruitment, receiving recombinant growth hormone therapy (10 mg/m^2/week) were included. Participants were randomized to oxandrolone (0.05 mg/kg/day, maximum 2.5 mg/day) or placebo from 9 years of age. Those with evidence of ovarian failure at 12 years were further randomized to oral ethinylestradiol in a controlled dose schedule or placebo; participants who received placebo and those recruited after the age of 12.25 years started ethinylestradiol at age 14. Final height was the main outcome measure.

Results: 106 participants were recruited, of whom 14 withdrew and 82/92 reached final height. Both oxandrolone and late pubertal induction increased final height: by 4.6 (95% confidence interval 1.9–7.2) cm (p = 0.001, n = 82) for oxandrolone and 3.8 (0.0–7.5) cm (p = 0.05, n = 48) for late pubertal induction with ethinylestradiol. In the 48 children who were randomized twice, the effects on final height (compared with placebo and early induction of puberty) of oxandrolone alone, late induction alone, and oxandrolone plus late induction were similar, averaging 7.1 (3.4–10.8) cm (p < 0.001). No cases of virilization were reported.

Conclusion: Oxandrolone had a positive effect on final height in girls with Turner's syndrome treated with growth hormone, as did late pubertal induction with ethinylestradiol at age 14 years. However, these effects were not additive, so using both had no advantage. Oxandrolone could, therefore, be offered as an alternative to late pubertal induction for increasing final height in Turner's syndrome.

This study shows convincingly that oxandrolone promotes longitudinal growth in girls with Turner's syndrome treated with growth hormone. Delaying puberty by later start of estrogen therapy in these patients treated with oxandrolone had no further effect on their final height. Oxandrolone thus allows an early start of pubertal induction without compromising final height. This is good news since many young adult Turner patients report they did suffer more from the delayed puberty in their teen age rather than the loss of a few centimeters in final height.

New genes (and old)

Etiology of hypospadias: a systematic review of genes and environment

Van der Zanden LF, van Rooij IA, Feitz WF, Franke B, Knoers NV, Roeleveld N
Department of Epidemiology, Biostatistics and HTA, Radboud University Nijmegen Medical Centre, Nijmegen, The Netherlands
Hum Reprod Update 2012;18:260–283

Background: Hypospadias is a common congenital malformation of the male external genitalia and a sign of undermasculinization during prenatal development. Most cases have an unknown etiology, which is probably a mix of monogenic and multifactorial forms, implicating both genes and environmental factors.

Method: The authors reviewed the current knowledge about the etiology of hypospadias. PubMed was used to identify studies on hypospadias etiology published between January 1995 and February 2011. Reference lists of the selected articles were also searched to identify additional studies, including those published before 1995.

Results: The search provided 922 articles and 169 were selected for this review. Studies screening groups of patients with hypospadias for single gene defects found mutations in WT1, SF1, BMP4, BMP7, HOXA4, HOXB6, FGF8, FGFR2, AR, HSD3B2, SRD5A2, ATF3, MAMLD1, MID1 and BNC2. However, most investigators were convinced that single mutations do not cause the majority of isolated hypospadias cases. Indeed, associations were found with common polymorphisms in FGF8, FGFR2, AR, HSD17B3, SRD5A2, ESR1, ESR2, ATF3, MAMLD1, DGKK, MID1, CYP1A1, GSTM1 and GSTT1. In addition, gene expression studies identified CTGF, CYR61 and EGF as candidate genes. Environmental factors consistently implicated in hypospadias were low birth weight, maternal hypertension and preeclampsia, suggesting that placental insufficiency may play an important role in hypospadias etiology. Exogenous endocrine-disrupting chemicals have the potential to induce hypospadias, but it is unclear whether human exposure is high enough to exert this effect. Other environmental factors have also been associated with hypospadias but, for most, the results are inconsistent.
Conclusions: A number of contributors to the etiology of hypospadias have been identified, but the majority of risk factors still remain unknown.

Despite its common nature and results of multiple extensive studies searching for causes, the etiology of hypospadias still remains an enigma in most cases. Due to poor reporting it has been difficult to find hard evidence that the incidence of hypospadias is increasing although some studies point to such trends, at least in certain geographical regions. This may implicate a role for environmental factors in the pathogenesis and most focus has been on endocrine-disrupting chemicals with antiandrogenic actions, hypothetically operating at critical time windows of male embryonic and fetal development. More studies looking for causative links of hypospadias are highly warranted.

FOXL2 impairment in human disease

Verdin H, De Baere E
Center for Medical Genetics, Ghent University Hospital, Ghent, Belgium
Horm Res Paediatr 2012;77:2–11

Missense mutation outside the forkhead domain of FOXL2 causes a severe form of BPES type II

Haghighi A, Verdin H, Haghighi-Kakhki H, Piri N, Gohari NS, Baere ED
Wellcome Trust Centre for Human Genetics, University of Oxford, Oxford, UK
Mol Vis 2012;18:211–218

Background: FOXL2 encodes a forkhead transcription factor that plays important roles in the ovary during development and in postnatal, adult life. FOXL2 impairment will, in line with other forkhead transcription factors, result in constitutional genetic defects and a somatic mutation which will lead to developmental disease and cancer, respectively. More than 100 unique constitutional mutations and regulatory defects have been found in blepharophimosis syndrome (BPES), a complex eyelid malformation associated (type I) or not (type II) with premature ovarian failure (POF). In agreement with the BPES phenotype, FOXL2 is expressed in the developing eyelids and in fetal and adult ovaries.
Methods: Article 1: Review of known models and patients with FOXL impairment. Article 2: A clinical and molecular genetic investigation was performed in affected and unaffected members of an Iranian family with BPES. The FOXL2 coding region was sequenced in an index case. Targeted mutation testing was performed in 8 family members.
Results: Article 1: Only a few constitutional mutations have been described in nonsyndromic POF. A recurrent somatic mutation p.C134W was found to be specific for adult ovarian granulosa cell tumors. A conditional knockout of Foxl2 in the mouse induced somatic transdifferentiation of ovary into testis in adult mice, suggesting that Foxl2 has an anti-testis function in the adult ovary. Article 2: A heterozygous FOXL2 missense mutation c.650C→G (p.Ser217Cys) cosegregating with disease in members of a three-generation family with BPES type II was identified. Only few missense mutations have been reported outside the forkhead domain so far, which were all found in mild BPES. Unlike previous studies, affected members of the family studied here showed a severe BPES phenotype, with bilateral amblyopia due to uncorrected ptosis.

Conclusions: The transdifferentiation of the ovary into a testis has changed the view of the gonads as terminally differentiated organs in adult mammals. This result might have potential implications for the understanding and treatment of conditions such as POF and polycystic ovary syndrome.
A severe BPES phenotype resulting from a FOXL2 missense mutation outside the forkhead domain was demonstrated, expanding knowledge of the phenotypic consequences of missense mutations outside the forkhead domain.

These two articles present FOXL2 as an important gene for which an impairment has important clinical consequences resulting in human disease. Not all BPES syndromes are accompanied by POF in female patients, although the gene is expressed in the eyelids and ovarian tissues. It is clear that FOXL2 has an important function for differentiation of the gonads.

Important for clinical practice

The physiology and timing of male puberty

Tinggaard J, Mieritz MG, Sorensen K, Mouritsen A, Hagen CP, Aksglaede L, Wohlfahrt-Veje C, Juul A
Department of Growth and Reproduction, Rigshospitalet, Faculty of Health Sciences, University of Copenhagen, Copenhagen, Denmark
Curr Opin Endocrinol Diabetes Obes 2012;19:197–203

Background: An earlier start of puberty during the past few decades been implicated and associated with environmental factors such as the obesity epidemic. However, the evidence base for such secular trends and environmental associations is greater in girls than in boys and more studies on gender differences are therefore warranted.
Methods: The authors aimed to describe available markers of male puberty, discuss associations between adiposity and pubertal timing and to review recent evidence of a possible secular trend in male pubertal timing.
Results: An expert panel reviewed existing American pubertal data from boys in 2005 and could not confirm a secular trend in male pubertal timing. National Health and Nutrition Examination Survey III findings have been confirmed by the National Institute of Child Health and Human Development study reporting a mean age of 10.4 years for Caucasian boys entering Tanner stage G2. Furthermore, the Copenhagen Puberty Study reported a 3-month decline in pubertal onset during a 15-year period (from 11.92 years in 1991 to 11.66 years in 2008). A negative association between obesity and early puberty was found in the National Institute of Child Health and Human Development study, in contrast to the positive association found in a Danish study. Other studies have not been able to document an association between prepubertal BMI and age at pubertal onset.
Conclusions: Evaluation of Tanner stage and especially assessment of testicular volume should both be used in epidemiological studies. The authors speculate that the association between fat mass and pubertal timing may be nonlinear and recent studies may indicate a small decline in age at pubertal onset in boys.

This review addresses the gender difference in the recently observed secular trend to earlier onset of puberty. Most studies have investigated this phenomenon in girls but not in boys, and studies addressing boys have conflicting results. This difference may have a methodological explanation due to the greater difficulties to examine boys than girls for such studies. However a difference in biology between boys and girls with respect to onset of puberty cannot be neglected, also displayed by the well-known gender differences in the incidences of precocious and delayed puberty. Speculatively, from a biological point of view, it makes more sense that overnutrition (with or without obesity) in boys results in delayed puberty reflecting less physical fitness in obese men whereas obese women may be nutritionally fit for reproduction.

Sertoli cell markers in the diagnosis of pediatric male hypogonadism

Grinspon RP, Loreti N, Braslavsky D, Bedecarras P, Ambao V, Gottlieb S, Bergada I, Campo SM, Rey RA
Centro de Investigaciones Endocrinológicas (CEDIE, CONICET), Hospital de Niños Ricardo Gutiérrez, Buenos Aires, Argentina
J Pediatr Endocrinol 2012;25:3–11

Background: During childhood, the pituitary-testicular axis is partially dormant: testosterone secretion decreases following a drop in luteinizing hormone (LH) levels; follicle-stimulating hormone (FSH) levels also go down. Conversely, Sertoli cells are most active, as revealed by the circulating levels of anti-müllerian hormone (AMH) and inhibin B. Therefore, hypogonadism can best be evidenced, without stimulation tests, if Sertoli cell function is assessed.

Methods: This paper reviews markers of testicular function in children and discusses their clinical implications.

Results: Serum AMH levels in boys are high from fetal life until midpuberty. Testicular AMH production increases in response to FSH and is potently inhibited by androgens. Inhibin B is high in the first years of life, then decreases partially while remaining clearly higher than in females, and increases again at puberty. Serum AMH and inhibin B are undetectable in anorchid patients. In primary or central hypogonadism affecting the whole gonad established in fetal life or childhood, all testicular markers are low. Conversely, when hypogonadism only affects Leydig cells, serum AMH and inhibin B are normal. In males of pubertal age with central hypogonadism, AMH and inhibin B are low. Treatment with FSH provokes an increase in serum levels of both Sertoli cell markers, whereas human chorionic gonadotrophin (hCG) administration increases testosterone levels.

Conclusions: Measurements of serum AMH and inhibin B are helpful in assessing testicular function, without need for stimulation tests, and orientates the etiological diagnosis of pediatric male hypogonadism.

> This review is a helpful summary of circulating biomarkers of testicular function to be used in clinical practice. AMH and inhibin B are markers of Sertoli cell function, which show age- and maturational stage-specific patterns in blood samples. By combining these factors with classical endocrine tests (gonadotropins) and Leydig cell markers (testosterone, INSL3) it is possible to get a good overview of testicular function without performing more cumbersome investigations including endocrine stimulation tests. See also the paper below by Dennis et al. in this chapter, discussing the role of vitamin D in AMH production.

Children and adolescents with gender identity disorder referred to a pediatric medical center

Spack NP, Edwards-Leeper L, Feldman HA, Leibowitz S, Mandel F, Diamond DA, Vance SR
Division of Endocrinology, Children's Hospital Boston, Boston, MA, USA
norman.spack@childrens.harvard.edu
Pediatrics 2012;129:418–425

Background: An increasing number of children and adolescents are seeking medical and psychological help for gender dysphoria. This paper aims at describing patients with gender identity disorder (GID) referred to a pediatric medical center. The authors identified changes in patient profiles and numbers after creation of a multidisciplinary gender management service by expanding the disorders of sex development clinic to include transgender patients.

Methods: Data were collected on 97 consecutive patients aged <21 years, with initial visits between January 1998 and February 2010, who fulfilled the following criteria: long-standing cross-gender behaviors, provided letters from current mental health professional and parental support. Main descriptive measures included gender, age, Tanner stage, history of gender identity development, and psychiatric comorbidity.

Results: Genotypic male:female ratio was 43:54 (0.8:1); there was a slight preponderance of female patients but not significantly different from 1:1. Age of presentation was 14.3 ± 3.4 years (mean ± SD) without sex difference (p = 0.11). Tanner stage at presentation was 4.1 ± 1.4 for genotypic female patients and 3.6 ± 1.5 for genotypic male patients (p = 0.02). Age at start of medical treatment was 15.6 ± 2.8 years. 43 patients (44%) presented with significant psychiatric history, including 20 reporting self-mutilation (21%) and suicide attempts (9%).

Conclusions: After establishment of a multidisciplinary gender clinic, the GID population increased 4-fold. Complex clinical presentations required additional mental health support as the patient population grew. Mean age and Tanner stage were too advanced for pubertal suppressive therapy to be an effective option for most patients. Two-thirds of patients were started on cross-sex hormone therapy. Greater awareness of the benefit of early medical intervention is needed. Psychological and physical effects of pubertal suppression and/or cross-sex hormones in our patients require further investigation.

Young patients with GID often report they are misunderstood or neglected by the healthcare system. These patients often show various forms of comorbidity and behavioral disturbances including self-destructive activities and drug abuse that may be related to the lack of adequate care. It is therefore important to recognize this condition and offer psychiatric and endocrine expertise. This paper describes a dramatic increase in the number of GID patients after opening a specific clinic for such problems. The gender balance of these young patients shows more female to male rather than male to female transgenderism which is opposite to that reported for adult patients. The reason for this is unknown. The role of the pediatric endocrinologist for these patients is to be responsible for the work-up to reveal 'cryptic' disorders of sexual development, e.g. 5α-reductase deficiency, and to care for the endocrine treatment before adult age has been reached.

New mechanisms

Targeted pituitary overexpression of pituitary adenylate-cyclase activating polypeptide alters postnatal sexual maturation in male mice

Moore JP Jr, Yang RQ, Winters SJ
Department of Anatomical Sciences and Neurobiology, University of Louisville, School of Medicine, Louisville, KY, USA
jpmoor03@louisville.edu
Endocrinology 2012;153:1421–1434

Background: The mechanisms behind pubertal onset and its molecular background are yet to be fully understood although many downstream signals and pathways have been discovered. The neuropeptide pituitary adenylate cyclase-activating polypeptide (PACAP) is present in high concentrations within the hypothalamus, suggesting a trophic role to the pituitary, whereas pituitary expression suggests a paracrine function. PACAP is known to stimulate gonadotropin secretion and enhances GnRH responsiveness. PACAP increases gonadotropin α-subunit (α-GSU), lengthens LH-β, but reduces FSH-β mRNA levels in adult pituitary cell cultures in part by increasing follistatin. PACAP stimulates LH secretion in rats, however the acceptance of PACAP as a regulator of reproduction has been limited by lack of results from in vivo studies.

Methods: The authors created a transgenic mouse model of pituitary PACAP overexpression using the α-GSU subunit promoter. Real-time PCR was used to evaluate PACAP, follistatin, GnRH receptor, and the gonadotropin subunit mRNA in male transgenic and wild-type mice of various ages.

Results: Transgenic mice had greater than 1,000-fold higher levels of pituitary PACAP mRNA, and immunocytochemistry, Western blot, and ELISA analyses confirmed high peptide levels. FSH, LH, and testosterone levels were significantly suppressed, and the timing of puberty was substantially delayed in PACAP transgenic mice in which gonadotropin subunit and GnRH receptor mRNA levels were reduced and pituitary follistatin expression was increased. Microarray analyses revealed 1,229 of 45,102 RNA probes were significantly ($p < 0.01$) different in pituitaries from PACAP transgenic mice, of which 83 genes were at least 2-fold different. Genes involved in small molecule biochemistry, cancer, and reproductive system diseases were the top associated networks. The GnRH signaling pathway was the top canonical pathway affected by pituitary PACAP excess.

Conclusions: These results provide the first evidence that PACAP affects gonadotropin expression and sexual maturation in vivo. Clinical implications of these findings await further studies.

PACAP is yet another factor that may be involved in the regulation of time of onset and tempo of puberty. This peptide seems to suppress the start and halt the progress on of pubertal development although its clinical role is yet to be defined. Its action seems to be more paracrine than endocrine, so unfortunately it is difficult to believe that circulating PACAP levels could be informative with regard to pubertal timing. However, a pharmacological role of PACAP in disorders of puberty may be worth exploring.

The level of serum anti-müllerian hormone correlates with vitamin D status in men and women but not in boys

Dennis NA, Houghton LA, Jones GT, van Rij AM, Morgan K, McLennan IS
Department of Anatomy (N.A.D., K.M., I.S.M.), Otago School of Medical Sciences and Departments of Human Nutrition (L.A.H.), Psychology (K.M.), and Surgery (G.T.J., A.M.v.R.), Dunedin School of Medicine, and Brain Health Research Centre (N.A.D., I.S.M.), University of Otago, Dunedin, New Zealand
J Clin Endocrinol Metab 2012;97:2450–2455

Background: Anti-müllerian hormone (AMH) is a gonad-specific hormone, which is increasingly used as a marker of gonadal status. The level of serum AMH has a high variance in similar individuals for reasons that are unknown. The AMH gene promoter contains a vitamin D response element that may cause vitamin D status to influence serum AMH levels. The objective of this study was to determine whether serum levels of AMH are related to 25-hydroxyvitamin D ([25(OH)D)] status.
Methods: Three cohorts of participants were analyzed in this observational and intervention study. The cohorts were mature men (n = 113), premenopausal women (n = 33), and 5- to 6-year-old boys (n = 74). Women were given a daily supplement of ergocalciferol, cholecalciferol, or a placebo for 6 months and provided baseline and posttreatment blood samples. Serum AMH and 25(OH)D were measured and analyzed for covariation.
Results: Serum AMH positively correlated with 25(OH)D in men (r = 0.22, p = 0.02) but not boys. Both 25(OH)D and AMH levels exhibited seasonal variation in women, with an 18% decrease in AMH levels in winter compared with summer (p = 0.01). Change in AMH level correlated with the initial AMH level and the magnitude of change in vitamin D levels (r = 0.36, p = 0.004). Cholecalciferol supplementation prevented seasonal AMH change.
Conclusion: Vitamin D may be a positive regulator of AMH production in adults, and vitamin D deficiency may confound clinical decisions based on AMH. Vitamin D status should be considered when serum AMH levels are obtained for diagnosis.

This paper demonstrates that vitamin D amongst many other functions is also involved in reproductive endocrinology, more specifically in regulation of AMH production. The message is that vitamin D status should be checked and any deficiency corrected before results of AMH analyses are interpreted. As the authors point out, the present findings may at least partially explain the great variability in AMH levels in different subjects with similar medical conditions. Further studies are required to understand better the specific physiological role of vitamin D in AMH regulation and gonadal function, if any, both prenatally and at different postnatal maturational stages.

Ten novel mutations in the NR5A1 gene cause disordered sex development in 46,XY and ovarian insufficiency in 46,XX individuals

Camats N, Pandey AV, Fernandez-Cancio M, Andaluz P, Janner M, Toran N, Moreno F, Bereket A, Akcay T, Garcia-Garcia E, Munoz MT, Gracia R, Nistal M, Castano L, Mullis PE, Carrascosa A, Audi L, Fluck CE
Pediatric Endocrinology (C.E.F.), Department of Pediatrics and Department of Clinical Research, University Children's Hospital Bern, Bern, Switzerland
J Clin Endocrinol Metab 2012;97:E1294–E1306

Background: Steroidogenic factor-1 (SF-1/NR5A1) is a nuclear receptor that regulates adrenal and reproductive development and function. NR5A1 mutations have been detected in 46,XY individuals with disorders of sexual development (DSD) but apparently normal adrenal function and in 46,XX women with normal sexual development but yet primary ovarian insufficiency (POI).

Methods: A group of 100 46,XY DSD and 2 POI patients were studied for NR5A1 mutations and their impact. Clinical, biochemical, histological, genetic, and functional characteristics of the patients with NR5A1 mutations are reported. Patients were referred from different centers in Spain, Switzerland, and Turkey. Histological and genetic studies were performed in Barcelona, Spain. In vitro studies were performed in Bern, Switzerland. A total of 65 Spanish and 35 Turkish patients with 46,XY DSD and 2 Swiss 46,XX patients with POI were investigated.

Results: Ten novel heterozygote NR5A1 mutations were detected and characterized (5 missense, 1 nonsense, 3 frameshift mutations, and 1 duplication). The novel NR5A1 mutations were tested in vitro by promoter transactivation assays showing grossly reduced activity for mutations in the DNA-binding domain and variably reduced activity for other mutations. The dominant negative effect of the mutations was excluded. The authors demonstrated high variability and thus no apparent genotype-structure-function-phenotype correlation. Histological studies of testes revealed vacuolization of Leydig cells due to fat accumulation.

Conclusions: SF-1/NR5A1 mutations are frequently found in 46,XY DSD individuals (9%) and manifest with a broad phenotype. Testis histology is characteristic for fat accumulation and degeneration over time, similar to findings observed in patients with lipoid congenital adrenal hyperplasia (due to StAR mutations). Genotype-structure-function-phenotype correlation remains elusive.

The SF1/NR5A1 gene is an important regulator of prenatal sex differentiation affecting both adrenal and gonadal functions. An increasing number of mutations of this gene are being discovered and such involvement should be considered in cases of DSD with unknown background. In contrast to other well-studied genes with more defined functions, such as 21-hydroxylase in congenital adrenal hyperplasia, mutations of SF1/NR5A1 are much more difficult to interpret with respect to their functional consequences. Such lack of genotype-phenotype correlation also makes family counseling difficult and challenging.

Food for thought

The science of sex – novel series in *EMBO* Reports

Breithaupt H (ed)
EMBO Rep 2012;13:394

Science & Society Series on Sex and Science

Sexual reproduction has facilitated the evolution of higher life forms and has had a profound influence on human history, culture and society. This series of invited papers in *EMBO Reports* explores the attempts to understand the influence of sex in the natural world, and the biological, medical and cultural aspects of sexual reproduction, gender and sexual pleasure.

Sperm counts and fertility in men: a rocky road ahead

Sharpe RM
MRC Centre for Reproductive Health, University of Edinburgh, The Queen's Medical Research Institute, Edinburgh, UK
EMBO Rep 2012;13:398–403

Synopsis of review: Both sperm counts and testosterone levels have been declining in men in recent decades which may suggest that male health might have also declined. There is a great incentive to understand what has caused lower sperm counts in men, and to establish whether this trend can be reversed or prevented. Falling sperm counts have been discussed as a scary story about environmental chemical pollution and unhealthy lifestyle changes but the evidence base for such conclusions is weak and the causes remain unknown. The fact that sperm counts have fallen across a short timescale of 50–70 years is indeed a strong indication that the causes are related to lifestyle and environment, rather than genetic.

This also means that the decline is probably preventable, and possibly reversible. For this to happen, the problem has to be recognized, its causes elucidated and appropriate intervention or prevention implemented. To identify the causes requires that one knows where and when to look. Sperm count probably matters more today than a few decades ago when most women had their children at an earlier age. But sperm count also matters for men for reasons even more fundamental than fertility. It is a sign of overall health; the lower your sperm count the greater your risk of dying. The other marker of healthy testis function – testosterone levels in blood – shows a similar relationship. Perhaps the most disturbing conclusion is that the evidence for low and falling sperm counts points to a wider issue of the subtle dysfunction of the process that makes men male. If this process is affected by maternal lifestyle and environmental exposures, which a growing body of evidence suggests is the case, then what other consequences for the programming of behavior and disease risks will it also bring?

This paper is an excellent review of the issue of decreasing sperm quality in Western societies during the past more than half a century. It brings up most of the relevant issues related to this important topic for critical discussion and points to important and necessary roads for future research. The paper is also the first in a series on Sex & Science published in *EMBO Reports*, with a scientific approach to different aspects of sex that promises interesting reading. It is highly recommended for the pediatric endocrinologist who wants to remain updated on these important and interesting issues.

Food for thought
Beware of the mattress!

Corncob bedding alters the effects of estrogens on aggressive behavior and reduces estrogen receptor-α expression in the brain

Landeros RV, Morisseau C, Yoo HJ, Fu SH, Hammock BD, Trainor BC
Department of Psychology and Center for Neuroscience, University of California, Davis, Davis, CA, USA

Endocrinology 2012;153:949–953

Background: Estrogen signaling pathways can be modulated by naturally occurring environmental compounds such as phytoestrogens and xenoestrogens. Many researchers studying the effects of estrogens on brain function or behavior in animal models choose to use phytoestrogen-free food for this reason. Corncob bedding is commonly used in animal facilities across the United States and has been shown to inhibit estrogen-dependent reproductive behavior in rats. The mechanism for this effect was unclear, because the components of corncob bedding mediating this effect did not bind estrogen receptors.
Methods: The California mouse *(Peromyscus californicus)* was used and housed either on cardboard or corncob bedding.
Results: Estrogens decreased aggression when cardboard-based bedding was used, but this effect was absent when corncob bedding was used. California mice housed on corncob bedding also had fewer estrogen receptor-α-positive cells in the bed nucleus of the stria terminalis and ventromedial hypothalamus compared with mice housed on cardboard-based bedding. In addition, corncob bedding suppressed the expression of phosphorylated ERK in these brain regions as well as in the medial amygdala and medial preoptic area.
Conclusion: The present observations on the effects of corncob bedding on behavior and brain function should draw attention to the importance that cage bedding can exert on neuroendocrine research.

This study lifts a warning flag worth noticing. A lot of effort has been put into reducing the impact from hormonal substances in food and cell medium to experimental animal and in vitro cultures. However, the cage bedding as well as the amusement toys for enrichment have not been thoroughly evaluated for unwanted hormonal side effects. The study by Landeros et al. is important to remind researchers that also cage inventories have to be cautiously chosen when doing studies where hormonal input might change the outcome. To pull these results a bit further and extrapolate to humans, one should be very careful when choosing bed material. Not many have mattresses stuffed with corncobs at home, but there are plenty of other materials which could very well contain, or be contaminated with, phytoestrogens or xenoestrogens. Since we spend almost a third of our lives in bed, the exposure time for the material is very high. Modern mattresses usually contain stuffing such as latex, viscoelastic or other flexible polyurethane foams. Mattresses may also be filled with air or water, or a variety of natural fibers. Futons, the Japanese beds, are often stuffed with cotton, wool or synthetic batting. The pillows are filled with beans, buckwheat chaff or plastic beads. The plastics could contain estrogenic substances which could meddle with the neuroendocrine system, as could phytoestrogens, e.g. in beans. Next time you change your matrass – consider the options thoroughly!

Food for thought
The scientific evidence for the good outcome of a weekend trip!

Short-term enrichment makes male rats more attractive, more defensive and alters hypothalamic neurons

Mitra R, Sapolsky RM
School of Biological Sciences, Nanyang Technological University, Singapore, Singapore
PloS One 2012;7:e36092

Background: Innate behaviors are shaped by contingencies built during evolutionary history. On the other hand, environmental stimuli play a significant role in shaping behavior. Environmental enrichment is known to improve physiology and behavior at multiple levels in a variety of species. A short period of environmental enrichment (EE) can enhance cognitive behavior, modify effects of stress on learned behaviors and induce brain plasticity.
Methods: The authors investigated whether modulation by environment can extend to innate behaviors that are preserved by intense selection pressure, by studying effects of relatively short (14-day) environmental enrichment on two prominent innate behaviors in rats: avoidance of predator odors and ability of males to attract mates.
Results: Enrichment had strong effects on both the innate behaviors. The enriched males were more avoidant of a predator odor than nonenriched controls, and had a greater rise in corticosterone levels in response to the odor. The enriched males also had higher testosterone levels and were more attractive to females. A decrease in dendritic length of neurons of ventrolateral nucleus of hypothalamus was demonstrated. These neurons are important for reproductive mate choice and an increase of the same neurons in the dorsomedial nucleus is important also for defensive behavior. The possibility that these two sets of changes in neuronal cytoarchitecture are plausibly coupled (i.e. that increased predator avoidance is an adaptive compensation for the conspicuousness of increased sexual attraction) is exciting, and awaits further investigations.
Conclusions: Behavioral and hormonal observations provide evidence that a short period of EE can alter innate behaviors, providing a good example of gene-environment interaction.

What can we learn from this study? The EE was shown to have a strong impact on innate behaviors like attraction to females and avoidance of predators. If a female gives her partner a short-term enrichment, the result might be that he turns out to be more attractive to her. Thus, in the long run a recreational break like a weekend trip, could be what is needed for any long relationship to work out. The female will, besides enjoying the trip in itself, find the partner more attractive, although this might be a farfetched conclusion to draw from studies on rats.

Ovarian control of nectar collection in the honey bee (*Apis mellifera*)

Siegel AJ, Freedman C, Page RE Jr
School of Life Sciences, Arizona State University, Tempe, AZ, USA
PloS One 2012;7:e33465

Background: Honey bees are a model system for the study of division of labor. Worker bees demonstrate a foraging division of labor (DOL) by biasing collection towards carbohydrates (nectar) or protein (pollen). There is a reproductive ground-plan hypothesis proposing that foraging DOL is regulated by the networks that controlled foraging behavior during the reproductive life cycle of honey bee ancestors.

Methods: A proposed mechanism was tested, through which the ovary of the facultatively sterile worker impacts foraging bias. The proposed mechanism suggests that the ovary has a regulatory effect on sucrose sensitivity, and sucrose sensitivity impacts nectar loading. This mechanism was tested by measuring worker ovary size (ovariole number), sucrose sensitivity, and sucrose solution load size collected from a rate-controlled artificial feeder. Three nonsimultaneous replicates were performed using 10 and 30% sucrose solutions.

Results: A significant interaction between ovariole number and sucrose sensitivity on sucrose solution load size was found when using low concentration nectar. This supports the proposed mechanism. As nectar and pollen loading are not independent, a mechanism impacting nectar load size would also impact pollen load size.

Conclusion: The results of this study demonstrate a link between ovariole number, sucrose sensitivity and nectar collection. These results support a proposed foraging DOL control mechanism where the ovary impacts sucrose responsiveness in honey bees. Sucrose responsiveness, in turn, impacts the loading of sugar-rich nectar. This mechanism fits well into the evolutionary hypothesis that mechanisms controlling food collection during the life cycle of solitary ancestors of honey bees have been coopted and remodeled to control foraging decisions in extant honey bees.

From this study it is evident that the ovary modulates sucrose perception, which in turn affects the volume of nectar collected. Bees with different numbers of ovarioles demonstrated different responses to sucrose concentration and this impacted on their foraging decisions regarding nectar loading. Extrapolating this into the human situation puts forward the possibility of ovarian regulation of sugar sensitivity and storage of calories. It is since long known that ovariectomized rats have higher body weight and increased appetite than their intact controls, a behavior that can be counteracted by estradiol treatment [1]. Similarly, postmenopausal women are more prone to gain weight than women before menopause [2]. Thus, from bees to women the ovaries are involved in keeping the metabolic balance.

Pubertal Stage and Brain Anatomy in Girls

Blanton RE, Cooney RE, Joormann J, Eugene F, Glover GH, Gotlib IH
Department of Psychiatry, Yale University, New Haven, CT, USA
Neuroscience 2012;217:105–112

Background: Studies of puberty have focused primarily on changes in hormones and on observable physical bodily characteristics. Little is known, however, about the nature of the relation between pubertal status and brain physiology and morphology. This is particularly important given findings that have linked the onset of puberty with both changes in cognitive functioning and increases in the incidence of depression and anxiety.

Methods: The study examined relationships between pubertal stage, assessed by Tanner staging, and brain anatomy in a sample of 54 girls aged 9–15 years. Brain morphometric analysis was conducted using high-resolution magnetic resonance imaging (MRI). The hippocampus and amygdala were manually traced on MRI scans in all participants. Stepwise regression analyses were conducted with total intracranial volume (ICV), age, and pubertal status as the predictor variables and hippocampus and amygdala volumes as outcome variables.

Results: Pubertal status was significantly associated with left amygdala volume, after controlling for both age and intracranial volume (ICV). In addition, puberty was related to right hippocampus and amygdala volumes, after controlling for ICV. In contrast, no significant associations were found between age and hippocampal and amygdala volumes after controlling for pubertal status and ICV.

Conclusions: These findings highlight the importance of the relation between pubertal status and morphometry of the hippocampus and amygdala, and of limbic and subcortical structures that have been implicated in emotional and social behavior.

Sex matters during adolescence: testosterone-related cortical thickness maturation differs between boys and girls

Bramen JE, Hranilovich JA, Dahl RE, Chen J, Rosso C, Forbes EE, Dinov ID, Worthman CM, Sowell ER
Developmental Cognitive Neuroimaging Laboratory, Children's Hospital Los Angeles, Los Angeles, CA, USA
PloS One 2012;7:e33850

Background: Age-related changes in brain cortical thickness have been observed during adolescence, including thinning in frontal and parietal cortices, and thickening in the lateral temporal lobes. Studies have shown sex differences in hormone-related brain maturation when boys and girls are age-matched, however, because girls mature 1–2 years earlier than boys, these sex differences could be confounded by pubertal maturation.

Methods: To address puberty effects directly, this study assessed sex differences in testosterone-related cortical maturation by studying 85 boys and girls in a narrow age range and matched on sexual maturity. The authors expected that testosterone-by-sex interactions on cortical thickness would be observed in brain regions known from the animal literature to be high in androgen receptor (AR) expression.

Results: There were sex differences in associations between circulating testosterone and thickness in left inferior parietal lobule, middle temporal gyrus, calcarine sulcus, and right lingual gyrus, all regions known to be high in AR expression. Visual areas increased with testosterone in boys, but decreased in girls. All other regions were more impacted by testosterone levels in girls than boys.

Conclusions: The regional pattern of sex-by-testosterone interactions may have implications for understanding sex differences in behavior and adolescent-onset neuropsychiatric disorders.

These two papers add fuel to the longstanding discussion on gender differences in brain function and morphology. Some investigators still argue such differences are sparse or nonexistent but the present two papers clearly demonstrate such differences in addition to those related to the maturational stage. Although up-to-date methodology was employed for these noninvasive investigations, the techniques are still crude when compared with more invasive and less safe methods that may be used in animal experiments. Future more refined imaging techniques will allow more detailed studies and will most certainly take this field further in the not so far future. For the clinician the papers help to set references for morphometric analyses that may be of importance in investigations of patients with, e.g., pubertal and gender identity disorders.

Lena Sahlin/Olle Söder

Sexual dimorphism in the early life programming of serum leptin levels in European adolescents: the HELENA study

Labayen I, Ruiz JR, Huybrechts I, Ortega FB, Rodriguez G, Dehenauw S, Breidenassel C, Jimenez-Pavon D, Vyncke KE, Censi L, Molnar D, Widhalm K, Kafatos A, Plada M, Diaz LE, Marcos A, Moreno LA, Gottrand F
Department of Nutrition and Food Science, University of the Basque Country, Vitoria, Spain
idoia.labayen@ehu.es
J Clin Endocrinol Metab 2011;96:E1330–1334

Background: Concentration of hormones, metabolites, and neurotransmitters during critical periods of early development has been suggested to preprogram brain development and metabolism later in life. Leptin is a hormone mainly produced and secreted into the circulation by the adipose tissue and plays a key role in the chronic control of energy balance and insulin sensitivity. In this study it was tested if a lower birth weight, as an indicator of adverse intrauterine environment, may be associated with higher serum leptin levels in European adolescents.
Methods: Fasting serum leptin was measured in 757 (429 females) European adolescents born at term aged 14.6 ± 1.2 years. Weight and height, was measured and body mass index was calculated. Birth weight, duration of pregnancy, and duration of breast-feeding were obtained from parental records. Duration of pregnancy and breast-feeding, pubertal status, center, body mass index, and physical activity were entered as confounders in the analyses.
Results: There was a significant interaction effect between sex and birth weight on serum leptin levels. Body weight at birth was negatively and significantly associated with serum leptin levels only in female adolescents. The association persisted after further controlling for physical activity.
Conclusions: These findings provide further evidence for a sex-specific programming effect of birth weight on serum leptin levels. The results could also contribute to explain the detrimental health effects associated with lower birth weight, such as long-term increased risk of developing obesity and type 2 diabetes.

Postterm birth is associated with greater risk of obesity in adolescent males

Beltrand J, Soboleva TK, Shorten PR, Derraik JG, Hofman P, Albertsson-Wikland K, Hochberg Z, Cutfield WS
Liggins Institute, University of Auckland, Auckland, New Zealand
J Pediatr 2012;160:769–773

Background: Individuals who were born preterm appear to be more prone to insulin resistance, and small size at birth is associated with a variety of adult diseases, including type 2 diabetes, ischemic heart disease, and obesity. Postterm birth has no known associated long-term sequelae, but it has been linked to greater perinatal mortality and morbidity. However, it is known that prolonged gestation may lead to a suboptimal fetal environment through inadequate nutrition or physiological stress, resulting in long-term postnatal alterations in body composition.
Methods: To test the hypothesis that postterm birth (at >42 completed weeks of gestation or >293 days from the first day of the last menstrual period) adversely affects longitudinal growth and weight gain throughout childhood a total of 525 children (including 17 boys and 20 girls born postterm) were followed from birth to the age of 16 years. Weight and height were recorded prospectively throughout childhood, and the respective velocities from birth to end of puberty were calculated using a mathematical model.
Results: At birth, postterm girls were slimmer than term girls. At 16 years of age, postterm boys were 11.8 kg heavier than term boys. The rate of obesity was 29% in postterm boys and 7% in term boys, and the combined rate of overweight and obesity was 47% in postterm boys and 13% in term boys. BMI was higher in postterm boys at already 3 years of age, with the difference increasing thereafter. BMI and growth were similar in postterm and term girls.
Conclusion: In this postterm birth cohort, boys, but not girls, demonstrated accelerated weight gain during childhood, leading to greater risk of obesity in adolescence.

There are many studies indicating that individuals exposed to metabolic and nutritional alterations in the fetal environment may have increased risk of developing obesity and type 2 diabetes in adulthood. A recent article in *Nature Reviews Endocrinology* [3] highlighted two studies which reported female-specific effects of fetal programming on later risk of developing obesity or type 2 diabetes mellitus. One of those studies was by Labayen et al., see above. The other study showed that high insulin levels at birth were associated with a slow rate of growth in the first year of life in girls, but not in boys [4]. Thus, the uterine environment reflected as both hormonal and nutritional status of the mother will impact on adult life and health of offspring – especially for the daughters. On the other hand, the current study by Beltrand et al. showed that postterm boys, but not girls, experienced increased weight gain during childhood and higher risk of obesity in adolescence. It is clear that the uterine environment and fetal programming is important for future health, but to what extent there is a sexual dimorphism varies between studies and the endpoints that are examined.

Diet-induced paternal obesity in the absence of diabetes diminishes the reproductive health of two subsequent generations of mice

Fullston T, Palmer NO, Owens JA, Mitchell M, Bakos HW, Lane M
Research Centre for Reproductive Health Discipline of Obstetrics and Gynaecology, Level 3 Medical School South, Robinson Institute, University of Adelaide, Adelaide, SA, Australia

Hum Reprod 2012;27:1391–1400

Background: Obesity and related conditions, notably subfertility, are increasingly prevalent. Paternal influences are known to affect the health of the offspring, but the impact of paternal obesity and subfertility on the reproductive health of subsequent generations is not known.

Methods: A high-fat diet (HFD) was used to induce obesity (but not diabetes) in male mice, which were subsequently mated to normal-weight females. First-generation offspring were raised on a control diet and their gametes were investigated for signs of subfertility. Second-generation offspring were generated from both first-generation sexes and their gametes were similarly assessed.

Results: HFD-induced paternal initiation of subfertility was found in both male and female offspring of two generations of mice. Furthermore, diminished reproductive and gamete functions were found to be transmitted through the first-generation paternal line to both sexes of the second generation and via the first-generation maternal line to second-generation males. Previous findings that male obesity alters the epigenome of sperm could provide a basis for the developmental programming of subfertility in subsequent generations.

Conclusions: This observation of paternal transmission of diminished reproductive health to future generations could have significant implications for the transgenerational amplification of subfertility observed worldwide in humans.

Nature, nurture or nutrition? Impact of maternal nutrition on maternal care, offspring development and reproductive function

Connor KL, Vickers MH, Beltrand J, Meaney MJ, Sloboda DM
Liggins Institute, University of Auckland, Grafton, Auckland, New Zealand
d.sloboda@auckland.ac.nz

J Physiol 2012;590:2167–2180

Background: Offspring of mothers fed a high-fat (HF) diet during pregnancy and lactation have been shown to enter puberty early and to be hyperleptinemic, hyperinsulinemic and obese as adults. Poor maternal care and bonding can also impact offspring development and disease risk. This study hypothesized that prenatal nutrition would affect maternal care and that an interaction may exist between a maternal HF diet and maternal care, subsequently impacting on offspring phenotype.

Methods: Wistar rats were mated and randomized to control dams fed a control diet (CON) or dams fed a HF diet from conception until the end of lactation (HF). Maternal care was assessed between postnatal day (P)3 and P8. Postweaning (P22), offspring were fed a control CON or HF diet. From P27, pubertal onset was assessed. At ~P105, estrous cyclicity was investigated.

Results: Maternal HF diet reduced maternal care; HF-fed mothers licked and groomed pups less than CON dams. Both female and male offspring of HF dams were lighter from birth to P11 than offspring of CON dams, but by P19 HF offspring were heavier than controls. Pups from HF-fed dams went into puberty early and this effect was exacerbated by a postweaning HF diet. Maternal and postweaning HF diets independently altered estrous cyclicity in females: female offspring of HF-fed mothers were more likely to have prolonged or persistent estrus, whilst female offspring fed a HF diet postweaning were more likely to have irregular estrous cycles and were more likely to have prolonged or persistent estrus.

Conclusion: Maternal HF nutrition during pregnancy and lactation results in a maternal obese phenotype and has a significant impact on maternal care during lactation. Maternal and postweaning nutritional signals, independent of maternal care, alter offspring body fat in prepuberty and female reproductive function in adulthood, which may be associated with advanced ovarian ageing and altered fertility.

In these animal studies it is shown that obese fathers affect the coming generations and give rise to subfertility among both male and female offspring. Obese mothers seem to affect reproductive function in daughters only, even if both male and female offspring went into puberty earlier and showed increased body weight after P19. These results indicate that the early nutritional environment can influence offspring development in a manner that alters reproductive potential and long-term health.

Concepts revised and follow-up on a *Yearbook 2009* (p. 79) paper

Oocyte formation by mitotically active germ cells purified from ovaries of reproductive-age women

White YA, Woods DC, Takai Y, Ishihara O, Seki H, Tilly JL
Vincent Center for Reproductive Biology, Massachusetts General Hospital Vincent Department of Obstetrics and Gynecology, Massachusetts General Hospital, Boston, MA, USA
Nat Med 2012;18:413–421

Background: Germline stem cells that produce oocytes in vitro and fertilization-competent eggs in vivo have been identified in and isolated from adult mouse ovaries.

Methods: A fluorescence-activated cell sorting-based protocol that can be used with adult mouse ovaries and human ovarian cortical tissue to purify rare mitotically active cells that have a gene expression profile that is consistent with primitive germ cells was described and validated.

Results: Once established in vitro, these primitive germ cells could be expanded for months and spontaneously generated 35- to 50-μm oocytes, as determined by morphology, gene expression and haploid (1n) status. Injection of the human germline cells, engineered to stably express GFP, into human ovarian cortical biopsies lead to formation of follicles containing GFP-positive oocytes 1–2 weeks after xenotransplantation into immunodeficient female mice.

Conclusions: Ovaries of reproductive-age women, similar to adult mice, possess rare mitotically active germ cells that can be propagated in vitro as well as generate oocytes in vitro and in vivo.

In the 2009 issue of the *Yearbook* we reported on a finding that juvenile and adult mouse ovaries possess mitotically active germ cells, which completely objected to the current dogma that females of most mammalian species have lost their capacity for oocyte production at birth. A neonatal mouse female fetal stem cell line (FGSC) was established and cultured for more than 15 months. These FGSCs were infected with GFP virus and transplanted into ovaries of infertile mice. Transplanted cells underwent oogenesis and the mice produced offspring that had the GFP transgene. Thus, there is a possibility for oocyte renewal after birth! This year we can report that isolated egg-producing stem cells from the ovaries of reproductive age women were obtained and these cells were shown to produce what appear to be normal egg cells or oocytes. It seems to be possible also for human ovaries to produce new oocytes postnatally!

This controversial result was highlighted in several journals and web pages, e.g. *Science Daily*, please see http://www.sciencedaily.com/releases/2012/02/120226153641.htm and MDNEWS.com, please see http://www.mdnews.com/news/hd/2012_10/hd_662066. In *Biology of Reproduction*, Oatley and Hunt [5] describe what they consider to be the first evidence that oogonial stem cells can also be isolated from human ovaries, with similar technique as was used to obtain the mouse oogonial stem cells. The results from White's paper definitely challenge the old dogma of girls being born with their final number of oocytes.

Neural Progestin Receptors and Female Sexual Behavior

Mani SK, Blaustein JD
Department of Molecular & Cellular Biology, Department of Neuroscience, Center on Addiction, Learning and Memory, Baylor College of Medicine, Houston, TX, USA
Neuroendocrinology 2012 (E-pub ahead of print)

Background: The steroid hormone, progesterone, modulates neuroendocrine functions in the central nervous system resulting in integration of reproduction and reproductive behaviors in female mammals. Although it is widely recognized that progesterone's effects on female sex behavior are mediated by the classical neural progestin receptors (PRs) functioning as 'ligand-dependent' transcription factors to regulate genes and genomic networks, additional mechanisms of PR activation also contribute to the behavioral response. PRs can be activated in a ligand-independent manner by neurotransmitters, growth factors, cyclic nucleotides, progestin metabolites and mating stimuli. The rapid responses of progesterone may be mediated by a variety of PR types, including membrane-associated PRs or extranuclear PRs. Furthermore, these rapid, nonclassical progesterone actions involving cytoplasmic kinase signaling and/or extranuclear PRs also converge with the classical PR-mediated, transcription-dependent pathway to regulate reproductive behaviors.

Method and Results: This review summarizes some of the history of the study of the role of PRs in reproductive behaviors, and update the status of PR-mediated mechanisms involved in the facilitation of female sex behavior. An integrative model of PR activation via cross-talk and convergence of multiple signaling pathways is presented.

Conclusions: The original two-step classical model of PR activation has undergone substantial modifications and evolved into a highly complex integrative model involving multiple signaling pathways. Recent studies have provided insights into ligand-dependent and ligand-independent mechanisms of receptor activation and provided a blueprint for the integrative model for PR activation in the regulation of female sexual behavior. It is also becoming abundantly clear that multiple intra- and intercellular mechanisms share signaling components that potentially amplify and integrate signals from a variety of stimuli to achieve neuroendocrine integration required for complex processes like reproductive behaviors. Future studies will likely reveal further insights into the mechanisms by which the multiple signals converge and reinforce neuronal responses to environmental and behavioral events to alter steroid hormone effects on female reproductive behavior.

The classical nuclear progesterone receptor is present in two isoforms, A and B, which are transcribed from two different initiation sites of the same gene. Progesterone-facilitated lordosis (a behavior of crucial importance for female reproduction in rats) is completely eliminated in the PR-A null mutant mouse. PR-B null mutant mice showed a trend of suppression of P-facilitated sexual behavior. Taken together, the data suggest that PR-A is essential for progesterone-facilitated lordosis, and both isoforms are required for optimal facilitation by progesterone. Today the increasing number of reports on alternative signaling pathways, e.g. nonligand-activated receptors, membrane-bound receptors, neurotransmitters and growth factors, have amplified the complexity in progesterone responses and the pathways regulating sexual behavior.

References

1. Wade GN: Gonadal hormones and behavioral regulation of body weight. Physiol Behav 1972;8:523–534.
2. Pasquali R, Casimirri F, Labate AM, Tortelli O, Pascal G, Anconetani B, et al: Body weight, fat distribution and the menopausal status in women. The VMH Collaborative Group. Int J Obes Relat Metab Disord 1994;18:614–621.
3. Wilson C: Reproductive endocrinology: sex-specific early life effects on metabolism. Nat Rev Endocrinol 2011;7:500.
4. Regnault N, Botton J, Heude B, Forhan A, Hankard R, Foliguet B, et al: Higher cord C-peptide concentrations are associated with slower growth rate in the first year of life in girls but not in boys. Diabetes 2011;60:2152–2159.
5. Oatley J, Hunt PA: Of mice and (wo)men: purified oogonial stem cells from mouse and human ovaries. Biol Reprod 2012;86:196.

Adrenals

Erica L.T. van den Akker[a] and Evangelia Charmandari[b]

[a]Department of Pediatric Endocrinology, Erasmus Medical Center, Rotterdam, The Netherlands
[b]Department of Endocrinology, Metabolism and Diabetes, University of Athens Medical School, 'Aghia Sophia' Children's Hospital, and Division of Endocrinology and Metabolism, Clinical Research Center, Biomedical Research Foundation of the Academy of Athens, Athens, Greece

For this year's chapter on 'Adrenals', we have searched the PubMed for articles on 'adrenal' and 'steroidogenesis' published in English between June 1, 2011 and May 31, 2012. Our search yielded more than 6500 citations. We have examined all citations individually and selected the following collection of basic research and clinical articles. Whenever possible, we have avoided topics that have been discussed in the Yearbook 2011, unless progress in the field has been incremental. Emerging themes for this year's chapter include the role of minichromosome maintenance 4 (MCM4) gene in adrenal function, novel mechanisms that control adrenal steroidogenesis, and a novel, dual-release formulation of hydrocortisone for the treatment of adrenal insufficiency and congenital adrenal hyperplasia.

Mechanism of the Year
MCM4 mutations are a cause of adrenal insufficiency, growth failure and natural killer cell deficiency in humans

MCM4 mutation causes adrenal failure, short stature and natural killer cell deficiency in humans

Hughes CR, Guasti L, Meimaridou E, Chuang CH, Schimenti JC, King PJ, Costigan C, Clark AJ, Metherell LA
Queen Mary University of London, Centre for Endocrinology, William Harvey Research Institute, Barts and the London School of Medicine and Dentistry, London, UK
J Clin Invest 2012;122:814–820

Background: A variant of familial glucocorticoid deficiency (FGD) is characterized by adrenal insufficiency, growth failure, increased chromosomal breakage and natural killer (NK) cell deficiency.
Methods and Results: Targeted exome sequencing in 8 patients with this condition identified a variant (c.71-1insG) in minichromosome maintenance-deficient 4 (MCM4) gene that was predicted to result in a severely truncated protein (p.Pro24ArgfsX4). Western blotting of patient samples revealed that the major 96-kDa isoform present in unaffected human controls was absent, while the presence of the minor 85-kDa isoform was preserved. Histological studies with Mcm4 knock-out mice showed grossly abnormal adrenal morphology. Given that MCM4 is one part of a MCM2-7 complex recently confirmed as the replicative helicase essential for normal DNA replication and genome stability in all eukaryotes, it is possible that these patients may have an increased risk of neoplastic change.
Conclusions: This study identified the first human mutation in MCM4, which is associated with adrenal insufficiency, short stature and NK cell deficiency.

Familial glucocorticoid deficiency (FGD) is an autosomal recessive condition characterized by adreno-corticotropic hormone (ACTH) resistant glucocorticoid deficiency [1]. The condition is relatively common in the Irish Traveler community, a genetically isolated population with increased rates of consanguinity. In addition to adrenal insufficiency, a subgroup of patients have evidence of increased chromosomal breakage, growth failure and NK cell deficiency. In this study, Hughes and colleagues investigated children with adrenal insufficiency from three kindreds within the Irish Traveler community. Known causes of adrenal insufficiency were excluded clinically and biochemically, and mutations in MC2R, MRAP, and STAR were not detected. Since the clinical features cosegregated and inheritance patterns were suggestive of an autosomal recessive mode of trasmission, the authors sought common areas of homozygosity and subsequently interrogated these areas using exon capture and high-throughput sequencing. They demonstrated a mutation in the MCM4 gene, which leads to adrenal insufficiency, short stature and NK cell deficiency. Patients demonstrate a phenotype similar to other DNA repair and replication disorders, including increased chromosomal fragility, pre- and postnatal growth retardation, and variable immune deficiency. In addition, this disorder includes adrenal insufficiency. MCM4, a component of the MCM2-7 complex, is part of the pre-replicative complex, which licenses origins for DNA synthesis in the S phase. These findings indicate that defects in replication licensing might lead to disorders with similar growth retardation phenotypes but distinct developmental abnormalities. Therefore, other components of the MCM complex represent prime potential candidates for other undiagnosed cases of chromosomal instability or adrenal insufficiency.

Partial MCM4 deficiency in patients with growth retardation, adrenal insufficiency and natural killer cell deficiency

Gineau L, Cognet C, Kara N, Lach FP, Dunne J, Veturi U, Picard C, Trouillet C, Eidenschenk C, Aoufouchi S, Alcaïs A, Smith O, Geissmann F, Feighery C, Abel L, Smogorzewska A, Stillman B, Vivier E, Casanova JL, Jouanguy E
Laboratory of Human Genetics of Infectious Diseases, Necker Branch, Institut National de la Santé et de la Recherche Médicale U980, Paris, France
J Clin Invest 2012;122:821–832

Background: Natural killer (NK) cells are circulating cytotoxic lymphocytes that exert potent and non-redundant antiviral activity and anti-tumoral activity in the mouse; however, their function in host defense in humans is not clear. In the present study, the authors investigated 6 related patients with autosomal recessive adrenal insufficiency, growth retardation and a selective NK cell deficiency characterized by a lack of the CD56(dim) NK subset.

Methods and Results: Using linkage analysis and fine mapping, they identified the disease-causing gene, MCM4, which encodes a component of the MCM2-7 helicase complex required for DNA replication. A splice-site mutation in the patients produced a frameshift, but the mutation was hypomorphic due to the creation of two new translation initiation methionine codons downstream of the premature termination codon. The patients' fibroblasts exhibited genomic instability, which was rescued by expression of the wild-type MCM4.

Conclusions: Partial MCM4 deficiency results in a genetic syndrome of growth retardation, adrenal insufficiency and selective NK deficiency. The clinical manifestations of growth retardation and adrenal insufficiency likely reflect the ubiquitous but heterogeneous impact of the MCM4 gene mutation in various tissues.

Natural killer (NK) cells are circulating cytotoxic lymphocytes lacking antigen-specific Tcell and Bcell receptors. They exert potent and non-redundant antiviral activity and anti-tumoral activity in the mouse model; however, their function in host defense in humans remains unclear. Several children with a specific quantitative circulating NK cell defect but normal Tcell counts have been reported. In the present study, Gineau and colleagues investigated six related patients with autosomal recessive adrenal insufficiency, growth retardation and a selective NK cell deficiency characterized by a lack of the CD56dim NK subset. Using linkage analysis and fine mapping, they confirmed that the MCM4 was the disease-causing gene. Partial MCM4 deficiency is the first genetic etiology of a human disorder associated with selective NK cell deficiency to be described. In humans, the MCM4 deficit selectively affects the CD56dim subset of NK cells, which account for 90% of the mature circulating NK cells. The NK CD56dim subset originates from the NK CD56bright subset and the transition between these two subsets is associated with a decrease in the capacity of NK cells to proliferate. The concomitant observation of a lack of proliferation of NK CD56bright cells and of the loss of the NK CD56dim subset in the patients suggests that the final stage of NK differentiation requires the proliferation of NK CD56bright cells. Thus, the identification of this MCM4 deficiency sheds light not only on the genetic deficiency in these patients, but also on the mechanisms of NK cell differentiation, providing the first genetic evidence for the differentiation of CD56bright cells into CD56dim NK cells in humans.

BDNF and glucocorticoids regulate corticotrophin-releasing hormone homeostasis in the hypothalamus

Jeanneteau FD, Lambert WM, Ismaili N, Bath KG, Lee FS, Garabedian MJ, Chao MV
Department of Cell Biology, Skirball Institute of Biomolecular Medicine, New York University School of Medicine, New York, NY, USA

Proc Natl Acad Sci USA 2012;109:1305–1310

Background: Regulation of the hypothalamic-pituitary-adrenal (HPA) axis is critical for adaptation to environmental changes. Corticotrophin-releasing hormone (CRH), the principle regulator of the HPA axis, is an important target of negative feedback by glucocorticoids. Disruption of normal HPA axis activity is a major risk factor of neuropsychiatric disorders, in which decreased expression of the glucocorticoid receptor (GR) has been documented.

Methods and Results: Impairment of GR function in the paraventricular nucleus (PVN) resulted in an enhancement of CRH expression, an up-regulation of hypothalamic levels of BDNF and disinhibition of the HPA axis. BDNF is a stress and activity-dependent factor involved in many activities modulated by the HPA axis. Ectopic expression of BDNF in vivo increased CRH, whereas reduced expression of BDNF, or its receptor TrkB, decreased CRH expression and normal HPA function. The differential regulation of CRH relies upon the cAMP response-element binding protein coactivator CRTC2, which serves as a switch for BDNF and glucocorticoids to direct the expression of CRH.

Conclusions: These findings revealed a homeostatic mechanism by which hypothalamic BDNF and glucocorticoid signaling maintain CRH and glucocorticoid bioavailability.

The HPA axis is regulated by CRH and glucocorticoids. Stress activates the HPA axis via polysynaptic circuits that converge on the hypothalamic paraventricular nucleus (PVN) to activate CRH-producing neurons. Endocrine feedback control is characterized by the down-regulation of CRH and ACTH by glucocorticoids to prevent further increase in glucocorticoid concentrations. Therefore, maintenance of the HPA axis involves a homeostatic equilibrium between activation and inhibitory feedback. Both activation and feedback regulation are dependent upon the glucocorticoid receptor (GR), which is expressed in brain structures that control HPA axis reactivity. Neurotrophic factors, such as BDNF (brain-derived neurotrophic factor), are involved in regulating many functions of the HPA axis [2]. BDNF and its receptor, TrkB, are both expressed in the PVN and other brain regions, and play an important role in neuroprotection and synaptic plasticity. In the present study, the authors demonstrated that genetic disruption of GR in the PVN disinhibited both the HPA axis and the expression of hypothalamic BDNF. BDNF and glucocorticoid signaling intersect upon CRH. These findings provide a unique mechanism involving cAMP response-element binding protein (CREB) and its coactivator protein, CRTC2, which explains how BDNF can balance the ability of glucocorticoids to influence CRH expression specifically in the PVN. These findings revealed a homeostatic mechanism by which hypothalamic BDNF and glucocorticoid signaling maintain CRH and glucocorticoid bioavailability.

Reconciling the nutritional and glucocorticoid hypotheses of fetal programming

Cottrell EC, Holmes MC, Livingstone DE, Kenyon CJ, Seckl JR
Faculty of Human and Medical Sciences, University of Manchester, Manchester, UK
FASEB J 2012;26:1866–1874

Background: Fetal growth restriction is associated with an increased risk of cardiometabolic and neuropsychiatric disorders in adulthood. Both maternal malnutrition (notably a low-protein (LP) diet) and stress/glucocorticoid exposure reduce fetal growth and cause persisting abnormalities in adult offspring. Deficiency of placental 11β-hydroxysteroid dehydrogenase-2 (11β-HSD2) is reduced by an LP diet and has been proposed as a unifying mechanism. The aim of the present study was to explore the role of glucocorticoids and placental 11β-HSD2 in dietary programming.
Methods and Results: Pregnant mice were fed a control or isocaloric LP diet throughout gestation. The LP diet first elevated fetal glucocorticoid levels, then reduced placental growth and finally decreased fetal weight near term by 17%. Whereas the LP diet reduced placental 11β-HSD2 activity near term by 25%, the activity was increased between 20 and 40% at earlier ages, implying that glucocorticoid overexposure in LP fetuses occurs via 11β-HSD2-independent mechanisms. Heterozygous 11β-HSD2$^{(+/-)}$ crosses showed that although both LP and 11β-HSD2 deficiency reduced fetal growth, LP indeed acted independently of 11β-HSD2. Instead, the LP diet induced the fetal hypothalamic-pituitary-adrenal axis per se.
Conclusions: Maternal malnutrition and placental 11β-HSD2 deficiency act via distinct processes to retard fetal growth, which both involve fetoplacental overexposure to glucocorticoids but from distinct sources.

Fetal growth restriction reflects an adverse intrauterine environment and is associated with a substantially increased risk of metabolic, cardiovascular, and behavioral disorders in adult life [3]. Maternal malnutrition or psychological stress and glucocorticoid exposure during pregnancy have been shown to constrain fetal growth and also to have long-term effects on adult health [4]; this phenomenon is called developmental programming. In both humans and rodents, circulating maternal glucocorticoid (cortisol in humans and corticosterone in rodents) concentrations during mid to late gestation are 5- to 10-fold higher than those in the fetus. The enzyme 11β-hydroxysteroid dehydrogenase type 2 (11β-HSD2) catalyzes the inactivation of cortisol and corticosterone to inert cortisone and 11-dehydrocorticosterone (11-DHC), respectively, and is highly expressed in the placenta, where it protects the developing fetus from the deleterious effects of excess maternal glucocorticoids. Inhibition of 11β-HSD2 or its bypass through administration of dexamethasone, which is poorly metabolized by 11β-HSD2, reduces offspring birth weight and causes adult programming outcomes. Maternal malnutrition in humans reduces birth weight and placental size at term, which correlate with reduced placental 11β-HSD2. In the present study, the authors directly tested the hypothesis that the maternal low-protein (LP) diet effects are mediated by increased fetal glucocorticoid exposure, specifically via a reduction in placental 11β-HSD2. They showed that maternal protein malnutrition causes placental and then late fetal growth restriction. The growth restriction was preceded and accompanied by fetal glucocorticoid excess, which correlated closely and negatively with fetal growth by late gestation. Although 11β-HSD2 deficiency also causes fetal growth restriction, placental insufficiency, and developmental programming, this was not the cause of LP-induced fetal growth restriction and, by implication, of programming by maternal malnutrition. Instead, the fetal HPA axis is prematurely activated in the LP fetus alongside fetoplacental IGF-II deficiency. It is clear that glucocorticoids are important in both models, yet the likely source and underlying processes differ.

     Erica L.T. van den Akker/Evangelia Charmandari

Genotype-phenotype analysis in congenital adrenal hyperplasia due to P450 oxidoreductase deficiency

Krone N, Reisch N, Idkowiak J, Dhir V, Ivison HE, Hughes BA, Rose IT, O'Neil DM, Vijzelaar R, Smith MJ, MacDonald F, Cole TR, Adolphs N, Barton JS, Blair EM, Braddock SR, Collins F, Cragun DL, Dattani MT, Day R, Dougan S, Feist M, Gottschalk ME, Gregory JW, Haim M, Harrison R, Olney AH, Hauffa BP, Hindmarsh PC, Hopkin RJ, Jira PE, Kempers M, Kerstens MN, Khalifa MM, Köhler B, Maiter D, Nielsen S, O'Riordan SM, Roth CL, Shane KP, Silink M, Stikkelbroeck NM, Sweeney E, Szarras-Czapnik M, Waterson JR, Williamson L, Hartmann MF, Taylor NF, Wudy SA, Malunowicz EM, Shackleton CH, Arlt W
Centre for Endocrinology, Diabetes, and Metabolism, School of Clinical and Experimental Medicine, University of Birmingham, Birmingham, UK

J Clin Endocrinol Metab 2012;97:E257–267

Background: P450 oxidoreductase deficiency (PORD) is a form of congenital adrenal hyperplasia that manifests with glucocorticoid deficiency, disordered sex development (DSD) and skeletal malformations. The aim of this study was to determine the genotype-phenotype correlation in a large cohort of subjects with PORD.

Methods: Thirty patients with PORD from 11 countries were recruited to participate in the study. Subjects underwent clinical, biochemical and genetic assessment, including multiplex ligation-dependent probe amplification (MLPA).

Results: Twenty-three P450 oxidoreductase (POR) mutations (14 novel) including an exonic deletion and a partial duplication were detected by MLPA. Only 22% of unrelated patients carried homozygous POR mutations. p.A287P was the most common mutation identified in 43% of unrelated alleles. Urinary steroid profiling showed characteristic PORD metabolomes with variable impairment of 17α-hydroxylase and 21-hydroxylase. Adrenal insufficiency was diagnosed in 89% of patients using a short cosyntropin test. DSD was present in 15 of 18 46,XX and seven of 12 46,XY individuals. Homozygosity for p.A287P was invariably associated with 46,XX DSD but normal genitalia in 46,XY individuals. The majority of patients with mild to moderate skeletal malformations were compound heterozygous for missense mutations, whereas nearly all patients with severe malformations carried a major loss-of-function defect on one of the affected alleles.

Conclusions: MLPA is a useful addition to POR mutation analysis. Homozygosity for the most frequent mutation in Caucasians, p.A287P, allows for prediction of genital phenotype and moderate malformations. Adrenal insufficiency is frequent, easily overlooked, but readily detectable by cosyntropin testing.

P450 oxidoreductase deficiency (PORD) is a congenital adrenal hyperplasia variant owing to mutations affecting POR, which serves as mandatory electron donor enzyme to all microsomal cytochrome P450 (CYP) enzymes [5]. In PORD, deficient steroidogenesis is caused by indirect impairment of key enzymes involved in glucocorticoid and sex steroid synthesis, including 17α-hydroxylase, 21-hydroxylase and P450 aromatase. In the present study, Krone and colleagues described in great detail the clinical, biochemical and genetic findings in a large Caucasian PORD cohort. They established the usefulness of MLPA as an addition to molecular genetic analysis of the POR gene, and provided a novel scoring system for standardized assessment of PORD-associated malformations. They showed that major loss-of-function mutations on one of the affected alleles are associated with severe malformations, whereas homozygosity or compound heterozygosity for missense mutations predicts a mild to moderate malformation phenotype. Importantly, homozygosity for the most common mutation in Caucasians, p.A287P, allows for prediction of the genital phenotype and is associated with mild to moderate malformations. Finally, adrenal insufficiency is present in the majority of patients and cannot be predicted by genotype.

18-Hydroxycorticosterone, 18-hydroxycortisol, and 18-oxocortisol in the diagnosis of primary aldosteronism and its subtypes

Mulatero P, di Cella SM, Monticone S, Schiavone D, Manzo M, Mengozzi G, Rabbia F, Terzolo M, Gomez-Sanchez EP, Gomez-Sanchez CE, Veglio F

Department of Medicine and Experimental Oncology, Division of Internal Medicine and Hypertension Unit, University of Torino, and Clinical Chemistry Laboratory, San Giovanni Battista University Hospital, Torino, Italy

J Clin Endocrinol Metab 2012;97:881–889

Background: The diagnosis of primary aldosteronism (PA) is made following a three-step procedure comprising of screening, confirmation testing, and subtype diagnosis. However, some tests are costly and unavailable in most hospitals. The aim of the study was to evaluate the role of serum 18-hydroxycorticosterone (s18OHB), urinary and serum 18-hydroxycortisol (u- and s18OHF), and urinary and serum 18-oxocortisol (u- and s18oxoF) in the diagnosis of PA and its subtypes, aldosterone-producing adenoma (APA) and bilateral adrenal hyperplasia (BAH).

Methods: 26 patients with low-renin essential hypertension (EH), 81 patients with PA (20 APA, 61 BAH), 24 patients with glucocorticoid-remediable aldosteronism, 16 patients with adrenal incidentaloma, and 30 normotensive subjects were recruited to participate in the study. s18OHB, s18OHF, and s18oxoF before and after saline load test (SLT) and 24-h u18OHF and u18oxoF were determined in all subjects.

Results: PA patients displayed significantly higher concentrations of s18OHB, u18OHF, and u18oxoF compared to EH and normal subjects. Patients with APA displayed significantly higher s18OHB, u18OHF, and u18oxoF concentrations than BAH patients. Similar results were obtained for s18OHF and s18oxoF. SLT significantly reduced s18OHB, s18OHF, and s18oxoF in all groups, but steroid reduction was much less for APA patients compared to BAH and EH. The s18OHB/aldosterone ratio after SLT more than doubled in EH but remained unchanged in APA patients.

Conclusions: u18OHF, u18oxoF, and s18OHB measurements in patients with a positive aldosterone/plasma renin activity ratio correlate with confirmatory tests and adrenal vein sampling in PA patients. If verified, these steroid assays would refine the diagnostic workup for PA.

Primary aldosteronism (PA) is the most common form of secondary hypertension. The detection of PA is of particular importance because affected subjects are more prone to cardiovascular events and target organ damage than patients with essential hypertension. According to the Endocrine Society Guidelines, the diagnosis of PA is made following a three-step procedure comprising screening, confirmation/exclusion testing, and subtype diagnosis [6]. The most common screening test for PA is the measurement of the aldosterone/plasma renin activity (PRA) ratio (ARR); a positive ARR is followed by a confirmatory test, preferably using a saline load, to definitively confirm/exclude PA. However, there is no agreement on which of four accepted confirmatory tests should be performed because each test displays both advantages and potential pitfalls. Adrenal vein sampling (AVS) is the only reliable method to differentiate unilateral from bilateral PA; however, this test is expensive, requires a dedicated and expert radiologist, and is not available in most hospitals.

18-Hydroxycorticosterone (18OHB) is an intermediate precursor in aldosterone biosynthesis that originates from the conversion of corticosterone by the aldosterone synthase, although small amounts may be produced by the 11β-hydroxylase. 18-Hydroxycortisol (18OHF) and 18-oxocortisol (18oxoF), known as "hybrid steroids" are produced by aldosterone synthase using 11-deoxycortisol as substrate, although 18OHF can also be produced by 11β-hydroxylase. Given that aldosterone synthase expression is normally limited to the zona glomerulosa, and 17α-hydroxylase and 11β-hydroxylase necessary for cortisol synthesis occur in the zona fasciculata, production of 18OHF and 18oxoF is normally very low. Their synthesis is dramatically increased in glucocorticoid-remediable aldosteronism (GRA) due to the availability of substrate to the aldosterone synthase expressed in the zona fasciculata in GRA. Levels of 18OHF and 18oxoF were shown to be better than the dexamethasone suppression test for the diagnosis of GRA. In the present study, the authors evaluated the role of 18OHB, 18OHF, and 18oxoF in the diagnosis of PA and its subtypes. This is the largest study addressing the role of 18OHF, 18oxoF, and 18OHB in the diagnosis of PA and its subtypes. It demonstrated that none of the steroid assays were sensitive or specific enough to replace a confirmatory test and/or AVS in all patients. AVS is still the only reliable way to distinguish unilateral from bilateral forms of hyperaldosteronism.

Recovery of the hypothalamic-pituitary-adrenal axis in children and adolescents after surgical cure of Cushing's disease

Lodish M, Dunn SV, Sinaii N, Keil MF, Stratakis CA
Program on Developmental Endocrinology and Genetics and Pediatric Endocrinology Inter-Institute Training Program, Eunice Kennedy Shriver National Institute of Child Health and Human Development, National Institutes of Health, Bethesda, MD, USA

J Clin Endocrinol Metab 2012;97:1483–1491

Background: Recovery of the hypothalamic-pituitary-adrenal (HPA) axis after transsphenoidal surgery (TSS) for Cushing's disease (CD) in children has not been adequately studied. The aim of this study was to assess the time to recovery of the HPA axis after TSS in children with CD.
Methods: 57 patients with CD (age range: 6–18 yr, mean: 13.0 ± 3.1 yr) given a standard regimen of glucocorticoid tapering after TSS were studied. ACTH (250 µg) stimulation tests were administered at 6-month intervals for up to 36 months. Age, sex, pubertal status, body mass index, length of disease, midnight cortisol, and urinary free cortisol at diagnosis were analyzed for effects on recovery. The main outcome measure was complete recovery of the HPA axis as defined by a cortisol concentration of at least 18 µg/dl in response to 250 µg ACTH.
Results: Full recovery of the HPA axis was documented in 43 (75.4%) of 57 patients, with 29 of the 43 (67.4%) and 41 of the 43 (95.3%) recovering by 12 and 18 months, respectively. The overall mean time to recovery was 12.6 ± 3.3 months. By receiver operating characteristic curve assessment, the cutoff of at least 10–11 µg/dl of cortisol as the peak of ACTH stimulation testing at 5 months after TSS yielded the highest sensitivity (70–80%) and specificity (64–73%) to predict full recovery of the HPA axis at 12 months. Two of the four patients that recovered fully within 6 months had recurrent CD.
Conclusions: This study presents a standardized tapering regimen for glucocorticoid replacement after TSS that led to recovery of the HPA axis in most patients within the first postoperative year. Although multiple factors may affect this process, an early recovery may indicate disease recurrence.

Recovery of normal pituitary function is essential for resumption of growth and development of children that undergo transsphenoidal surgery (TSS) for Cushing's disease (CD). Hypercortisolism suppresses hypothalamic and pituitary functions preoperatively. Unless TSS was complicated by multiple procedures and other untoward effects, hypercortisolism (and not surgery) appears to be mostly responsible for the pituitary hormone deficiencies seen postoperatively. This study proposes that an empirically made but standardized regimen for replacement and tapering of glucocorticoid replacement after TSS for CD leads to safe recovery of HPA axis function within 12 months after TSS in most patients. The standardized tapering regimen consisted of a starting dose of hydrocortisone of at 8–12 mg/m^2/day in two divided doses with the larger dose (approximately two thirds of the total dose) administered in the morning. After 4 months, the hydrocortisone dose was reduced by 2.5 mg every 4–6 wk until the patients were on only 5 mg/d. This slow tapering method aimed at avoiding undertreatment with possible adrenal crises and overtreatment leading to HPA axis suppression. The data of this study also indicate that the severity of hypercortisolism before TSS is a factor that influences recovery, whereas early recovery is highly suspicious for failed surgical treatment.

Urine steroid metabolomics as a biomarker tool for detecting malignancy in adrenal tumors

Arlt W, Biehl M, Taylor AE, Hahner S, Libé R, Hughes BA, Schneider P, Smith DJ, Stiekema H, Krone N, Porfiri E, Opocher G, Bertherat J, Mantero F, Allolio B, Terzolo M, Nightingale P, Shackleton CH, Bertagna X, Fassnacht M, Stewart PM
Centre for Endocrinology, Diabetes, and Metabolism, School of Clinical and Experimental Medicine, University of Birmingham, Birmingham, UK

J Clin Endocrinol Metab 2011;96:3775–3784

Background: Adrenal tumors have a prevalence of approximately 2% in the general population. Adrenocortical carcinoma (ACC) is rare but accounts for 2–11% of incidentally discovered adrenal masses. The differentiation of ACC from adrenocortical adenoma (ACA) represents a diagnostic challenge in patients with adrenal incidentalomas. The aim of this study was to examine the diagnostic value of a novel steroid metabolomic approach (mass spectrometry-based steroid profiling followed by machine learning analysis) for the detection of adrenal malignancy.

Methods: Quantification of 32 distinct adrenal derived steroids was carried out by gas chromatography/ mass spectrometry in 24-h urine samples from 102 ACA patients (age range 19–84 yr) and 45 ACC patients (20–80 yr). The underlying diagnosis was ascertained by histology and metastasis in ACC and by clinical follow-up (median duration 52 (range 26–201) months) without evidence of metastasis in ACA. Steroid excretion data were subjected to generalized matrix learning vector quantization (GMLVQ) to identify the most discriminative steroids.

Results: Steroid profiling revealed a pattern of predominantly immature, early-stage steroidogenesis in ACC. GMLVQ analysis identified a subset of nine steroids that performed best in differentiating ACA from ACC. Receiver-operating characteristics analysis of GMLVQ results demonstrated sensitivity = specificity = 90% employing all 32 steroids and sensitivity = specificity = 88% when using only the nine most differentiating markers.

Conclusions: Urine steroid metabolomics is a novel, highly sensitive, and specific biomarker tool for discriminating benign from malignant adrenal tumors, with obvious promise for the diagnostic work-up of patients with adrenal incidentalomas.

Adrenocortical carcinoma (ACC) is a rare tumor, however, it accounts for 2–11% of incidentally discovered adrenal masses. Even when basing the histopathological assessment on the entire tumor specimen, the differentiation between benign and malignant lesions represents a major diagnostic challenge. In this study, Arlt and colleagues undertook steroid metabolite excretion analysis by mass spectrometry followed by computational analysis, and investigated the performance of this novel biomarker tool in detecting malignancy and hormone excess in a large cohort of patients with adrenal tumors. They demonstrated that this method has a sensitivity and specificity of 90% for discriminating ACCs from ACAs. They also identified the 11-deoxycortisol metabolite THS to be the most discriminative steroid in differentiating ACC from ACA. THS was significantly increased in both ACA and ACC patients compared with controls, but excretion levels were significantly higher in ACC than in ACA, suggesting inhibition or lack of expression of 11β-hydroxylase, the enzyme that converts the glucocorticoid precursor 11-deoxycortisol to active cortisol. These data clearly indicate that urine steroid metabolomics represents a novel and highly promising biomarker approach to the differential diagnosis of adrenal tumors. Before implementation of this novel approach as a diagnostic test in routine clinical practice, prospective validation in large cohorts of patients with adrenal tumors is recommended.

Clinical trials – new treatments
A dual-release formulation of hydrocortisone for the treatment of adrenal insufficiency

Improved cortisol exposure-time profile and outcome in patients with adrenal insufficiency: a prospective randomized trial of a novel hydrocortisone dual-release formulation

Johannsson G, Nilsson AG, Bergthorsdottir R, Burman P, Dahlqvist P, Ekman B, Engström BE, Olsson T, Ragnarsson O, Ryberg M, Wahlberg J, Biller BM, Monson JP, Stewart PM, Lennernäs H, Skrtic S
Department of Endocrinology, Sahlgrenska Academy, University of Gothenburg, Gothenburg, Sweden
J Clin Endocrinol Metab 2012;97:473–481

Background: Patients with adrenal insufficiency (AI) have increased morbidity and mortality rate on standard replacement therapy. The aim of this study was to compare the pharmacokinetics and metabolic outcome between a once-daily (OD) oral hydrocortisone dual-release tablet and the same daily dose of thrice-daily (TID) dose of conventional hydrocortisone tablets.

Methods: An open, randomized, two-period, 12-wk crossover multicenter trial with a 24-wk extension was conducted at five university hospital centers. The trial enrolled 64 adults with primary AI; 11 had concomitant diabetes mellitus (DM). The same daily dose of hydrocortisone was administered as OD dual-release or TID.

Results: Compared with conventional TID, OD provided a sustained serum cortisol profile 0–4 h after the morning intake and reduced the late afternoon and the 24-h cortisol exposure. The mean weight (difference: –0.7 kg, p = 0.005), systolic blood pressure (difference: –5.5 mm Hg, p = 0.0001), diastolic blood pressure (difference: –2.3 mm Hg; p = 0.03), and glycated hemoglobin (absolute difference: –0.1%, p = 0.0006) were all decreased after OD compared with TID at 12 wk. Compared with TID, a reduction in glycated hemoglobin by 0.6% was observed in patients with concomitant DM during OD (p = 0.004).

Conclusions: The OD dual-release tablet provided a more circadian-based serum cortisol profile and was associated with reduced body weight, reduced blood pressure and improved glucose metabolism. Furthermore, glucose metabolism improved in patients with concomitant DM.

Although glucocorticoid replacement has been available for over a half-century, there have been few new developments in the oral preparations for treatment of patients with adrenal insufficiency (AI). Oral hydrocortisone in daily divided doses is the most widely used glucocorticoid in cortisol replacement therapy. Studies in patients with AD have shown a more than double the standardized mortality rate despite contemporary optimal glucocorticoid replacement therapy [7]. Also, patients with hypopituitarism have a doubled standardized mortality rate, and young adults with AI as part of their hypopituitarism have a 7-fold excessive mortality rate [8]. Likely explanations include the supra-physiological maintenance doses, poor diurnal glucocorticoid exposure-time profile and inadequate rescue therapy in response to intercurrent illnesses. Patients with AI also have increased cardiovascular risk factors, reduced health-related quality of life (QoL) and decreased bone mineral density. In an attempt to improve patient outcome, studies in which both the dose and the dosing strategies were adjusted have been performed and demonstrated that the pattern of hydrocortisone delivery and the serum cortisol exposure-time profile may be as crucial for patient outcome as the total daily dose. A novel once-daily (OD) dual-release hydrocortisone tablet, based on an immediate-release coating together with an extended-release core, was developed to obtain a more physiological circadian-based serum cortisol exposure-time profile. The cortisol time-exposure profile achieved using the OD dual-release hydrocortisone treatment improved cardiovascular risk factors, glucose metabolism and QoL in comparison with conventional treatment. The OD dosing achieved a high and reliable bio-availability and consistent-exposure serum cortisol profile more resembling normal physiology, avoiding the last two peaks during TID, all of which may be of importance for improving outcome in AI patients.

New Mechanisms
Novel mechanisms that control adrenal steroidogenesis

Transcriptional control of adrenal steroidogenesis: novel connection between Janus kinase 2 protein and protein kinase A through stabilization of cAMP response element-binding protein transcription factor

Lefrancois-Martinez AM, Blondet-Trichard A, Binart N, Val P, Chambon C, Sahut-Barnola I, Pointud JC, Martinez A
CNRS UMR6247, Génétique Reproduction et Développement, Clermont Université, Aubière, France
J Biol Chem 2011;286:32976–32985

Background: In the adrenal gland, adrenocorticotropin (ACTH) acts through the cAMP protein kinase (PKA) transduction pathway and represents the main regulator of genes involved in glucocorticoid synthesis. The present study investigated the influence of JAK/STAT signaling on the steroidogenic activity of adrenocortical cell cultures.

Methods and Results: Pharmacological or siRNA-mediated inhibition of Janus kinase 2 (JAK2) reveals its essential role in both basal and ACTH/cAMP-induced steroidogenesis. In addition, nuclear JAK2 regulates the amount of active transcription factor CREB (cAMP response element-binding protein) through tyrosine phosphorylation and prevention of proteasomal degradation, which in turn leads to transcriptional activation of the rate-limiting steroidogenic Star gene.

Conclusions: These findings demonstrate a novel link between PKA and JAK2, by which nuclear JAK2 signaling controls adrenal steroidogenesis by increasing the stability of CREB.

Steroidogenesis is regulated mainly through the adrenocorticotropin (ACTH) activation of the cAMP-dependent protein kinase A (PKA) signaling pathway. Chronic response to ACTH results in increased transcription of genes encoding steroidogenic enzymes and the proteins responsible for cholesterol mobilization and transport, such as the steroidogenic acute regulatory protein (STAR). cAMP-induced PKA activation results in the phosphorylation of the transcription factors GATA-4-binding protein, steroidogenic factor 1 (SF1), CAAT enhancer-binding protein (C/EBP) and cAMP response element-binding protein (CREB), which in turn stimulate the transcription of genes involved in steroidogenesis. Although cAMP is an essential inducer of steroidogenesis, other mechanisms triggered by paracrine and endocrine signals have been involved in the regulation of steroid synthesis in basal or stress-related conditions. They can either act independently or in synergy with the PKA signaling. In the present study, the authors demonstrated that Janus kinase 2 (JAK2), which is well known to be involved in GH, prolactin and leptin signaling, was also involved in basal and ACTH-induced steroidogenesis. In adrenocortical cells, activated JAK2 levels were not sensitive to ACTH. They exerted an essential control on basal and ACTH-induced steroidogenesis by interacting with the PKA through the modulation of CREB protein accumulation. CREB-induced Star transcription was dependent on JAK2 but was independent of signal transducer and activation of transcription 5 (STAT5). In adrenocortical cells, JAK2 acted in the nucleus to stabilize the Ser(P)133-CREB by preventing its early proteasomal degradation. This, in turn, allowed stimulation of Star gene transcription. These data demonstrate for the first time that STAT5-independent nuclear JAK2 signaling plays an essential role in adrenal steroidogenesis by increasing the stability of the transcriptionally active CREB protein, thereby allowing the expression of CREB steroidogenic target genes.

Inner mitochondrial translocase Tim50 interacts with 3β-hydroxysteroid dehydrogenase type 2 to regulate adrenal and gonadal steroidogenesis

Pawlak KJ, Prasad M, Thomas JL, Whittal RM, Bose HS
Mercer University School of Medicine, Savannah, GA, USA
J Biol Chem 2011;286:39130–39140

Background: In the adrenal glands, testes and ovaries, 3β-hydroxysteroid dehydrogenase type 2 (3βHSD2) catalyzes the conversion of pregnenolone to progesterone and dehydroepiandrostenedione (DHEA) to androstenedione. 3βHSD2 is synthesized in the cytosol and is imported into the inner mitochondrial membrane (IMM) by translocases. Steroidogenesis requires that 3βHSD2 acts as both a dehydrogenase and isomerase. To achieve this dual functionality, 3βHSD2 must undergo a conformational change; however, the underlying mechanisms remain unknown.

Methods and Results: Fractionation assays demonstrated that 3βHSD2 is associated with the IMM but did not integrate into the membrane. Mass spectrometry and Western blotting of mitochondrial complexes and density gradient ultracentrifugation showed that that 3βHSD2 formed a transient association with the translocases Tim50 and Tom22 with Tim23. Tim50 knockdown inhibited catalysis of DHEA to androstenedione and pregnenolone to progesterone. Although Tim50 knockdown decreased 3βHSD2 expression, restoration of expression via proteasome and protease inhibition did not rescue activity. In addition, protein fingerprinting and CD spectroscopy revealed the flexibility of 3βHSD2, a necessary characteristic for forming multiple associations.

Conclusions: Tim50 regulates the expression and activity of 3βHSD2, which represents a new role for translocases in steroidogenesis.

Most mitochondrial proteins are synthesized as precursors on cytosolic polysomes and imported across the outer (OMM) and inner mitochondrial membranes (IMM). Translocases are loosely associated protein complexes at the mitochondrial membranes, which mediate protein import and sorting. Translocase complexes found at the OMM are called Tom (translocase, outer membrane), while those at the IMM are called Tim (translocase, inner membrane).

The IMM-associated 3β-hydroxysteroid dehydrogenase (3βHSD2) catalyzes the conversion of pregnenolone to progesterone, 17α-hydroxy-pregnenolone to 17α-hydroxy-progesterone, and dehydroepiandostenedione (DHEA) to androstenedione in conjunction with NAD+ as a cofactor. 3βHSD2 has both dehydrogenase and isomerase activities. In this study, Pawlak and colleagues tested the hypothesis that the bifunctional activity of 3βHSD2 requires the protein to undergo a conformational change. They showed that 3βHSD2 associated with the IMM but did not integrate into it. This likely was the result of the interaction between 3βHSD2 and Tim50, resulting in a transient complex formation of 3βHSD2, Tom22, Tim23, and Tim50. Moreover, restoration of 3βHSD2 expression in the Tim50 knockdown cells via proteasome and protease inhibition did not rescue the steroidogenic activity. Therefore, the association of 3βHSD2 with the translocase appears to play a key role in the regulation of enzymatic activity. The absence of Tim50 inhibited the catalysis of DHEA to androstenedione and pregnenolone to progesterone but did not affect the expression of endoplasmic reticulum resident cytochrome P450c17.

New genes

Exome sequencing identifies MAX mutations as a cause of hereditary pheochromocytoma

Comino-Méndez I, Gracia-Aznárez FJ, Schiavi F, Landa I, Leandro-García LJ, Letón R, Honrado E, Ramos-Medina R, Caronia D, Pita G, Gómez-Graña A, de Cubas AA, Inglada-Pérez L, Maliszewska A, Taschin E, Bobisse S, Pica G, Loli P, Hernández-Lavado R, Díaz JA, Gómez-Morales M, González-Neira A, Roncador G, Rodríguez-Antona C, Benítez J, Mannelli M, Opocher G, Robledo M, Cascón A
Hereditary Endocrine Cancer Group, Spanish National Cancer Research Centre (CNIO), Madrid, Spain

Nat Genet 2011;43:663–667

Background: Hereditary pheochromocytoma (PCC) is often caused by germline mutations in one of nine susceptibility genes described to date, but there are familial cases without mutations in these known genes.

Methods and Results: Sequencing of the exomes of three unrelated individuals with hereditary PCC (cases) identified mutations in MAX, the MYCassociated factor X gene. Absence of MAX protein in the tumors and loss of heterozygosity caused by uniparental disomy supported the involvement of MAX alterations in the disease. A follow-up study of a selected series of 59 cases with PCC identified five additional MAX mutations and suggested an association with malignant outcome and preferential paternal transmission of MAX mutations.

Conclusions: These findings elucidate the mechanisms underlying the development of hereditary PCC, as well as those of metastatic potential.

Pheochromocytoma (PCC) is a rare neural crest cell tumor mainly localized within the adrenal medulla. Approximately 30–40% of individuals with PCC are familial cases, who show dominant autosomal inheritance caused by germline mutations affecting one of nine susceptibility genes: RET, VHL, SDHA, SDHB, SDHC, SDHD, SDHAF2, NF1 or TMEM127. A subset of tumors from familial cases with PCC without germline alterations in the susceptibility genes identified to date showed a homogeneous expression profile, suggesting that mutations in the same as yet unidentified gene could be responsible for these cases. Next-generation sequencing is an emerging new tool for discovering genes responsible for genetically heterogeneous diseases. In the present study, next-generation sequencing allowed the identification of MAX as a new PCC tumor suppressor gene. MAX is the most conserved dimerization component of the MYC-MAX-MXD1 network of basic helix-loop-helix leucine zipper (bHLHZip) transcription factors that regulate cell proliferation, differentiation and apoptosis. In this network, MAX plays an essential role, as it is the common interaction partner for both MYC and MXD1 proteins. The discovery of MAX germline mutations in individuals with a hereditary adrenal tumor suggests a role for the MYC-MAX-MXD1 network in the development and progression of neural crest tumors. Moreover, the malignant behavior of MAX-related PCCs supports the idea that MAX loss of function is correlated to metastatic potential. The results of this study elucidate the mechanisms underlying the development of hereditary PCCs, as well as those of their metastatic potential. In addition, they have clinical implications for genetic counseling and genetic testing algorithms. Further studies are required to determine the prevalence of MAX mutations in PCC and the phenotype associated with MAX mutations.

Development and function of the human fetal adrenal cortex: a key component in the feto-placental unit

Ishimoto H, Jaffe RB
Center for Reproductive Sciences, Department of Obstetrics, Gynecology and Reproductive Sciences, University of California, San Francisco, CA, USA
Endocr Rev 2011;32:317–355

The human fetal adrenal cortex plays a pivotal role in the regulation of intrauterine homeostasis and in fetal development and maturation. The steroidogenic activity is characterized by early transient cortisol biosynthesis, followed by its suppressed synthesis until late gestation, as well as extensive production of dehydroepiandrosterone and its sulfate, precursors of placental estrogen, during most of gestation. Recent studies revealed that the development and/or function of the fetal adrenal cortex may be regulated by a number of molecules, including transcription factors, extracellular matrix components, locally produced growth factors, and placenta-derived CRH, in addition to the primary regulator, fetal pituitary ACTH. The role of the fetal adrenal cortex in human pregnancy and parturition appears highly complex. The actions of hormones operating in the human feto-placental unit are most likely mediated by mechanisms including target tissue responsiveness, local metabolism and bioavailability, as well as changes in circulating concentrations. The comprehensive study of such molecular mechanisms and the newly identified factors implicated in adrenal development should enhance our understanding of the development and function of the human fetal adrenal cortex.

The human fetal adrenal (HFA) cortex shares its unique structural and functional organization with higher primates, such as the rhesus monkey and baboon. The HFA cortex is an active endocrine organ in which most steroidogenic activity is exerted in a specialized cortical compartment known as the fetal zone (FZ), a unique feature of fetal adrenals in humans and some higher primates, but not in other species, such as rodents and sheep. Accumulating evidence suggests that growth of the HFA appears to involve cellular proliferation, hypertrophy, apoptosis, and migration. Appropriate development and function of the fetal adrenal cortex are critical for fetal maturation and perinatal survival. Moreover, the fetal adrenal cortex must itself undergo maturation in preparation for its essential role postnatally, i.e., production of glucocorticoids, androgens, and mineralocorticoids for fetal intrauterine homeostasis, and to insure adrenal cortical autonomy once the placenta has separated. This article presents an overview of recent key observations that serve to gain a better understanding of the developmental processes and functional aspects of the HFA.

The syndrome of 17,20lyase deficiency

Miller WL
Department of Pediatrics, University of California, San Francisco, San Francisco, CA, USA
J Clin Endocrinol Metab 2012;97:59–67

Disorders of steroidogenesis have been instrumental in delineating human steroidogenic pathways. Since 1972, several patients have been reported as having '17,20lyase deficiency,' but there have been inconsistent genetic findings. A single enzyme, cytochrome P450c17, catalyzes both 17α-hydroxylase activity and 17,20lyase activity. The 17,20lyase activity is especially sensitive to the activities of the accessory proteins P450 oxidoreductase and cytochrome b_5. The first cases of genetically and biochemically proven 17,20lyase deficiency were reported in 1997, in which specific P450c17 mutations were identified that lost 17,20lyase activity but not 17α-hydroxylase activity. Subsequent work identified other P450c17 mutations and mutations in the genes encoding P450 oxidoreductase and cytochrome b₅. Recently, the initially reported cases from 1972 were found to carry mutations in two aldo-keto reductases, AKR1C2 and AKR1C4. These AKR1C isozymes catalyze 3α-hydroxysteroid dehydrogenase activity in the so-called 'backdoor pathway' by which the fetal testis produces dihydrotestosterone without the intermediacy of testosterone. 17,20Lyase deficiency should be considered a syndrome with multiple causes, and not a single disease. Study of this very rare disorder has substantially advanced our understanding of the pathways, mechanisms and control of androgen synthesis. Mutations in other as yet unidentified genes may also cause this phenotype.

Apparent 17,20lyase deficiency is a complex syndrome that can be caused by mutations in several genes. Although this disorder is rare, its study provides an excellent example of how the detailed study of a rare disorder has substantially improved our understanding of a basic physiological process: in this case, illustrating the key roles of POR and cytochrome b₅ in the synthesis of adrenal androgens, and leading to the discovery of the crucial role of AKR1C2 in fetal testicular synthesis of DHT and the role of fetal testicular DHT in normal male genital development. 17,20Lyase deficiency is an extremely difficult diagnosis to establish, so that endocrinologists must be skeptical about clinical case reports of this disorder that do not include a genetic diagnosis and proof that the identified mutation indeed reduces 17,20lyase activity while preserving 17α-hydroxylase activity. In addition, one might consider other genes, which, if disordered, might cause a clinically similar syndrome. This study reviews the biochemistry, genetics and clinical disorders of 17,20lyase activity, which converts 21-carbon precursors of glucocorticoids to 19-carbon precursors of sex steroids.

Autoimmune Addison disease: pathophysiology and genetic complexity

Mitchell AL, Pearce SH
Institute of Genetic Medicine, Newcastle University, International Centre for Life, Newcastle upon Tyne, UK
Nat Rev Endocrinol 2012;8:306–316

Autoimmune Addison disease is a rare autoimmune disorder with symptoms that typically develop over months or years. Following the development of serum autoantibodies to the key steroidogenic enzyme, 21-hydroxylase, patients have a period of compensated or preclinical disease, characterized by elevations in adrenocortcotropic hormone and renin, before overt, symptomatic adrenal failure develops. Local failure of steroidogenesis, causing breakdown of tolerance to adrenal antigens, might be a key factor in disease progression. The etiology of autoimmune Addison disease has a strong genetic component in man. Allelic variants of genes encoding molecules of both the adaptive and innate immune systems have now been implicated, with a focus on the immunological synapse and downstream participants in T lymphocyte antigen-receptor signaling. With the exception of MHC alleles, no major or highly penetrant disease alleles have been found to date. Future research into autoimmune Addison disease, using genome-wide association studies and next-generation sequencing technology, will elucidate our understanding of the etiology of this disease.

Autoimmune Addison disease (AAD) is a rare endocrine condition with a prevalence in white European populations of 110–140 cases per million [9], making it 30-fold less prevalent than type 1 diabetes (T1DM) and 200-fold rarer than autoimmune thyroid diseases. Like other autoimmune diseases, AAD is more frequent in women (female:male ratio 1.5–3.5:1) and often presents in individuals between the ages of 30 and 50 years, although it can affect individuals at any age. AAD is a condition that results from the interaction of currently unknown environmental factors with incompletely defined genetic factors in a susceptible individual. The number of susceptibility loci known to contribute to this disease is gradually increasing, but those discovered so far make only a modest contribution to disease susceptibility. Studies of larger cohorts of patients with AAD are required. In addition to the candidate-gene approach, genome-wide association studies and whole-genome sequencing could offer unique insights into the genetic etiology of AAD. With an increased understanding of the etiology of AAD and the biological pathways involved, new therapeutic targets and diagnostic tools could be developed that will offer an improved outcome in patients with the condition.

Familial longevity is marked by lower diurnal salivary cortisol levels: the Leiden Longevity Study

Noordam R, Jansen SW, Akintola AA, Oei NY, Maier AB, Pijl H, Slagboom PE, Westendorp RG, van der Grond J, de Craen AJ, van Heemst D; Leiden Longevity Study Group
Department of Gerontology and Geriatrics, Leiden University Medical Center, Leiden, The Netherlands
PLoS One 2012;7:e31166

Background: Research findings are inconsistent whether hypothalamic-pituitary-adrenal (HPA) signaling becomes hyperactive with increasing age, resulting in increasing cortisol concentrations. Recent evidence suggests that offspring from long-lived families are biologically younger. The aim of this study was to assess whether these offspring have a lower HPA axis activity, as indicated by lower concentrations of cortisol and higher cortisol feedback sensitivity.
Methods: In a cohort of subjects from the Leiden Longevity Study comprising 149 offspring and 154 partners, salivary cortisol concentrations were determined at four time points within the first hour upon awakening and at two time points in the evening. A dexamethasone suppression test was performed as a measure of cortisol feedback sensitivity. Age, gender and body mass index, smoking and disease history (type 2 diabetes and hypertension) were considered as possible confounding factors.
Results: Salivary cortisol secretion was lower in offspring compared to partners in the morning (area under the curve: 15.6 versus 17.1 nmol/l, respectively; p = 0.048) and in the evening (area under the curve: 3.32 versus 3.82 nmol/l, respectively; p = 0.024). Salivary cortisol concentrations were not different after dexamethasone (0.5 mg) suppression between offspring and partners (4.82 versus 5.26 nmol/l, respectively; p = 0.28).
Conclusions: Offspring of long-lived families display a lower HPA axis activity, but not a difference in cortisol feedback sensitivity; however, further studies are required to characterize the HPA axis in offspring and partners are needed.

In this study, Noordam and colleagues investigated the relation between cortisol concentrations and cortisol feedback sensitivity with familial longevity. They showed that salivary cortisol concentrations were lower in the offspring of long-lived families compared with their partners both in the morning and in the evening. The authors also showed that cortisol feedback sensitivity, as estimated by a dexamethasone suppression test, was similar between offspring and partners, suggesting that the difference between offspring and partners in salivary cortisol concentration is most likely not caused by a difference in cortisol feedback sensitivity. However, the dose of dexamethasone used in this study (0.5 mg) might have been too high for studying cortisol sensitivity in a general population, given that it leads to a near-complete suppression in most individuals. The range of cortisol concentrations following a lower dose of dexamethasone (e.g. 0.25 mg) is much wider, and may be more appropriate to identify differences in cortisol sensitivity among individuals.

Childhood adversity and epigenetic modulation of the leukocyte glucocorticoid receptor: preliminary findings in healthy adults

Tyrka AR, Price LH, Marsit C, Walters OC, Carpenter LL
Laboratory for Clinical Neuroscience, Mood Disorders Research Program, Butler Hospital, Providence, RI, USA
PLoS One 2012;7:e30148

Background: A history of early adverse experiences is an important risk factor for adult psychopathology. Alterations in stress sensitivity and functioning of the hypothalamic-pituitary-adrenal (HPA) axis may underlie the association between stress and risk for psychiatric disorders. The aim of this study was to examine whether early-life stress leads to epigenetic modifications of the glucocorticoid receptor (GR) gene in humans.
Methods: The degree of methylation of a region of the promoter of the human GR gene (NR3C1) was examined in leukocyte DNA from 99 healthy adults. Participants reported on their childhood experiences of parental behavior, parental death or desertion, and childhood maltreatment. On a separate day, participants completed the dexamethasone/corticotropin-releasing hormone (Dex/CRH) test.

Results: Disruption or lack of adequate nurturing, as measured by parental loss, childhood maltreatment, and parental care, was associated with increased NR3C1 promoter methylation (p<0.05). In addition, NR3C1 promoter methylation was linked to attenuated cortisol responses to the Dex/CRH test (p<005).

Conclusions: Childhood maltreatment or adversity may lead to epigenetic modifications of the human GR gene. Alterations in methylation of this gene could underlie the associations between childhood adversity, alterations in stress reactivity, and risk for psychopathology.

Research studies in rodents, non-human primates and humans have documented the impact of early life experiences on the neurobiological mechanisms regulating stress responses and mood and anxiety disorders. Young children are dependent on caregivers for their basic physical, social and emotional needs. When this is poorly provided, the child develops a strategy adaptive to stressful life. Such children undergo substantial developmental changes in neural pathways involved in regulating emotion and behavior. As a result, disruption of early care-giving can produce profound and long-lasting changes in these neurobiological and behavioral systems. Early-life stress is a risk factor for major depression, post-traumatic stress disorder, and drug abuse, among other conditions. In this study, Tyrka and colleagues demonstrated that early-life stress, in the form of loss of a parent during childhood, maltreatment, and low parental care, was associated with epigenetic changes to the promoter region of the glucocorticoid receptor gene. Furthermore, methylation of the promoter region of this gene was linked to alterations in HPA axis function. These findings provide preliminary support for the hypothesis that altered expression of the GR due to cytosine methylation of the gene promoter could be a mechanism of the neuroendocrine effects of early-life stress, and could predispose to the development of major depression and post-traumatic stress disorder. Further work is needed to determine whether these findings are specific to lymphocytes and whether this reflects changes in central regulation of the glucocorticoid receptor in brain regions involved in stress responses and mood and anxiety disorders.

Follow-up on *Yearbook 2011*
K⁺ channel mutations are a cause of early-onset familial hypertension

Hypertension with or without adrenal hyperplasia due to different inherited mutations in the potassium channel KCNJ5

Scholl UI, Nelson-Williams C, Yue P, Grekin R, Wyatt RJ, Dillon MJ, Couch R, Hammer LK, Harley FL, Farhi A, Wang WH, Lifton RP
Departments of Genetics and Internal Medicine and Howard Hughes Medical Institute, Yale University School of Medicine, New Haven, CT, USA
Proc Natl Acad Sci USA 2012;109:2533–2538

Background: Mutations in the KCNJ5 (potassium inwardly rectifying channel, subfamily J, member 5) gene are implicated in primary hyperaldosteronism and in autonomous glomerulosa cell proliferation in humans. These mutations alter the channel selectivity filter, producing increased Na⁺ conductance and membrane depolarization, the signal for aldosterone production and proliferation of adrenal glomerulosa cells.

Methods and Results: The members of four kindreds with early onset primary aldosteronism of unknown cause were studied. Sequencing of KCNJ5 gene revealed that affected members of two kindreds had KCNJ5(G151R) mutations. These individuals had severe progressive aldosteronism and hyperplasia requiring bilateral adrenalectomy in childhood to control arterial blood pressure. Affected members of the other two kindreds had KCNJ5(G151E) mutations. These subjects had easily controlled hypertension and no evidence of hyperplasia. Electrophysiological studies of channels expressed in 293T cells demonstrated that KCNJ5(G151E) was the more extreme mutation, producing a much larger Na⁺ conductance than KCNJ5(G151R), resulting in rapid Na⁺-dependent cell lethality.

Conclusions: These findings demonstrate striking variations in the phenotype and clinical outcome resulting from different mutations of the same amino acid in KCNJ5 and have implications for the diagnosis and pathogenesis of primary aldosteronism with and without adrenal hyperplasia.

Prevalence, clinical, and molecular correlates of KCNJ5 mutations in primary aldosteronism

Boulkroun S, Beuschlein F, Rossi GP, Golib-Dzib JF, Fischer E, Amar L, Mulatero P, Samson-Couterie B, Hahner S, Quinkler M, Fallo F, Letizia C, Allolio B, Ceolotto G, Cicala MV, Lang K, Lefebvre H, Lenzini L, Maniero C, Monticone S, Perrocheau M, Pilon C, Plouin PF, Rayes N, Seccia TM, Veglio F, Williams TA, Zinnamosca L, Mantero F, Benecke A, Jeunemaitre X, Reincke M, Zennaro MC
Institut National de la Santé et de la Recherche Médicale, Unité Mixte de Recherche Scientifique 970, Paris Cardiovascular Research Center, Paris, France
Hypertension 2012;59:592–598

Background: Mutations in the KCNJ5 gene have been described recently in aldosterone-producing adenomas (APAs). The aim of this study was to investigate the prevalence of KCNJ5 mutations in patients with primary aldosteronism and their correlation with clinical, biological and molecular findings.
Methods and Results: KCNJ5 sequencing was performed on somatic (APA, n=380) and peripheral (APA, n=344; bilateral adrenal hyperplasia, n=174) DNA of patients with primary aldosteronism, collected through the European Network for the Study of Adrenal Tumors. Transcriptome analysis was performed in 102 tumors. Somatic KCNJ5 mutations (p.Gly151Arg or p.Leu168Arg) were found in 34% of APA. They were significantly more prevalent in females (49%) than males (19%; p<0.001) and in younger patients (42.1±1.0 *vs.* 47.6±0.7 years; p<0.001) and were associated with higher preoperative aldosterone levels (455±26 *vs.* 376±17 ng/l; p = 0.012) but not with therapeutic outcome after surgery. Germline KCNJ5 mutations were found neither in patients with APA nor those with bilateral adrenal hyperplasia. Somatic KCNJ5 mutations were specific for APA, since they were not identified in 25 peritumoral adrenal tissues or 16 cortisol-producing adenomas.
Conclusions: Although a large proportion of sporadic APAs harbors somatic KCNJ5 mutations, germline mutations are not similarly causative for bilateral adrenal hyperplasia. KCNJ5 mutation carriers are more likely to be females; younger age and higher aldosterone concentrations at diagnosis suggest that KCNJ5 mutations may be associated with a more florid phenotype of primary aldosteronism.

Primary hyperaldosteronism (PA) is the most common cause of secondary hypertension. Its prevalence is estimated to be approximately 10% within the hypertensive population and higher among patients with hypertension refractory to medical treatment. Early diagnosis and treatment of patients with PA is of fundamental importance because they have significantly higher incidence of stroke, myocardial infarction, and atrial fibrillation compared with age-, sex-, and BP-matched patients with essential HTN. Familial hyperaldosteronism (FH)-III is an autosomal dominant condition characterized by early-onset hypertension, non glucocorticoid-remediable hyperaldosteronism and hypokalemia. The genetic cause of FH-III is attributed to mutations in the KCNJ5 gene encoding the potassium channel Kir-3.4 [10]. The clinical spectrum of the condition in the limited number of families reported to date appears to be broad, ranging from mild or moderate hypertension, which is responsive to medical therapy, to more severe and refractory to medical treatment hypertension that requires bilateral adrenalectomy. The above studies demonstrate the striking variations in the phenotype and clinical outcome resulting from different mutations in KCNJ5 in subjects with PA with and without adrenal hyperplasia. They also showed that the absence of adrenal hyperplasia in subjects with genetically confirmed FH-III is thought to arise as a result of mutations in the KCNJ5 gene that produce a much larger Na^+ conductance, leading to rapid Na^+-dependent cell lethality.

References
1. Clark AJ, Weber A: Adrenocorticotropin insensitivity syndromes. Endocr Rev 1998;19:828–843.
2. Minichiello L, Calella AM, Medina DL, Bonhoeffer T, Klein R, Korte M: Mechanism of TrkB-mediated hippocampal long-term potentiation. Neuron 2002;36:121–137.
3. Barker DJ: The developmental origins of adult disease. J Am Coll Nutr 2004;23:588S–595S.
4. Barker DJ, Gluckman PD, Godfrey KM, Harding JE, Owens JA, Robinson JS: Fetal nutrition and cardiovascular disease in adult life. Lancet 1993;341:938–941.

5. Arlt W, Walker EA, Draper N, Ivison HE, Ride JP, Hammer F, Chalder SM, Borucka-Mankiewicz M, Hauffa BP, Malunowicz EM, Stewart PM, Shackleton CH: Congenital adrenal hyperplasia caused by mutant P450 oxidoreductase and human androgen synthesis: analytical study. Lancet 2004;363:2128–2135.
6. Funder JW, Carey RM, Fardella C, Gomez-Sanchez CE, Mantero F, Stowasser M, Young WF Jr, Montori VM: Case detection, diagnosis, and treatment of patients with primary aldosteronism: an Endocrine Society Clinical Practice Guideline. J Clin Endocrinol Metab 2008;93:3266–3281.
7. Bergthorsdottir R, Leonsson-Zachrisson M, Odén A, Johannsson G: Premature mortality in patients with Addison's disease: a population-based study. J Clin Endocrinol Metab 2006;91:4849–4853.
8. Tomlinson JW, Holden N, Hills RK, Wheatley K, Clayton RN, Bates AS, Sheppard MC, Stewart PM: Association between premature mortality and hypopituitarism. West Midlands Prospective Hypopituitary Study Group. Lancet 2001;357:425–431.
9. Laureti S, Vecchi L, Santeusanio F, Falorni A: Is the prevalence of Addison's disease underestimated? J Clin Endocrinol Metab 1999;84:1762.
10. Choi M, Scholl UI, Yue P, Björklund P, Zhao B, Nelson-Williams C, Ji W, Cho Y, Patel A, Men CJ, Lolis E, Wisgerhof MV, Geller DS, Mane S, Hellman P, Westin G, Åkerström G, Wang W, Carling T, Lifton RP: K$^+$ channel mutations in adrenal aldosterone-producing adenomas and hereditary hypertension. Science 2011;331:768–772.

Oncology and Chronic Disease

Thomas M.K. Völkl[a], Tilman Rohrer[b] and Helmuth-Günther Dörr[a]

[a]Pediatric Endocrinology, Department of Pediatrics, University of Erlangen, Erlangen, Germany
[b]Pediatric Endocrinology, Department of Pediatrics and Neonatology, University Medical Centre, Homburg/
Saar, Germany

This chapter on oncology and chronic disease has been integrated for the first time in the *Yearbook of Pediatric Endocrinology*. In developed countries, 1:250 of the adult population is a long-term survivor of childhood cancer. Thus, a dramatic paradigm shift has occurred in pediatric oncology during the last 40 years. For example, the meaning of 'outcome' after tumor therapy has changed and includes not only the counting of the number of therapy survival rates but also the importance of analyzing the consequences of tumor therapy or, in other words, the study of the late effects of tumor therapy. The identification and analysis of late effects, especially endocrine sequelae after cancer therapy, has generated many interesting publications during the last years. The topic 'Chronic Disease' will be regarded here from a different perspective, e.g. analyzing growth and pubertal development of affected patients and analyzing side effects of the respective therapy on the endocrine system.

Late effects of childhood cancer therapy
Important for clinical practice

Hypothyroidism following childhood cancer therapy – an underdiagnosed complication

Brabant G, Toogood AA, Shalet SM, Frobisher C, Lancashire ER, Reulen RC, Winter DL, Hawkins MM
Department of Endocrinology, The Christie NHS Foundation Trust, Manchester, UK
georg.brabant@manchester.ac.uk
Int J Cancer 2012;130:1145–1150

Objective: To determine the prevalence of hypothyroidism amongst most adult survivors of childhood cancer in Britain using the British Childhood Cancer Survivor Study (BCCSS). The BCCSS is a population-based cohort of individuals diagnosed with childhood cancer between 1940 and 1991, and who survived at least 5 years from diagnosis (n = 17,981). 10,483 (71%) of those survivors aged at least 16 years, returned a completed questionnaire, which asked if hypothyroidism had been diagnosed.
Results: Of the whole cohort, 7.7% reported hypothyroidism with the highest risk among patients treated for Hodgkin's disease (HD) (19.9%), CNS neoplasms (15.3%), non-Hodgkin's lymphoma (6.2%) and leukemia (5.2%). Survivors were more likely to develop hypothyroidism if they had received radiotherapy for HD (p = 0.0001) or a CNS neoplasm (p < 0.00005) but not leukemia (p = 0.3). In these three patient groups, the frequency of hypothyroidism was similar in men and women. Survivors of irradiated CNS tumors reported a prevalence of hypothyroidism, which was substantially lower if discharged to primary care compared with being on hospital follow-up and which declined substantially with increased follow-up in both primary care (p = 0.004) and hospital follow-up (p = 0.023) settings.
Conclusions: Hypothyroidism is a common finding amongst adult survivors of childhood malignancy. The substantial differences in reported hypothyroidism prevalence after irradiated CNS neoplasms suggests substantial underdiagnosis, which increased with increased follow-up, and which increased among those followed-up in primary care compared with hospital settings.

Patients of the British Childhood Cancer Survivor Study were asked by questionnaire if hypothyroidism had been diagnosed. The approach of the study to send the questionnaire at first to the primary care physician with a request to forward it on to the survivor was an excellent move as reflected by the impressive number of completed questionnaires. The authors confirm and extend knowledge on hypothyroidism as a major endocrine complication after childhood cancer therapy. Survivors of Hodgkin's lymphoma and CNS tumors had a two- to threefold greater risk of developing hypothyroidism than survivors of other cancers. Their data also suggest that hypothyroidism may be substantially underdiagnosed in childhood cancer survivors. Therefore, it is necessary to raise the awareness of hypothyroidism in the care of these patients, and periodically test for thyroid functions.

Endocrine health problems detected in 519 patients evaluated in a pediatric cancer survivor program

Patterson BC, Wasilewski-Masker K, Ryerson AB, Mertens A, Meacham L
Emory University School of Medicine, Department of Pediatrics, M.S., Emory Children's Center, Atlanta, GA, USA
bcpatte@emory.edu
J Clin Endocrinol Metab 2012;97:810–818

Context: Survivors of pediatric cancer frequently develop endocrine conditions. National guidelines recommend surveillance of these patients for late endocrine effects after alkylating agents, steroids, methotrexate, and radiation. The study was conducted to analyze endocrine outcomes in surviving patients.

Methods: The study included pediatric and young adult survivors of noncentral nervous system childhood malignancies followed up in the Comprehensive Cancer Survivor Program, an academic pediatric oncology program based on national screening guidelines, from January 1, 2001, until December 15, 2005. Patients were evaluated with history, physical examinations, and evaluations recommended in the Children's Oncology Group's Long-Term Follow-Up Guidelines for Survivors of Childhood, Adolescent and Young Adult Cancers. Their medical records were reviewed for the types and frequencies of endocrine conditions.

Results: In total, 519 survivors were included in the analysis and 480 endocrine conditions were observed in 299/519 (57.6%) survivors. The most common endocrine conditions were problems with weight and gonadal function. A Cox regression model identified stem cell transplant, radiation, and older age at cancer diagnosis as being associated with higher hazard of an endocrine condition. Radiation, stem cell transplant, and sarcoma diagnosis were associated with growth problems.

Conclusion: Endocrine disorders were common sequelae of pediatric cancers. Endocrinologists should be aware of national guidelines, anticipate referral of pediatric cancer survivors, and participate in further research to optimize screening for, and treatment of, endocrine effects of cancer therapy.

In the past decades there has been a marked increase in the survival rates of pediatric cancer patients. However, survivors are at risk for long-term complications of cancer therapy throughout their lives. The authors add further evidence in support of the association between radiation and stem cell transplantation therapy and the occurrence of endocrine conditions. In this study, radiation therapy was independently associated with the development of classical endocrine disorders, including thyroid disease, short stature, and gonadal problems. The study did not allow for stratification of subjects by radiation site or radiation dose. Limitations of the study included selection bias in that not all survivors were evaluated in the program. Moreover, some endocrine conditions might be underrepresented due to defining the presence of disease by the need for hormonal replacement. Thus, Sertoli cell dysfunction and small testicular volume were not represented in this study cohort.

Antimüllerian hormone is a marker of gonadotoxicity in pre- and postpubertal girls treated for cancer: a prospective study

Brougham MF, Crofton PM, Johnson EJ, Evans N, Anderson RA, Wallace WH
Department of Paediatric Oncology (M.F.H.B., E.J.J., W.H.B.W.), Department of Paediatric Biochemistry (P.M.C.), Royal Hospital for Sick Children, Edinburgh, UK; Medical Research Council Human Reproductive Sciences Unit (N.E.), Edinburgh, UK, and Medical Research Council Centre for Reproductive Health (R.A.A.), University of Edinburgh, Edinburgh, UK
J Clin Endocrinol Metab 2012;97:2059–2067

Background: Cytotoxic treatment may accelerate depletion of the primordial follicle pool, leading to impaired fertility and premature menopause. Assessment of ovarian damage in prepubertal girls is not currently possible, but antimüllerian hormone (AMH) is a useful marker of ovarian reserve in adults.

Objective: The objective of the study was to prospectively evaluate AMH measurement in children as a marker of ovarian toxicity during cancer treatment.

Design and Setting: This was a prospective, longitudinal study at a university hospital.

Patients: 22 females (17 prepubertal), median age 4.4 years (range 0.3–15), were recruited before treatment for cancer.

Main Outcome Measures: AMH, inhibin B, and FSH at diagnosis, after each chemotherapy course and during follow-up, were measured. Risk of gonadotoxicity was classified as low/medium (n = 13) or high (n = 9) based on chemotherapy agent, cumulative dose, and radiotherapy involving the ovaries.

Results: Pretreatment AMH was detectable across the age range studied. AMH decreased progressively during chemotherapy (p < 0.0001) in both prepubertal and pubertal girls, becoming undetectable in 50% of patients, with recovery in the low-/medium-risk groups after completion of treatment. In the high-risk group, AMH became undetectable in all patients and showed no recovery. Inhibin B was undetectable in most patients before treatment and, with FSH, showed no clear relationship to treatment.

Conclusions: AMH is detectable in girls of all ages and falls rapidly during cancer treatment in both prepubertal and pubertal girls. Both the fall during treatment and recovery thereafter varied with risk of gonadotoxicity. AMH is therefore a clinically useful marker of damage to the ovarian reserve in girls receiving treatment for cancer.

Inhibin B and antimüllerian hormone as markers of gonadal function after treatment for medulloblastoma or posterior fossa ependymoma during childhood

Cuny A, Trivin C, Brailly-Tabard S, Adan L, Zerah M, Sainte-Rose C, Alapetite C, Brugieres L, Habrand JL, Doz F, Brauner R
Université Paris Descartes and AP-HP, Hôpital Bicêtre, Unité d'endocrinologie pédiatrique. Le Kremlin Bicêtre, France
J Pediatr 2011;158:1016–1022 e1

Objective: To evaluate the roles of hypothalamic-pituitary and spinal irradiations and chemotherapy in gonadal deficiency after treatment for medulloblastoma or posterior fossa ependymoma by measuring levels of plasma inhibin B and antimüllerian hormone (AMH).

Patients and Methods: A total of 34 boys and 22 girls were classified as having normal levels of plasma follicle-stimulating hormone (FSH; <9 IU/l), or abnormal levels of FSH (>9 IU/l) and luteinizing hormone (LH; <5 or >5 IU/l).

Results: Two boys had partial gonadotropin deficiency, combined with testicular deficiency in 1 boy. Six boys had increased levels of FSH, indicating tubular deficiency, combined with Leydig cell deficiency in 5 boys. The 7 boys with inhibin B levels <100 ng/ml included the 1 with combined deficiencies and the 6 with testicular deficiency. Puberty did not progress in 7 girls; 3 had gonadotropin deficiency, combined with ovarian deficiency in 1, and 4 had increased FSH levels, indicating ovarian deficiency. Inhibin B and AMH levels were low in the girl with combined deficiencies, in the 4 girls with ovarian deficiency, and in 4 girls with normal clinical-biological ovarian function, including 2 who underwent ovarian transposition before irradiation.

Conclusions: The plasma concentrations of inhibin B and AMH are useful means of detecting primary gonad deficiency in patients with no increase in their plasma gonadotropin levels because of radiation-induced gonadotropin deficiency.

In the 2011 issue of the *Yearbook of Pediatric Endocrinology*, Lena Sahlin and Olle Söder commented on two papers reporting antimüllerian hormone (AMH) levels in healthy female and male patients from birth to adulthood. Additionally, AMH levels were measured in patients with Turner syndrome (TS), showing that low or undetectable AMH levels correlate with ovarian failure in TS patients. They stated that 'the full potential of AMH measurements most certainly requires more time to develop'. A year later, and two independent groups published AMH data showing the usefulness of AMH measurement as a marker of gonadal damage. Since AMH is produced solely in the granulosa cells of growing ovarian follicles, the AMH serum levels correlate strongly with the number of growing follicles. Inhibin B is also a marker of ovarian reserve. The paper by Mark Brougham et al. shows that the extent of gonadal damage in female cancer survivors is better reflected by measurement of AMH than by inhibin B levels. In boys, inhibin B is produced by Sertoli cells, and its plasma concentration is positively correlated with spermatogenesis and negatively correlated with FSH levels. The paper by Ariane Cuny et al. shows that inhibin B can be used as a marker of gonadal damage in boys after brain tumor therapy.

AMH and AFC (antral follicle counts) – sensitive measures of ovarian reserve

Impact of cancer therapies on ovarian reserve

Gracia CR, Sammel MD, Freeman E, Prewitt M, Carlson C, Ray A, Vance A, Ginsberg JP
Department of Obstetrics/Gynecology, Children's Hospital of Philadelphia, Philadelphia, PA, USA
cgracia@obgyn.upenn.edu
Fertil Steril 2012;97:134–140 e1

Objective: To determine whether measures of ovarian reserve differ between females exposed to cancer therapies in a dose-dependent manner as compared with healthy controls of similar age and late reproductive age.
Design: Cross-sectional analysis of data from a prospective cohort study.
Setting: University medical center.
Patients: 71 cancer survivors aged 15–39 years, 67 healthy, similarly aged unexposed subjects, and 69 regularly menstruating women of late reproductive age (40–52 years).
Intervention(s): None.
Main outcome measure(s): Early follicular-phase hormones (FSH, E_2, inhibin B, antimüllerian hormone (AMH)) and ovarian ultrasound measurements (ovarian volume and antral follicle counts (AFC)) were compared using multivariable linear regression.
Results: In adjusted models, FSH, AMH, and AFC differed between exposed vs. unexposed subjects (FSH 11.12 vs. 7.25 mIU/ml, AMH 0.81 vs. 2.85 ng/ml, AFC 14.55 vs. 27.20). In participants with an FSH <10 mIU/ml, survivors had lower levels of AMH and AFC compared with controls. Alkylating agent dose score was associated with increased levels of FSH and decreased levels of AMH. Exposure to pelvic radiation was associated with impairment in FSH, AMH, AFC, and ovarian volume. Antimüllerian hormone was similar in women previously exposed to high-dose cancer therapy and 40- to 42-year-old controls.
Conclusions: Measures of ovarian reserve are impaired in a dose-dependent manner among cancer survivors compared with unexposed females of similar age. Reproductive hormone levels in menstruating survivors exposed to high-dose therapy are similar to those in late-reproductive-age women. The predictive value of measures for pregnancy and menopause must be studied.

It has been shown the risk of ovarian failure to be dependent on the dose of alkylating agents and pelvic radiotherapy. The paper by Mark Brougham et al. (see p. 119) correlated the risk of gonadotoxicity with the used therapeutic regimen and found that AMH levels recovered only in the low-/ medium-risk groups after completion of treatment, and not in the high-risk group. Clarisa Gracia et al. studied female cancer survivors together with a control group of healthy, similarly aged unexposed subjects. They found that ovarian reserve was significantly impaired in cancer survivors. Even cancer survivors with regular menstrual cycles or those with normal FSH levels had significantly lower levels of AMH and AFC compared with controls supporting subclinical follicular depletion. Cancer survivors with greater exposure to alkylators, pelvic radiotherapy, or bone marrow transplantation with total body irradiation had the most impaired ovarian reserve. The authors showed that ovarian reserve is impaired in a dose-dependent fashion in subjects exposed to cancer therapies. Current methods of ovarian follicle preservation need to be entertained more seriously before a girl is subject to these devastating therapies.

Puzzling result
Testicular size is a better predictor of fertility

Semen quality and fertility in adult long-term survivors of childhood acute lymphoblastic leukemia

Jahnukainen K, Heikkinen R, Henriksson M, Cooper TG, Puukko-Viertomies LR, Makitie O
Division of Hematology-Oncology and Stem Cell Transplantation, Hospital for Children and Adolescents, University of Helsinki, Helsinki, Finland
kirsi.jahnukainen@ki.se

Fertil Steril 2011;96:837–842

Objective: To assess testicular function and its determinants in adult survivors of childhood acute lymphoblastic leukemia (ALL) at a median time of 20 years after ALL therapy.

Design: Prospective investigation.

Setting: University hospital.

Patient(s): 51 male long-term survivors and 56 age-matched controls (median age of survivors at ALL diagnosis was 5 years, range 1–15 years, and at the study 29 years, range 26–38 years).

Intervention(s): None.

Main outcome measure(s): Testicular size (mean value of both testicular volumes), serum hormone concentrations, semen quality, and number of children fathered correlated with ALL therapy.

Result(s): Survivors treated with 0–10 g/m^2 of cyclophosphamide had sperm quality and fertility rates comparable with those of controls, but the serum-free testosterone in the survivors treated with cyclophosphamide was lower than in controls (median 213 pmol/l, range 189–260 vs. 296 pmol/l, range 242–338, respectively). Cranial irradiation without cyclophosphamide did not affect semen quality, fertility, or testosterone levels. None of the survivors of a high cumulative dose of cyclophosphamide (>20 g/m^2) and testicular irradiation (10–24 Gy) had fathered a child. Testicular size was shown to be better than serum inhibin B in predicting nonazoospermic semen samples or fertility.

Conclusion(s): Treatment of childhood ALL with 0–10 g/m^2 of cyclophosphamide and cranial irradiation does not affect fertility or semen quality but may impair long-term Leydig cell function.

Nice to hear good news: long-term survivors of ALL therapy who had been treated with cyclophosphamide in a dose of <10 g/m^2 had sperm quality and fertility rates comparable with those of controls, whereas the serum-free testosterone levels were lower. The result that testicular size is a better predictor of normal semen quality or fertility than serum inhibin B is surprising and not confirmed in the literature. We have some concerns with regard to measurement of the testicular size with a ruler (longitudinal and transverse axis in centimeters). In the literature, there is consensus that inhibin B is the best plasma marker of spermatogenesis, but those of us who do not have access to the new assays may resort to clinical evaluation using a Prader orchiometer. According to the study of subfertile men, the inhibin B concentrations allow accurate differentiation between competent and impaired spermatogenesis [1]. Nevertheless, the study is important and shows that long-term surveillance of the testicular function should be implemented for childhood ALL survivors.

Risk factors for obesity in adult survivors of childhood cancer: a report from the Childhood Cancer Survivor Study

Green DM, Cox CL, Zhu L, Krull KR, Srivastava DK, Stovall M, Nolan VG, Ness KK, Donaldson SS, Oeffinger KC, Meacham LR, Sklar CA, Armstrong GT, Robison LL
Department of Epidemiology and Cancer Control, St Jude Children's Research Hospital, Memphis, TN, USA
daniel.green@stjude.org
J Clin Oncol 2012;30:246–255

Objective: Survivors of childhood cancer are at increased risk for obesity, the etiology of which is not well understood and is likely to be multifactorial.
Methods: The study analyzed demographic, lifestyle, treatment, and intrapersonal factors and self-reported use of pharmaceuticals for their potential contribution to obesity (body mass index $\geq$30 kg/m^2) in 9,284 adult participants aged >18 years in the CCSS. Multivariable regression models were used to identify independent predictors of obesity. Interrelationships were determined by means of structural equation modeling (SEM).
Results: Independent risk factors for obesity included cancer diagnosed at age 5–9 years (relative risk (RR) 1.12; 95% confidence interval (CI) 1.01–1.24; p = 0.03), abnormal Short Form-36 physical function (RR 1.19; 95% CI 1.06–1.33; p < 0.001), hypothalamic/pituitary radiation doses of 20–30 Gy (RR 1.17; 95% CI 1.05–1.30; p = 0.01), and the use of the antidepressant paroxetine (RR 1.29; 95% CI 1.08–1.54; p = 0.01). Risk of obesity was reduced by meeting guidelines for vigorous physical activity issued by the US Centers for Disease Control and Prevention (RR 0.90; 95% CI 0.82–0.97; p = 0.01) and by a medium amount of anxiety (RR 0.86; 95% CI 0.75–0.99; p = 0.04). The hierarchical impact of the direct predictors, moderators, and mediators of obesity was described by the results of SEM (n = 8,244; comparative fit index = 0.999; Tucker Lewis index = 0.999; root mean square error of approximation = 0.014; weighted root mean square residual = 0.749).
Conclusions: Treatment, lifestyle, and intrapersonal factors, as well as the use of specific antidepressants, may be factors contributing to obesity among survivors of childhood cancer. Multifaceted intervention, including alternative drug and other treatments for depression and anxiety, may be required to reduce the risk of obesity in these patients.

The study by Green et al. reports hitherto unknown risk factors for later obesity in survivors of childhood cancer. In particular, it provides evidence that in these patients obesity is associated with a sedentary lifestyle, and the use of antidepressants. In this context, self-reported cancer-related anxiety and cancer-related pain are important confounders next to 'poor physical activity'. The use of an antidepressant (paroxetine) contributed to the development of obesity, as did low social status (less education), older age at survey, cranial irradiation and low family income.

Distinct impact of imatinib on growth at prepubertal and pubertal ages of children with chronic myeloid leukemia

Shima H, Tokuyama M, Tanizawa A, Tono C, Hamamoto K, Muramatsu H, Watanabe A, Hotta N, Ito M, Kurosawa H, Kato K, Tsurusawa M, Horibe K, Shimada H
Department of Pediatrics, Keio University School of Medicine, Tokyo, Japan
J Pediatr 2011;159:676–681

Objective: Imatinib side effects are generally mild to moderate but the drug's long-term effects remain unknown. Effects on growth are a major concern when treating children and growth deceleration after imatinib has been reported. This study aimed to determine the extent of imatinib-related growth impairment in children with chronic myeloid leukemia (CML).

Methods: Clinical records of 48 chronic-phase CML children who received first-line treatment with imatinib during 2001–2006 were analyzed retrospectively. Cumulative change in height was assessed using the height standard deviation score (SDS) and converted height data from age- and sex-adjusted Japanese norms.

Results: Height SDS was decreased in 72.9% of children; median maximum reduction in height SDS was 0.61 during imatinib treatment. Patients were followed up for a median (range) of 34 (10–88) months. Growth impairment was predominantly seen in children who started imatinib before pubertal onset compared with those who started treatment after reaching puberty. Growth velocity tended to recover as prepubertal children with growth impairment reached puberty, suggesting that imatinib had little impact on growth during puberty.

Conclusions: Growth impairment was a major adverse effect of long-term imatinib treatment in children with CML. The study revealed a distinct inhibitory effect of imatinib on growth in prepubertal and pubertal children with CML. The authors call for awareness of growth deceleration in children, especially in young children, given imatinib before puberty and subjected to prolonged exposure.

Imatinib is a specific inhibitor of several tyrosine kinases (TKs). By occupying the TK-active site it causes a decrease in activity. There are many different TK enzymes present in the body, including the insulin receptor. The authors demonstrated an association between imatinib treatment and growth impairment and postulated a negative effect of imatinib on GH secretion and function. Unfortunately, no IGF-1 data were reported in this study. A further limitation of the study results from short follow-up periods in the majority of cohort patients who showed no late effects on growth. To detect iatrogenically induced GH deficiency resulting from TK inhibitor therapy, the authors recommended careful monitoring of growth velocity, bone metabolic markers, and serum IGF-1. Performing GH stimulation tests before and during treatment with TK inhibitors would provide new insights into the dynamics of growth under such treatment.

Clinical trial
Endocrine outcomes after childhood NHL therapy

Endocrine late sequelae in long-term survivors of childhood non-Hodgkin lymphoma

Van Waas M, Neggers SJ, Te Winkel ML, Beishuizen A, Pieters R, van den Heuvel-Eibrink MM
Department of Pediatric Oncology/Hematology, Erasmus Medical Center-Sophia Children's Hospital, Rotterdam, The Netherlands

Ann Oncol 2012;23:1626–1632

Objective: Studies investigating the late endocrine sequelae of treatment in survivors of childhood non-Hodgkin lymphoma (NHL) are scarce. Available studies are often limited by small sample size or combination of NHL survivors with survivors of other malignancies. This study therefore undertook to investigate the long-term endocrine effects of childhood NHL treatment.

Methods: Included in this retrospective analysis of single-center data from 84 (males/females 62/22 females) survivors (median (range) age: 21 (9–40) years; time since cessation of therapy: 12 (4–30) years). Study assessments included height, weight, body mass index (BMI), percentage of body fat (% fat), lean body mass (LBM), bone mineral content (BMC), and bone mineral density of total body (BMD(TB)) and lumbar spine (BMD(LS)). Endocrine evaluation included thyroid-stimulating hormone (TSH), free thyroxine (fT$_4$), insulin-like growth factor-1 (IGF-1), inhibin B, and antimüllerian hormone (AMH). Results were compared with Dutch control groups of children and young adults.

Results: Survivors had significantly decreased height (mean standard deviation score (SDS): –0.36, p = 0.002), but closer analysis revealed that shorter stature had already been present at diagnosis (mean SDS –0.28, p = 0.023). BMI, % fat, BMC, BMD(TB), and BMD(LS) did not differ significantly from controls. LBM was lower in survivors (mean SDS –0.47, p = 0.008). TSH, fT$_4$ and IGF-1 levels were normal in all survivors. Low AMH levels were noted in 3 of 20 adult females, and inhibin B levels were decreased in 23/42 adult males.

Conclusions: Twelve years after the end of treatment, no NHL survivors of either sex had developed obesity, osteoporosis or thyroid disease. Male survivors may be at risk for infertility.

In long-term childhood NHL survivors, especially males, shorter stature seems to be determined by height at diagnosis rather than treatment-related side effects. This was a retrospective study and therefore IGF-1 levels were analyzed in the absence of data on dynamic stimulations tests. Since NHL, as a rule, is treated by chemotherapy, and occasionally by local irradiation, the study confirmed that treatment-related damage primarily affects the testes and does not cause central deficiencies, i.e. hypothalamic or pituitary damage. In addition, the study showed that long-term childhood NHL survivors appear not to be at risk for endocrine late sequelae such as osteoporosis, obesity, or hypothyroidism. However, males might be especially at risk for gonadal damage possibly related to cumulative doses of cytarabine. This is the first study to demonstrate such a cumulative effect of cytarabine. Usually, alkylating chemotherapeutic agents, e.g. cyclophosphamide, or abdominal irradiation are responsible for gonadal damage. By adjusting for these factors the authors were able to demonstrate the effect of cytarabine.

Endocrine tumors
Extremely rare but important for clinical practice

Ectopic ACTH syndrome in children and adolescents

More J, Young J, Reznik Y, Raverot G, Borson-Chazot F, Rohmer V, Baudin E, Coutant R, Tabarin A
Department of Endocrinology, University Hospital of Bordeaux, Pessac, France
J Clin Endocrinol Metab 2011;96:1213–1222

Objective: Ectopic ACTH syndrome (EAS) in youngsters has seldom been reported and is poorly known.
Setting: We conducted a multicenter retrospective study involving 18 French tertiary hospitals. Cases of EAS presenting Cushing's syndrome before the age of 20 during the period from 1985 to 2008 were analyzed.
Patients: Ten patients aged 14–20 years were identified and compared to 20 age-matched patients with Cushing's disease diagnosed during the same period.
Main Outcome Measures: Etiologies, clinical, biochemical and radiological features, prognosis, and treatment were described.
Results: Seven patients had well-differentiated neuroendocrine tumors (5 bronchial carcinoids, 1 mediastinal lymph node, and 1 thymic), 1 had a poorly differentiated thymic carcinoma, 1 had a pleural Ewing's sarcoma, and 1 had a liver nested stromal epithelial tumor. At presentation, seven tumors were identified with computed tomography scanning and somatostatin receptor scintigraphy, and one with ^{18}F-L-dihydroxyphenylalanine positron emission tomography scan. Two carcinoids were occult and were identified during follow-up. Cushing's syndrome was more intense in EAS, but the clinical and biological spectrum overlapped with that of Cushing's disease. No dynamic test achieved 100% accuracy, whereas petrosal sinus sampling provided correct diagnosis in all patients tested. Medical treatment of hypercortisolism was successful in 6 of the 8 patients with whom it was attempted, and bilateral adrenalectomy had to be performed in only 2 cases. Prognosis was good; 9 patients with curative resection of the tumor were alive and cured (median follow-up 6.5 years), whereas 1 patient died.
Conclusions: EAS in youngsters displays many similarities to that described in adults. The diagnostic and therapeutic algorithms recommended in adults can be used in this population.

This paper summarizes the experiences of different tertiary hospitals in France with ectopic ACTH syndrome (EAS) in 10 patients aged 10–20 years. Endogenous Cushing syndrome is rare in children, but as one can see – not unheard of. Etiologically, cortisol-producing adrenocortical tumors are more common in children than ACTH-producing pituitary tumors whereas ectopic ACTH production is extraordinarily rare. There are some case reports in the literature on infants with neuroblastomas or other neuroendocrine tumors, and adolescents with carcinoids. The most important messages of the paper are: (1) clinical overlap with Cushing's disease, and (2) diagnostic and therapeutic algorithms recommended in adults can be used in this population. Since most patients with EAS had neuroendocrine tumors, it is necessary to consider MEN1 syndrome, as is the case with any childhood pituitary adenoma.

Sporadic and genetic forms of pediatric somatotropinoma: a retrospective analysis of seven cases and a review of the literature

Nozières C, Berlier P, Dupuis C, Raynaud-Ravni C, Morel Y, Chazot FB, Nicolino M
Fédération d'Endocrinologie du Pole Est, Groupement Hospitalier Lyon Est, Bron, France
cecile.nozieres@chu-lyon.fr
Orphanet J Rare Dis 2011;6:67

Objective: Somatotropinoma is extremely rare in childhood. This pituitary adenoma is characterized by excessive growth hormone (GH) production. In some cases, involvement of genetic defects has been demonstrated, including multiple endocrine neoplasia type 1 (MEN1), Carney complex, McCune-Albright syndrome, and aryl hydrocarbon receptor-interacting protein (AIP). The study reports on 7 pediatric patients, placing a particular focus on the differences between genetic and sporadic forms of somatotropinoma.

Methods: The study retrospectively analyzed the clinical data of children aged <18 years who presented to a French regional pediatric endocrinology network during 1992–2008. First-line treatment consisted in somatostatin (SMS) analogs or transsphenoidal surgery. Endocrine control was defined as insulin-like growth factor-1 (IGF-1) levels within the age-appropriate normal range at 6 months after initiation of therapy in conjunction with a decrease in tumor volume.

Results: Included were 7 patients (6 males, 1 female) aged 5–17 years. Four patients had an identified genetic mutation (McCune-Albright syndrome (1 patient), MEN1 (1) and AIP (2)) whereas the other 3 had a sporadic form of somatotropinoma. Accelerated growth rate was reported as the first clinical sign in 4 patients. Macroadenoma was diagnosed in 5 patients, invasion being noted in 4 of these patients, 1 with a sporadic form and 3 with genetic forms of somatotropinoma. Six patients received SMS analogs; normalization of IGF-1 occurred in 1 patient with sporadic intrasellar macroadenoma. All patients with an identified genetic mutation required several different types of treatment (1 patient received 4 types, 2 patients had 3 types, and 1 patient had 2 types), whereas 2 of the 3 sporadic somatotropinoma patients needed only one type of therapy.

Conclusions: This is the first series that analyzes the therapeutic response of somatotropinoma in pediatric patients with identified genetic defects. In children, genetic forms of somatotropinoma are more invasive than the sporadic forms. Furthermore, SMS analogs appear to be less effective against genetic forms than against sporadic forms of somatotropinoma.

In both adults and children, conventional treatment of somatotropinoma consists in transsphenoidal surgery. In cases of intracavernous extension or incomplete surgery, SMS analog treatment may be administered preoperatively and/or postoperatively to suppress GH release. The study shows that SMS analogs are effective without surgery and can normalize IGF-1 levels and reduce tumor size. The observational nature of the study and the small sample size however weaken the authors' conclusions concerning the influence of genetic forms of somatotropinoma on the effect of SMS analogs.

Management of medullary thyroid carcinoma and MEN2 syndromes in childhood

Waguespack SG, Rich TA, Perrier ND, Jimenez C, Cote GJ
The Department of Endocrine Neoplasia and Hormonal Disorders, Houston, TX, USA
swagues@mdanderson.org
Nat Rev Endocrinol 2011;7:596–607

Objective: Medullary thyroid carcinoma (MTC) and the multiple endocrine neoplasia (MEN) type 2 syndromes are rare but important endocrine diseases that are increasingly managed by pediatric providers. MTC is generally associated with a favorable prognosis when diagnosed during childhood, where it frequently occurs secondary to activating mutations in the RET proto-oncogene and arises from preexisting C-cell hyperplasia.

Results: MEN2A accounts for 90–95% of childhood MTC cases and is most commonly due to mutations in codon 634 of RET. MEN2B is associated with the most aggressive clinical presentation of MTC and is almost always due to the Met918Thr mutation of RET. Surgery is the primary treatment and only chance of cure, although the advent of targeted therapies seems to be improving progression-free survival in advanced cases. Since the discovery of the role of RET in MEN2A, considerable advances in the management of this syndrome have occurred, and most of the children with MEN2A who have undergone early thyroidectomy will now lead full, productive lives. Strong genotype-phenotype correlations have facilitated the development of guidelines for interventions. Contemporary approaches for deciding the appropriate age at which surgery should take place incorporate data from ultrasonography and calcitonin measurements in addition to the results of genotyping.

Conclusions: To optimize care and to facilitate ongoing research, children with MTC and the MEN2 syndromes are optimally treated at tertiary centers with multidisciplinary expertise.

This is an excellent overview on the current management of children with medullary thyroid carcinoma (MTC) and multiple endocrine neoplasia (MEN) type 2 – genetic syndromes caused by germline mutations in the RET proto-oncogene. The best strategy is to prevent MTC by early surgical thyroidectomy. The authors make the important note that to understand rare diseases, it is important that such children are managed in networked disease-specific research clinics, so that the knowledge gained from each case is utilized in an optimal manner. Referring patients to such networks requires both organization and good will. An example of that approach is provided in the next abstract.

Prognostic factors of disease-free survival after thyroidectomy in 170 young patients with a RET germline mutation: a multicenter study of the Groupe Français d'Etude des Tumeurs Endocrines

Rohmer V, Vidal-Trecan G, Bourdelot A, Niccoli P, Murat A, Wemeau JL, Borson-Chazot F, Schvartz C, Tabarin A, Chabre O, Chabrier G, Caron P, Rodien P, Schlumberger M, Baudin E
Centre hospitalier universitaire Angers, Endocrinologie, Faculté de médecine, Université Angers, Angers, France
virohmer@chu-angers.fr
J Clin Endocrinol Metab 2011;96:E509–518

Background: In hereditary medullary thyroid carcinoma (HMTC), prophylactic surgery is the only curative option, which should be properly defined both in time and extent.

Objectives: To identify and characterize prognostic factors associated with disease-free survival (DFS) in children from HMTC families.

Design: We conducted a retrospective analysis of a multicenter cohort of 170 patients below age 21 at surgery. Demographic, clinical, genetic, biological data (basal and pentagastrin-stimulated calcitonin

(CT and CT/Pg, respectively)), and tumor node metastasis (TNM) status were collected. DFS was assessed based on basal CT levels. Kaplan-Meier curves, Cox regression, and logistic regression models were used to determine factors associated with DFS and TNM staging.

Results: No patients with a preoperative basal CT <31 ng/ml had persistent or recurrent disease. Medullary thyroid carcinoma defined by a diameter ≥10 mm (hazard ratio (HR) 6.0, 95% confidence interval (CI) 1.8–19.8) and N1 status (HR 20.8, 95% CI 3.9–109.8) were independently associated with DFS. Class D genotype (odds ratio (OR) 48.5, 95% CI 10.6–225.1), preoperative basal CT >30 ng/l (OR 43.4, 95% CI 5.2–359.8), and age >10 (OR 5.5, 95% CI 1.4–21.8) were associated with medullary thyroid carcinoma ≥10 mm. No patient with a preoperative basal CT <31 ng/ml had a N1 status. Class D genotype (OR 48.6, 95% CI 8.6–274.1), and age >10 (OR 4.6, 95% CI 1.1–19.0) were associated with N1 status.

Conclusions: In HMTC patients, DFS is best predicted by TNM staging and preoperative basal CT level <30 pg/ml. Basal CT, class D genotype, and age constitute key determinants to decide preoperatively timely surgery.

By analyzing a large group of patients with hereditary MTC the authors could identify various important key factors (basal calcitonin, class D genotype, chronological age) which should be considered to determine the optimal time point of surgery.

Endocrine aspects of chronic disease
Trisomy 21 – Sertoli and Leydig cell dysfunction soon after birth

Early onset of primary hypogonadism revealed by serum antimüllerian hormone determination during infancy and childhood in trisomy 21

Grinspon RP, Bedecarrás P, Ballerini MG, Iñiguez G, Rocha A, Mantovani Rodrigues Reserde EA, Brito VN, Milani C, Figueroa Gacitúa V, Chiesa A, Keselman A, Gottlieb S, Borges MF, Ropelato MG, Picard JY, Codner E, Rey RA
Division de Endocrinologia, Centro de Investigaciones Endocrinológicas (CEDIE-CONICET), Hospital de Niños Ricardo Gutiérrez, Buenos Aires, Argentina
rgrinspon@cedie.org.ar
Int J Androl 2011;34:e487–498

Background: Primary hypogonadism, or testicular dysfunction, in male patients with an extra sex chromosome or autosome is expected to manifest at puberty owing to meiotic germ-cell failure. Relevant data on patients with trisomy 21, a frequent autosomal aneuploidy, are sparse. This study aimed to assess whether trisomy 21 in males presents with pubertal-onset, germ cell-specific, primary hypogonadism, or whether the condition is established earlier and affects other testicular cell populations.

Methods: The study evaluated 117 boys and young men with trisomy 21 aged 2 months to 20 years by assessing the pituitary-testicular axis for functional status, especially Sertoli cell function. To enable comparison with an appropriate control population, reference levels for serum antimüllerian hormone (AMH) were prospectively established in 421 males of normal karyotype aged 2 days to 52 years by means of a recently developed ultrasensitive assay.

Results: From early infancy, trisomy 21 was associated with lower than normal AMH levels, indicating Sertoli cell dysfunction, regardless of cryptorchidism. In infants with trisomy 21, overall prevalence of AMH below the 3rd percentile was 64.3%. Follicle-stimulating hormone was elevated at age <6 months and after the onset of puberty. Testosterone was within the normal range, but luteinizing hormone was elevated in most patients aged <6 months and after pubertal onset, indicating mild Leydig cell dysfunction.

Conclusions: In trisomy 21, primary hypogonadism involves combined dysfunction of both Sertoli and Leydig cells, which can be observed soon after birth independently of cryptorchidism. The authors expect their findings to trigger the search for new hypotheses explaining the pathophysiology of gonadal dysfunction in autosomal trisomy.

This cross-sectional study in a relatively large cohort of individuals with Down syndrome shows that males with this trisomic disorder develop primary hypogonadism soon after birth and that Sertoli and Leydig cell function are both impaired. The study thus demonstrates that both testosterone production and spermatogenesis are impaired from early childhood rather than puberty and are also independent of cryptorchidism. Even though other markers such as inhibin B for Sertoli cells and INSL-3 for Leydig cells are available today, the hormonal constellation of gonadotropins and testosterone provides a basis for a valid statement regarding Leydig cells. Hence AMH can be considered a marker of clinical relevance. The study of a trisomy provides a unique opportunity to understand the role of excess genetic material on specific endocrine mechanisms [2].

Cerebral palsy: important for clinical practice: weight-for-age charts

Low weight, morbidity, and mortality in children with cerebral palsy: new clinical growth charts

Brooks J, Day S, Shavelle R, Strauss D
Life Expectancy Project, San Francisco, CA, USA
brooks@lifeexpectancy.org
Pediatrics 2011;128:e299–307

Objective: To determine the percentiles of weight for age in cerebral palsy according to gender and Gross Motor Function Classification System (GMFCS) level and to identify weights associated with negative health outcomes.

Study Design: This study consists of a total of 102,163 measurements of weight from 25,545 children with cerebral palsy who were clients of the California Department of Developmental Services from 1988 through 2002. Percentiles were estimated using generalized additive models for location, scale, and shape. Numbers of comorbidities were compared using t tests. The effect of low weight on mortality was estimated with proportional hazards regression.

Results: Weight-for-age percentiles in children with cerebral palsy varied with gender and GMFCS level. Comorbidities were more common among those with weights below the 20th percentile in GMFCS levels I through IV and level V without feeding tubes (p < 0.01). For GMFCS levels I and II, weights below the 5th percentile were associated with a hazard ratio of 2.2 (95% CI 1.3–3.7). For children in GMFCS levels III through V, weights below the 20th percentile were associated with a mortality hazard ratio of 1.5 (95% CI 1.4–1.7).

Conclusions: Children with cerebral palsy who have very low weights have more major medical conditions and are at increased risk of death. The weight-for-age charts presented here may assist in the early detection of nutritional issues or other health risks in these children.

Unlike the longevity effect of low BMI in the general population, in chronic diseases low weight is associated with higher rates of comorbidities and mortality. This is also true for children and adolescents with cerebral palsy. However, it is difficult to define low weight within these patients because they do not follow growth and weight charts that were based on data of healthy children. Thus, Brooks et al. developed weight-for-age charts and, in addition, for each degree of severity of loss of motor function based on the Gross Motor Function Classification System (GMFCS). They could define the 5th percentile for GMFCS levels I and II and the 20th percentile for GMFCS levels III–V (without feeding tube) as cut-off values associated with higher degrees of chronic major medical conditions included, but were not limited to, diabetes mellitus, hypertension, congenital or arteriosclerotic heart disease, upper respiratory infections, etc. The authors showed how important it is to achieve a certain weight level when suffering from a chronic disease. Surprisingly, the authors did not find higher morbidity or mortality rates associated with overweight and obesity. This issue should be addressed in further long-term studies reaching adult ages.

Salivary cortisol levels in prepubertal children using inhaled corticosteroids with or without concurrent intranasal corticosteroids

Heijsman SM, de Vries TW, Wolthuis A, Kamps AW
Department of Paediatrics, Medical Centre Leeuwarden, Leeuwarden, The Netherlands

Pediatr Pulmonol 2011;46:1055–1061

Background: Inhaled corticosteroids (ICS) and intranasal steroids (INS) are frequently coadministered in children with asthma and rhinitis. In contrast to monotherapy with ICS or INS, little is known about the safety of concurrent use of topical steroids on hypothalamic-pituitary-adrenal (HPA) axis function in prepubertal children.

Objective: Comparison of morning salivary cortisol levels in prepubertal children using maintenance treatment with ICS with and without concurrent use of INS to steroid-naive control groups (healthy children, and children with constipation who are under pediatric care).

Study Design: Cross-sectional observational study in prepubertal children (6–12 years) using ICS alone (n = 41) or in combination with INS (n = 22), compared to different control groups with no steroid treatment (18 healthy children, and 28 children with constipation). Morning salivary cortisol levels were determined from saliva samples collected at home.

Results: The morning salivary cortisol levels of the healthy children (8.7 nmol/l; 95% CI 5.9–18.8), and the children with constipation (8.9 nmol/l; 8.0–11.3) were comparable. The salivary cortisol levels of prepubertal children using ICS (median 4.7 nmol/l; 95% CI 4.6–6.9) or a combination of ICS and INS (5.1 nmol/l; 4.2–7.6) were comparable, but significantly reduced compared to both control groups. There was no correlation between salivary cortisol level and age, duration of disease, or cumulative daily dose of topical steroids.

Conclusions: Salivary cortisol levels in prepubertal children using ICS, with or without concurrent use of INS, were comparable. However, salivary cortisol levels were significantly reduced compared to steroid-naive controls, irrespective of the cumulative daily dose of topical steroids.

Hypothalamic-pituitary-adrenal axis suppression in asthmatic children on inhaled and nasal corticosteroids: is the early-morning serum adrenocorticotropic hormone (ACTH) a useful screening test?

Zollner EW, Lombard C, Galal U, Hough S, Irusen E, Weinberg E
Paediatric Endocrine Unit, Tygerberg Children's Hospital, University of Stellenbosch, Cape Town, South Africa
zollner@sun.ac.za

Pediatr Allergy Immunol 2011;22:614–620

Background: Hypothalamic-pituitary-adrenal axis suppression (HPAS) in asthmatic children treated with inhaled corticosteroids (ICS), with or without nasal steroids (NS), may be more common than previously thought. Only dynamic testing will identify children at risk of adrenal crisis. It is impractical to test all asthmatic children for HPAS with a gold standard adrenal function test, i.e. the metyrapone or insulin tolerance test.

Objective: To determine which clinical or biochemical parameter is the most useful screening test for HPAS in asthmatic children.

Study design: 26 asthmatic children, 5–18 years old, on ICS ± NS, not treated with oral or topical steroids in the preceding year were recruited. Height, weight, height velocity, weight velocity and a change in systolic blood pressure from the recumbent to the standing position (ΔSBP) were recorded. Early-morning urine for urinary-free cortisol (UFC) and urinary cortisol metabolites (UCM) was collected. UFC was analyzed by both a chemiluminescent assay and gas chromatography/mass spectrometry (GC-MS). Morning serum cortisol and adrenocorticotropic hormone (ACTH) levels were measured. The overnight metyrapone test was performed if the fasting morning serum cortisol was >83 nmol/l. HPAS was diagnosed if the ACTH failed to rise >100 pg/ml after metyrapone. Spearman correlation coefficients (r) were calculated between the post-metyrapone ACTH and each variable. A receiver-operating characteristics (ROC) curve was drawn for the most promising test, and the diagnostic performance was calculated.

Results: All clinical and biochemical parameters investigated were weakly and nonsignificantly correlated with the post-metyrapone ACTH, except for the morning serum ACTH (r = 0.68; p <0.001). The best discrimination between those who have and those who do not have HPAS is a morning serum ACTH level of 11.7 pg/ml. This corresponds to a sensitivity of 0.89 (0.57–0.98), a specificity of 0.77 (0.53–0.90), a positive predictive value of 0.67 (0.39–0.87), a negative predictive value of 0.93 (0.69–0.99), an accuracy of 0.81 (0.61–0.94), a positive likelihood ratio of 3.78 (1.68–9.49) and a negative likelihood ratio of 0.15 (0.03–0.60).
Conclusions: The morning serum ACTH level was found to be the most useful screening test to detect HPAS in this sample of children receiving ICS ± NS. A larger study should be undertaken to refine the diagnostic precision of the morning serum ACTH level.

Suppression of the hypothalamic-pituitary-adrenal axis (HPA) in asthmatic children treated with inhaled corticosteroids (ICS), with or without nasal steroids (INS), is one of the major endocrine concerns among these patients. The debate has been around for many decades. Two recent papers address this issue. Up to 80% of children with asthma also suffer from concomitant allergic rhinitis which requires long-term treatment with a combination of inhaled (ICS) and intranasal corticosteroids (INS). Heijsman et al. studied morning salivary cortisol levels in prepubertal children and could not find an additional suppressive effect of combined glucocorticoid treatment on HPA axis function. However, cortisol levels have been decreased among treated children compared with steroid-naive controls, irrespective of the cumulative daily dose of topical steroids. None of the treated children had growth restrictions based on height SDS; data on height velocities were not provided. The authors speculate about an individual susceptibility for suppression of HPA axis. Relative hypocortisolemia may have other untoward effects such as fatigue, but mostly when a child needs his maximal adrenal capacity in extreme stress.

The second paper by Zöllner et al. focused on the important question how to screen for suppression of HPA axis among children with asthma. They compared morning urinary-free cortisol and serum levels of cortisol and ACTH with post-metyrapone ACTH levels as the gold standard (it is important to keep in mind this neglected test as the ultimate test for HPA axis activity). Only the morning ACTH was significantly correlated with post-metyrapone ACTH. Unfortunately, the better available salivary cortisol levels or 24 h urine measurements have not been performed. In line with the paper of Heijsman et al., further long-term studies addressing the question of diagnosis and clinical relevance based on robust parameters like final heights are necessary. The debate goes on.

Inflammatory bowel disease and vitamin D insufficiency

Treatment of Vitamin D Insufficiency in Children and Adolescents with Inflammatory Bowel Disease: A Randomized Clinical Trial Comparing Three Regimens

Pappa HM, Mitchell PD, Jiang H, Kassiff S, Filip-Dhima R, Difabio D, Quinn N, Lawton RC, Varvaris M, Van Straaten S, Gordon CM
Center for Inflammatory Bowel Diseases (H.M.P., S.K.); Clinical Research Center, Design and Analysis Core (P.D.M., H.J., R.F.D.); Clinical and Translational Study Unit (D.D., N.Q.), Children's Hospital Boston, Boston, MA; Northwestern University Feinberg School of Medicine (R.C.L.), Center for Psychosocial Research in Gastrointestinal Diseases, Chicago, IL; Johns Hopkins University (M.V.), Department of Psychiatry, Division of Medical Psychology, Baltimore, MD, USA; Academic Medical Center (S.V.S.), Amsterdam, The Netherlands, and Bone Health Program (C.M.G.), Children's Hospital Boston, Boston, MA, USA
J Clin Endocrinol Metab 2012;97:2134–2142

Background: Vitamin D insufficiency (serum 25-hydroxyvitamin D (25OHD) concentration <20 ng/ml) is prevalent among children with inflammatory bowel disease (IBD), and its treatment has not been studied.
Objective: The aim of this study was to compare the efficacy and safety of three vitamin D repletion regimens.

Study Design: We conducted a randomized, controlled clinical trial from November 2007 to June 2010 at the Clinical and Translational Study Unit of Children's Hospital Boston. The study was not blinded to participants and investigators. Eligibility criteria included diagnosis of IBD, age 5–21, and serum 25OHD concentration <20 ng/ml. 71 patients enrolled, 61 completed the trial, and 2 withdrew due to adverse events.

Intervention: Patients received orally for 6 weeks: vitamin D_2, 2,000 IU daily (arm A, control); vitamin D_3, 2,000 IU daily (arm B); vitamin D_2, 50,000 IU weekly (arm C), and an age-appropriate calcium supplement.

Main Outcome Measure: We measured the change in serum 25OHD concentration (Δ25OHD) (ng/ml). Secondary outcomes included change in serum intact PTH concentration (ΔPTH) (pg/ml) and the adverse event occurrence rate.

Results: After 6 weeks, Δ25OHD ± se was: 9.3 ± 1.8 (arm A); 16.4 ± 2.0 (arm B); 25.4 ± 2.5 (arm C); p (A vs. C) = 0.0004; p (A vs. B) = 0.03. ΔPTH ± se was −5.6 ± 5.5 (arm A); −0.1 ± 4.2 (arm B); −4.4 ± 3.9 (arm C); p = 0.57. No participant experienced hypercalcemia or hyperphosphatemia, and the prevalence of hypercalciuria did not differ among arms at follow-up.

Conclusions: Oral doses of 2,000 IU vitamin D_3 daily and 50,000 IU vitamin D_2 weekly for 6 weeks are superior to 2,000 IU vitamin D_2 daily for 6 weeks in raising serum 25OHD concentration and are well tolerated among children and adolescents with IBD. The change in serum PTH concentration did not differ among arms.

Besides the classical role of vitamin D, new evidence has been reported that vitamin D deficiency might be implicated in a host of other diseases including psoriasis, multiple sclerosis, inflammatory bowel disease, type 1 and 2 diabetes, hypertension, cardiovascular disease, the metabolic syndrome and various cancers. Pappa et al. conducted a randomized control trial (RCT) on different supplementation regimens in IBS patients. They postulate that 50,000 IU of oral vitamin D_2 weekly or 2,000 IU of oral vitamin D_3 daily for 6 weeks are sufficient to raise serum 25OHD concentration in children and adolescents with IBD and vitamin D insufficiency. The second finding was that PTH seems to play no role in diagnosis and treatment control, since PTH levels were low before initiation of substitution. The authors speculate about a potential involvement of antibodies against the calcium-sensing receptor which directly upregulate its expression driving downward the calcium level needed to stimulate PTH secretion. In agreement with the authors, one major limitation of this study was the lack of a healthy control group. These issues should be addressed in upcoming studies.

The role of growth hormone and insulin-like growth factor-1 in Crohn's disease: implications for therapeutic use of human growth hormone in pediatric patients

Vortia E, Kay M, Wyllie R
Department of Pediatric Gastroenterology and Nutrition, Children's Hospital, Cleveland Clinic, Cleveland, OH, USA
Curr Opin Pediatr 2011;23:545–551

Objective: This review evaluates the role of the growth hormone (GH) and insulin-like growth factor (IGF) in influencing linear growth in pediatric Crohn's disease. It also examines the current evidence concerning the use of recombinant human growth hormone (rhGH) as a potential therapy in achieving optimal growth and inducing mucosal healing for pediatric Crohn's disease.

Recent Findings: Current treatment strategies for Crohn's disease including antitumor necrosis factor-α (TNF-α) therapy have been demonstrated to improve growth velocity, but linear growth deficits persist despite optimization of therapy. By complex mechanisms, including the reduction of levels of IGF-1 and induction of systemic and hepatic GH resistance, cytokines such as TNF-α and interleukin-6 (IL-6), commonly elevated in active Crohn's disease, are important as mediators of linear growth delay. Recent evidence suggests that rhGH therapy is effective in improving short-term linear growth for a selected group of patients but of limited benefit as a therapy for improving mucosal disease and reducing clinical disease activity.

Summary and Conclusions: Crohn's disease interacts with the GH-IGF-1 axis in important ways. Recent studies evaluating rhGH use in pediatric Crohn's disease have demonstrated some efficacy in reversing persistent linear growth delay but limited benefits in terms of improving mucosal disease and clinical disease activity. Larger studies of adequate power are needed to confirm a true benefit in terms of growth, to examine a potential benefit with regard to modification of disease activity, and to evaluate long-term risks.

Growth failure and delayed puberty are particular comorbidities among children with inflammatory bowel disease such as Crohn's disease. Several studies with different patient numbers ranging between 3 and 37 have been conducted. However, to date there is no convincing evidence that there is a substantial role for rhGH in these patients on linear growth or disease activity. We agree with Vortia et al. that larger studies are needed examining disease activity and robust parameters of linear growth like final heights.

Endocrine and bone metabolic complications in chronic liver disease and after liver transplantation in children

Högler W, Baumann U, Kelly D
Department of Endocrinology and Diabetes, Birmingham Children's Hospital, Birmingham, UK
wolfgang.hogler@bch.nhs.uk

J Pediatr Gastroenterol Nutr 2012;54:313–321

Background: With improved survival of orthotopic liver transplantation (OLT) in children, prevention and treatment of pre- and posttransplant complications have become a major focus of care. End-stage liver failure can cause endocrine complications such as growth failure and hepatic osteodystrophy, and, like other chronic illnesses, also pubertal delay, relative adrenal insufficiency, and the sick euthyroid syndrome.

Results: Drug-induced diabetes mellitus post-OLT affects approximately 10% of children. Growth failure is found in 60% of children assessed for OLT. Despite optimization of nutrition, rarely can further stunting of growth before OLT be prevented. Catch-up growth is usually observed after steroid weaning from 18 months post-OLT. Whether growth hormone treatment would benefit the 20% of children who fail to catch up in height requires testing in randomized controlled trials. Hepatic osteodystrophy in children comprises vitamin D deficiency rickets, low bone mass, and fractures caused by malnutrition and malabsorption. Vitamin D deficiency requires aggressive treatment with ergocalciferol (D_2) or cholecalciferol (D_3). The active vitamin D metabolites alphacalcidol or calcitriol increase gut calcium absorption but do not replace vitamin D stores. Prevalence of fractures is increased both before OLT (10–28% of children) and after OLT (12–38%). Most fractures are vertebral, are associated with low spine bone mineral density, and frequently occur asymptomatically, but they may also cause chronic pain. Fracture prediction in these children is limited. OLT in children is also associated with a greater risk of developing avascular bone necrosis (4%) and scoliosis (13%–38%).

Summary: This article reviews the literature on endocrine and skeletal complications of liver disease and presents preventive screening recommendations and therapeutic strategies.

The number of long-term survivors after childhood liver transplantation is increasing. Thus, questions about long-term outcomes and disease/treatment associated comorbidities have to be asked. The excellent review by Högler et al. summarizes current knowledge on these issues. Short stature, a role for growth-promoting therapies like treatment with rhGH, 'sick thyroid syndrome' due to low thyroid hormone transport protein production in liver disease, and transient or persistent adrenal insufficiency are among them. As previously commented on rare diseases, this review underlines the need for collecting long-term data in (inter)national registries of patients after liver transplantation.

References
1. Pierik FH, Vreeburg JT, Stijnen T, De Jong FH, Weber RF: Serum inhibin B as a marker of spermatogenesis. J Clin Endocrinol Metab 1998;83:3110–3114.
2. Meyerovitch J, Antebi F, Greenberg-Dotan S, Bar-Tal O, Hochberg Z: Hyperthyrotropinaemia in untreated subjects with down's syndrome aged 6 months to 64 years: a comparative analysis. Arch Dis Child 2012 (E-pub ahead of print).

Type 1 Diabetes: Clinical and Experimental

M. Loredana Marcovecchio and Francesco Chiarelli

Department of Paediatrics, University of Chieti, Chieti, Italy

The continuous rise in the incidence of type 1 diabetes (T1D), particularly in younger children, has been a constant theme highlighted in all previous *Yearbook* chapters on T1D. It is impossible not to reiterate this concept this year, given that it represents a major epidemiological issue and the driving force for the studies reported in this chapter.

Several interesting basic and clinical studies have been published in 2011–2012 and some of the most interesting ones, dealing with a wide range of aspects associated with T1D, from pathogenesis to treatment, are presented. Progress has been made in terms of the understanding of the pathogenesis of T1D and how changes in environmental factors can interact with the individual genetic background in explaining the rising number of new cases of T1D. Changes in the immunophenotype of patients with T1D seem to have occurred over time, moving towards a more mature and aggressive immune response. Peripheral blood monocyte expression profiles have emerged to be a clinical useful marker to stratify patients with recent-onset T1D. New β-cell-specific markers, which could be invaluable for diagnostic and intervention purposes, have also been identified. Clinical trials have been assessing new potential treatment strategies, such as immune treatments as well as new insulin analogues. Genetic studies have become more and more complex, by including interaction models which allow a better understanding of the role of genetic changes at single or multiple loci. In addition, the potential role of epigenetic changes has also been explored. Exciting has been the discovery of genetic manipulations which can influence insulin secretion, or even turn some gut cells into insulin-producing cells.

From a clinical point of view, interesting findings have been the higher risk of T1D associated with cesarean section in combination with genetic susceptibility, the beneficial effect of intensive insulin treatment on glomerular filtration rate and the feasibility of behavioral interventions in the management of adolescents with T1D. Last but not least, the 'new hope' section is, as last year, dedicated to the progress in the field of islet transplantation.

Many articles presented in this chapter will be followed by new studies aiming at confirming specific findings or extending them and leading to more discoveries, which will hopefully help prevent T1D or at least improve management, reducing complication risks and improving the prognosis of people affected by this disease.

Mechanism of the year
Turning gut cells into β-cells

Generation of functional insulin-producing cells in the gut by Foxo1 ablation

Talchai C, Xuan S, Kitamura T, DePinho RA, Accili D
Naomi Berrie Diabetes Center, Columbia University Medical Center, New York, NY, USA
Nat Genet 2012;44:406–412

Background: Restoration of regulated insulin secretion is the ultimate goal of therapy for T1D.
Methods and Results: Somatic ablation of Foxo1 in Neurog3+ enteroendocrine progenitor cells gave rise to gut insulin-positive (Ins+) cells that expressed markers of mature β-cells and secreted bioactive insulin as well as C-peptide in response to glucose and sulfonylureas. Lineage tracing experiments showed that gut Ins+ cells arose from Foxo1-deficient cells. Inducible Foxo1 ablation in adult mice also resulted in the generation of gut Ins+ cells. Interestingly, after β-cell ablation by the toxin streptozotocin, gut Ins+ cells were able to regenerate and produce insulin, thus reversing hyperglycemia in mice.
Conclusions: The data indicate that Neurog3+ enteroendocrine progenitors require active Foxo1 to prevent differentiation into Ins+ cells. Foxo1 ablation in gut cells might become a key approach to restore insulin production in T1D.

Regeneration of β-cells and consequently insulin secretion is the fundamental goal for fighting T1D. Talchai et al. reports the very interesting finding on how loss of the transcriptional factor Foxo1 in Neurog3+ enteroendocrine progenitor cells can convert them into cells able to synthesize, process and secrete insulin as well as C-peptide. Following Foxo1 inactivation, enteric cells express markers typical of β-cells, such as Pdx1, MafA and Nkx6.1, and respond to β-cell secretagogues, such as glucose and sulfonylureas. Even more exciting was the finding that in mice gut, Ins+ cells derived from Neurog3+ progenitors can regenerate after streptozotocin treatment, differently from other cell lines previously shown to be able to convert into insulin-producing cells, but inexorably destroyed by streptozocin. Therefore, not only inactivation of Foxo1 converts the fate of a subset of gut cells into insulin-producing cells, but can even confer them the potential of regenerating after a toxic hit.

Overall these data suggest that Foxo1 is a key factor required for suppressing a pancreatic β-cell-like program in enteroendocrine cells and, modulation of this factor appears to be a promising way for regenerating β-cells in the context of T1D.

These findings are promising and highlight new potential resources to be used when attempting to regenerate β-cells.

New paradigms 1
A monocyte signature as a biomarker of T1D progression

Peripheral blood monocyte gene expression profile clinically stratifies patients with recent-onset type 1 diabetes

Irvine KM, Gallego P, An X, Best SE, Thomas G, Wells C, Harris M, Cotterill A, Thomas R
The University of Queensland Diamantina Institute, Brisbane, Qld., Australia
Diabetes 2012;61;1281–1290

Background: There is a great need to identify novel biomarkers of disease progression after T1D onset.

Methods: Peripheral blood (PB) monocyte gene expression was profiled in 6 healthy subjects and 16 children with T1D within 3 months from diagnosis.

Results: Monocyte expression profiles clustered into two distinct subgroups, representing mild and severe deviation from healthy control subjects. Patients with strongly divergent monocyte gene expression had significantly higher insulin dose-adjusted HbA$_{1c}$ levels during the first year, compared with patients with mild deviation. The diabetes-associated expression signature identified multiple perturbations in pathways controlling cellular metabolism and survival, including endoplasmic reticulum and oxidative stress. Quantitative PCR (qPCR) of a 9-gene panel correlated with glycemic control in 12 additional recent-onset patients. The qPCR signature was also detected in PB from healthy first-degree relatives.

Conclusion: A PB gene expression signature correlates with glycemic control in the first year after T1D diagnosis and is present in at-risk subjects. These data suggest that monocyte phenotype might be a candidate biomarker for disease progression pre- and post-onset. In addition, systemic stresses appear to be contributors to innate immune function in T1D.

Searching for biomarkers of progression after T1D onset is of utmost importance to identify patients with different levels of severity of the disease, which could determine faster or slower progression rates and different risk of complications. Such biomarkers could also be particularly useful for clinical trials aiming at preventing T1D progression.

In this context, the present study was able to demonstrate that monocyte gene expression can help in distinguishing newly diagnosed patients with a different progression rate. The same expression profile could predict progression in subjects at risk for T1D before the onset of the disease. A severe deviation from a healthy monocyte expression profile, which was found in 50% of newly diagnosed children, was associated with a worse glycemic control and higher insulin requirements during a follow-up period up to 1 year after diagnosis. This might also determine a higher risk of complications in the long-term. Interestingly, this monocyte profile was characterized by upregulation of genes implicated in cellular stress, mainly oxidative and endoplasmic reticulum stress, and downregulation of genes involved in cellular energy and metabolite production, thus highlighting an underlying high susceptibility or exposure to physiological stress.

Overall, these data suggest that monocyte phenotype might be a candidate biomarker for disease progression pre- and post-onset in T1D, which could allow a better patient stratification on the basis of different levels of progression risk and therefore potentially guide intervention strategies on a personalized basis.

New paradigms 2
Emerging new β-cell markers

Novel pancreatic β-cell-specific proteins: antibody-based proteomics for identification of new biomarker candidates

Lindskog C, Korsgren O, Ponten F, Eriksson JW, Johansson L, Danielsson A
Department of Immunology, Genetics and Pathology, Science for Life Laboratory, Uppsala University, Uppsala, Sweden
J Proteomics 2012;75:2611–2620

Background: β-Cell-specific surface targets are required for noninvasive monitoring of β-cell mass, which could be used for evaluation of new diabetes treatments as well as to help unravel pathogenic mechanisms underlying β-cell dysfunction.

Methods and Results: Antibody-based proteomics was used to identify and explore a set of islet cell-specific proteins. A search algorithm in the Human Protein Atlas was performed to identify islet-specific proteins. This led to the identification of 27 hits, of which 12 showed a clear membranous expression pattern or had predicted transmembrane regions. The specificity of the identified proteins was investigated by immunohistochemical staining of pancreas sections from diabetic and nondiabetic subjects. None of these antigens were expressed in the exocrine pancreas. Colocalization with insulin and glucagon was further determined by confocal microscopy using isolated human islets. All antibodies specifically stained human islets and colocalization analysis revealed that four proteins were exclusively expressed in β-cells. Of note, these antibodies were negative in sections from subjects with long-standing T1D.

Conclusions: The present study identified four specific β-cell proteins: DGCR2, GBF1, GPR44 and SerpinB10, the expression of which has not previously been described.

The identification of specific β-cell markers, which could allow the assessment of β-cells in a noninvasive manner, is of paramount importance in terms of diagnostic and therapeutic approaches. Up to now, several molecules have been tested as possible targets for β-cell assessment, without finding an ideal marker [1]. The best β-cell marker should be membrane-expressed and highly represented in order to allow discerning β-cells from the more abundant cells characterizing the exocrine pancreas. A surface β-cell-specific marker could be used as a target for tracers for imaging technique, or even as a target for interventions aiming at preserving β-cell mass/function or to monitor the effect of therapies on β-cells.

Antibody-based proteomics is an emerging approach which provides a strategy to explore protein expression patterns on a genome-wide scale [2]. The application of this approach is possible thanks to the Human Protein Atlas (HPA) project which has generated antibodies towards at least one major isoform of all human proteins encoded by the human genome [3]. These antibodies are then used to map protein expression in specific tissues under normal or pathological conditions.

In the present study, the antibody-based proteomic approach allowed the identification of four specific proteins: DGCR2, GBF1, GPR44 and SerpinB10, which all showed β-cell-specific immunoreactivity mainly localized to the plasma membrane in islets. This positivity was found in nondiabetic subjects and in those with diabetes and insulin-positive cells, but not in patients with diabetes and insulin-negative cells.

These results are of note and represent a step forwards in the process of a better characterization of β-cells.

Glycotoxin and autoantibodies are additive environmentally determined predictors of type 1 diabetes: a twin and population study

Beyan H, Riese H, Hawa MI, Beretta G, Davidson HW, Hutton JC, Burger H, Schlosser M, Snieder H, Boehm BO, Leslie RD

Centre for Diabetes and Metabolic Medicine, Blizard Institute, Queen Mary, University of London, London, UK
r.d.g.leslie@qmul.ac.uk

Diabetes 2012;61:1192–1198

Background: In T1D, diabetes-associated autoantibodies, including islet cell antibodies (ICAs), reflect adaptive immunity, while increased serum N^ε-carboxymethyl-lysine (CML), an advanced glycation end product (AGE), is associated with proinflammation. The aim of this study was to investigate whether serum CML and autoantibodies predicted T1D and to what extent they were determined by genetic or environmental factors.

Methods: Of 7,287 unselected screened schoolchildren, 115 were ICA+ and were tested for baseline CML and diabetes autoantibodies and followed (for median 7 years), whereas a random selection (n = 2,102) had CML tested. CML and diabetes autoantibodies were determined in twin pairs discordant for T1D (32 monozygotic, 32 dizygotic pairs).

Results: CML was increased in ICA+ and prediabetic schoolchildren and in diabetic and nondiabetic twins (all p < 0.001). Elevated levels of CML in ICA+ children were a persistent, independent predictor of diabetes progression, in addition to autoantibodies and HLA risk. In a twin model, shared familial environment explained 75% of CML variance, and nonshared environment explained all autoantibody variance.

Conclusions: Serum CML, a glycotoxin, emerged as an environmentally determined diabetes risk factor, in addition to autoimmunity and HLA genetic risk, and a potential therapeutic target.

In search for predictive markers of T1D, the present study assessed the predictive role of an AGE, such as CML, and autoantibodies. Starting with a population-based study, where autoantibody-positive children (ICA+, n 115) were identified and followed for diabetes development, one of the main findings was that not only autoantibodies, but also CML levels, were significantly increased in subjects who went into develop T1D. CML emerged to be an important predictor of T1D, in addition to autoantibodies and HLA predisposition. In addition, it was shown that environmental factors significantly contributed to the variability of both CML and autoantibodies. Interestingly, whereas shared (familial) environmental factors were an important determinant for CML, nonshared environmental factors mainly influenced autoantibodies.

This study adds a further detail to the 'AGE-T1D relationship'. From an original interest in AGEs mainly in relation to the development of vascular complications of diabetes, the focus is now on the role of AGEs in the pathogenesis of T1D. The next step is to understand the mechanisms responsible for increased AGEs, in order to identify a potential target for preventive and therapeutic strategies. Diet is a well-known important source of AGEs. Therefore, early life modifications in diet could represent a potential preventive strategy for T1D.

Mixed chimerism and growth factors augment β-cell regeneration and reverse late-stage type 1 diabetes

Wang M, Racine JJ, Song X, Li X, Nair I, Liu H, Avakian-Mansoorian A, Johnston HF, Liu C, Shen C, Atkinson M, Todorov I, Kandeel F, Forman S, Wilson B, Zeng D
Departments of Diabetes Research and Hematopoietic Cell Transplantation, Beckman Research Institute of City of Hope, Duarte, CA, USA

Sci Transl Med 2012;4:133ra59

Background: Islet transplantation is the only curative therapy for late-stage T1D, but the beneficial effect is limited in its duration, due to the effects of both auto- and alloimmunity. Another important limitation is the shortage of donor islets. The present study tested the effect of combining mixed chimerism with administration of gastrin and epidermal growth factor (EGF). These two strategies are known to be effective when applied individually in new onset by not late stages T1D.

Methods: Induction of mixed chimerism was associated with administration of gastrin and EGF in non-obese diabetic (NOD) mouse model of T1D.

Results: Combination therapy of induced mixed chimerism under a radiation-free nontoxic anti-CD3/CD8 conditioning regimen and administration of gastrin/EGF increased both β-cell neogenesis and replication, resulting in reversal of late-stage T1D in NOD mice.

Conclusions: If successfully translated into humans, this combination therapy could replace islet transplantation as a long-term curative therapy for T1D.

Improvement of islet function in a bioartificial pancreas by enhanced oxygen supply and growth hormone-releasing hormone agonist

Ludwig B, Rotem A, Schmid J, Weir GC, Colton CK, Brendel MD, Neufeld T, Block NL, Yavriyants K, Steffen A, Ludwig S, Chavakis T, Reichel A, Azarov D, Zimermann B, Maimon S, Balyura M, Rozenshtein T, Shabtay N, Vardi P, Bloch K, de Vos P, Schally AV, Bornstein SR, Barkai U
Department of Medicine III, University Hospital Carl Gustav Carus, Dresden, Germany

Proc Natl Acad Sci USA 2012;109:5022–5027

Background: Islet transplantation is a feasible therapeutic alternative for metabolically labile patients with T1D. However, the application of this methodology is still limited by several factors: shortage of donor organs, gradual loss in graft function over time, and chronic need for immunosuppression. In the present study a promising approach to address some of the limitations of islet transplantation was tested.

Methods: A macrochamber specially engineered for islet transplantation was implanted in streptozotocin-induced diabetic rats, in association with pretreatment of islet cells with the growth hormone-releasing hormone (GHRH) agonist JI-36.

Results: A subcutaneous implantable device was created allowing for controlled and adequate oxygen supply and providing immunological protection of donor islets against the host immune system. Pretreatment with the GHRH agonist, JI-36, significantly enhanced graft function by improving glucose tolerance and increasing β-cell insulin reserve and allowed a reduction in the transplanted islet mass required to achieve metabolic control. As a result of hypervascularization of the tissue surrounding the device, no relevant delay in insulin response to glucose changes was observed.

Conclusions: This system opens up a fundamental strategy for therapy of diabetes and may provide a promising avenue for future approaches to xenotransplantation.

Islet transplantation is considered the definitive cure for T1D, through the reconstitution of the pool of β-cells, destroyed by the autoimmune attack. The original very promising results of the Edmonton Protocol generated tremendous excitement over the application of pancreatic islet transplantation as a viable approach to achieve consistent insulin independence in patients with T1D [4]. However, soon after those initial highly promising results, it became clear that this is a treatment still far away from a potential wide application in patients with T1D. One of the main obstacles to overcome is finding 'islet donors'. In addition, it has become evident that islet transplants last only about 3 years. Several factors influence the success of this method, including the need of islets from more than one donor, prolonged immunosuppression therapies, the low rate of survival of transplanted islets, due to the different characteristics of the environment where they are implanted compared to the natural milieu in the pancreas. Therefore, there is ongoing research to overcome these limitations.

In this context, Wang et al. assessed a combination of radiation-free conditioning regimen to induce mixed chimerism associated with administration of growth factors, such as gastrin and EGF, to reverse late stage T1D in nonobese diabetic mice. Through a series of elegant experiments the authors clearly showed that the 'combination of two treatments is definitively better than one'. In animal models, mixed chimerism had already emerged as a valid approach to reverse autoimmunity, and eliminate insulinitis. However, those benefits occur in cases of new-onset diabetes but not in late cases. Similarly, gastrin/EGF can stimulate β-cell regeneration in animal models with new-onset diabetes but not in late-stage T1D. Combination therapy was effective in reversing late-stage diabetes and improved insulin sensitivity, highlighting that during late stages of diabetes it is important not only to control autoimmunity, but also to promote regeneration of β-cells, whose number is very limited at that stage.

Another exciting finding comes from the study by Ludwig et al., where the authors tried to improve oxygenation of encapsulated islets in order to increase their survival. Encapsulated islets are generally used to avoid the attack by the immune system. However, this process can limit oxygenation of transplanted islets and therefore contribute to cell death. In the present study an implantable subcutaneous bioartificial chamber system, specifically created for encapsulated islets, was developed. This system, which is designed for subcutaneous implantation, is minimally invasive and easily retrievable, and provided a good level of oxygenation of the islets, while creating an immune-barrier sufficient to prevent allogeneic immune response. Successful survival of transplanted islets was improved by conditioning of pancreatic islets with a GHRH agonist, given the high expression of receptors for this factor on pancreatic cells. This pretreatment reduced cells apoptosis and preserved β-cell proliferative capacity.

Although both treatments are based on animal studies, they are promising and represent tremendous progresses in the field of islet transplantation.

New concerns 1
Vitamin D and T1D: the prenatal origin of an association

Maternal serum levels of 25-hydroxyvitamin D during pregnancy and risk of type 1 diabetes in the offspring

Sørensen IM, Joner G, Jenum PA, Eskild A, Torjesen PA, Stene LC
Department of Pediatrics, Oslo University Hospital Ullevål, Oslo, Norway
i.m.sorensen@medisin.uio.no
Diabetes 2012;61:175–178

Background: Risk of T1D has been reported to be reduced after intake of vitamin D supplements during pregnancy or early childhood. The aim of this study was to assess whether lower maternal serum concentrations of 25-hydroxyvitamin D (25-OH-D) during pregnancy were associated with an increased risk of T1D in the offspring.

Methods: 25-OH-D levels were measured using a radioimmunoassay on samples from late pregnancy in 109 women delivering a child who developed T1D before 15 years of age (case subjects) and from 219 control women.

Results: There was a trend toward a higher risk of T1D with lower levels of 25-OH-D during pregnancy: the odds of T1D being 2.38 (1.12–5.07) for the offspring of women with the lowest levels of 25-OH-D (first quartile) compared to the offspring of women with levels in the highest quartile.

Conclusion: Reduced maternal 25-OH-D levels increase the risk of developing T1D in the offspring. If these results are confirmed, they could provide support for the initiation of a randomized intervention trial to prevent T1D in children by enhancing maternal 25-OH-D levels during pregnancy.

Over the last years there has been a growing interest in the immunomodulatory effect of vitamin D and in its association with the pathogenesis of autoimmune diseases, such as T1D [5]. Reduced levels of vitamin D have been reported in children and adults with T1D compared to healthy controls. In addition, there have also been studies assessing the potential role of polymorphisms in genes implicated in vitamin D metabolism in the pathogenesis of T1D [6].

This recent study reports an interesting association between reduced maternal serum vitamin D levels and risk of developing T1D in the offspring before the age of 15 years. Levels of vitamin D were reduced in mothers of offspring who developed T1D compared to controls (65.8 vs. 73.1 nmol/l). Of particular note was the finding that children born from women with a 25-OH-D level in the lowest quartile had a risk of developing T1D more than twofold higher than those born from women with a 25-OH-D level in the highest quartile. These findings suggest that vitamin D could influence T1D risk already during prenatal life, by influencing the immune system. In fact, although the exact mechanisms linking reduced vitamin D levels to T1D are not yet completely understood, there is evidence suggesting that vitamin D can enhance immunologic tolerance [7].

These results are of interest given that they provide further support for the potential role of vitamin D in the pathogenesis of T1D and, in the meantime, they confirm the role of environmental factors acting early in life in the pathogenesis of this autoimmune disease. If these results are confirmed by future studies, they could represent the driving force for trials with vitamin D supplementation during pregnancy as a preventive strategy for T1D.

New concerns 2
Secular changes in T1D immunophenotype

Rising incidence of type 1 diabetes is associated with altered immunophenotype at diagnosis

Long AE, Gillespie KM, Rokni S, Bingley PJ, Williams AJ
School of Clinical Sciences, University of Bristol, Bristol, UK
Diabetes 2012;61:683–686

Background: Over the last decades there has been a significant increase in the incidence of T1D in children. The aim of this study was to assess whether this trend is associated with changes in the patterns of humoral islet autoimmunity at diagnosis.

Methods: Autoantibodies to insulin (IAA), GAD (GADA), islet antigen-2 (IA-2A), and zinc transporter 8 (ZnT8A) were measured by radioimmunoassay in sera collected from children and young adults with newly diagnosed T1D between 1985 and 2002. The effect of date at diagnosis on prevalence and levels of these autoantibodies was assessed, with adjustments for age and HLA class II genetic risk.

Results: Over the study period there was a significant increase in the prevalence of IA-2A and ZnT8A together with increased levels of IA-2A, ZnT8A, and IA-2β autoantibodies. In contrast, no significant changes occurred in the prevalence and levels of IAA and GADA.

Conclusions: The increased prevalence and levels of IA-2A, ZnT8A, and IA-2β at diagnosis suggest that the process leading to T1D is now characterized by a more intense humoral autoimmune response.

The increasing incidence in childhood-onset T1D, particularly in younger children, is a worldwide established phenomenon. Changes in environmental factors have been claimed as the major determinant of the rise in T1D cases. Interestingly, there have been observations suggesting that the increasing incidence in T1D is associated with a reduced frequency of high-risk HLA-class II genotypes and a higher prevalence of low-risk genotypes [8].

The intriguing hypothesis tested in the present study was that the rising incidence in T1D could be associated with an altered immunophenotype at diagnosis. Indeed, this was the case, with a detected higher prevalence of autoantibodies, such as IA-2 and ZnT8A, as well as higher levels of these autoantibodies, over time, from 1985 to 2002. These autoantibodies are known to appear after GADA and IAA, whose levels and prevalence did not significantly change over time in this study. This finding along with the increased levels of IA-2βA, among IA-2A-positive patients, suggest a more intense and mature humoral autoimmunity in patients diagnosed during more recent years, which might lead to faster development of the disease in at-risk individuals. The association between date at diagnosis and changes in the immunophenotype was independent of age and HLA genotype. These results suggest the potential effect of changes in the environment and/or lifestyle on the humoral autoimmune response to islet antigens. Identifying the mechanisms underlining this link would help in understanding the rising trend in T1D incidence, and hopefully help in developing new potential preventive strategies.

Important for clinical practice 1
New important result from the landmark DCCT/EDIC studies

Intensive diabetes therapy and glomerular filtration rate in type 1 diabetes

De Boer IH, Sun W, Cleary PA, Lachin JM, Molitch ME, Steffes MW, Zinman B
Kidney Research Institute and Division of Nephrology, University of Washington, Seattle, WA, USA
deboer@u.washington.edu
N Engl J Med 2011;365:2366–2376

Background: An impaired glomerular filtration rate (GFR) leads to end-stage renal disease and increases the risks of cardiovascular disease and death. This study tested the effects of intensive insulin therapy on the development of impaired GFR.

Methods: The Diabetes Control and Complications Trial (DCCT) recruited 1,441 persons with T1D who were randomized to 6.5 years of intensive diabetes therapy or to conventional diabetes therapy. Subsequently, 1,375 participants were followed in the observational Epidemiology of Diabetes Interventions and Complications (EDIC) study. Serum creatinine levels were measured annually during the DCCT and EDIC studies. GFR was estimated with the use of the Chronic Kidney Disease Epidemiology Collaboration formula. Incident impaired GFR was defined as an estimated GFR of <60 ml/min/1.73 m^2 of body surface area at two consecutive study visits.

Results: Over a median follow-up period of 22 years, impaired GFR developed in 24 participants assigned to intensive therapy (IT) and in 46 assigned to conventional therapy (CT) (risk reduction with IT, 50% (95% CI 18–69); p = 0.006). End-stage renal disease developed in 8 participants in the IT group and in 16 in the CT group. IT was associated with a reduction in the mean estimated GFR of 1.7 ml/min/1.73 m^2 during the DCCT study compared to CT, but during the EDIC study was associated with a slower rate of reduction in the GFR and 2.5 ml/min/1.73 m^2 higher mean estimated GFR compared to CT (p < 0.001 for both comparisons). Adjustments for HbA$_{1c}$ or albumin excretion rate completely attenuated the beneficial effect of IT on GFR.

Conclusions: Intensive insulin therapy started early in the course of T1D and when compared with conventional diabetes therapy was associated with a significantly lower risk of impaired GFR.

Impaired GFR is an important risk factor for the progression to end-stage renal disease and for cardiovascular morbidity and mortality in patients with T1D [9]. Over previous years, the DCCT and EDIC studies have provided crucial evidence on the many benefits of good glycemic control, as achieved with an intensive insulin therapy, started early in the course of diabetes, in reducing risk for the development and progression of albuminuria, diabetic retinopathy, neuropathy as well as cardiovascular disease. This publication further adds to those previous findings, by assessing another important endpoint: GFR. Perturbations in GFR are common in patients with T1D, where during early stages hyperfiltration can be the main finding [9], whereas from, or even slightly before, the development of microalbuminuria, there is a progressive decrease in GFR, which can prelude to the stage of renal failure.

Epidemiological studies have shown the adverse prognostic effect of impaired GFR, although until now there has been a lack of long-term longitudinal studies assessing the effect of intensive insulin therapy on GFR. The DCCT/EDIC studies offer a unique source of data with up to 22 years of follow-up. Risk of impaired GFR was reduced by 50% in patients in the intensive treatment group. Similarly, cases of end-stage renal disease, although low in numbers, tended to be lower in the intensive treatment group. The differences in GFR between the two groups were mainly explained by differences in HbA$_{1c}$ and albuminuria. These data reiterate the importance of a strict glycemic control started early in the course of diabetes to prevent renal complications. The DCCT/EDIC data mainly explored the effect of intensive insulin therapy without assessing whether other treatment strategies with ACE inhibitors or other agents could have an additional beneficial effect on GFR. Further studies are required to test that.

Clinic-integrated behavioral intervention for families of youth with type 1 diabetes: randomized clinical trial

Nansel TR, Iannotti RJ, Liu A
Eunice Kennedy Shriver National Institute of Child Health and Human Development, Bethesda, MD, USA
nanselt@mail.nih.gov
Pediatrics 2012;129:e866–873

Background: The aim of this study was to test the effect of a low-intensity, clinic-integrated behavioral intervention for families of youth with T1D, on diabetes management outcomes.
Methods: A 2-year randomized clinical trial of a clinic-integrated behavioral intervention was performed and included 390 families of youth with T1D. The primary outcome was HbA_{1c}, which was measured at each clinic visit and assessed centrally. At each visit, blood glucose meter data were downloaded. In addition, treatment adherence was assessed by using a semistructured interview at baseline, mid-study, and follow-up.
Results: The behavioral intervention was associated with a significant improvement in glycemic control from baseline to 24 months (p = 0.03). A significant intervention by age interaction (p < 0.001) was detected such that whereas among participants aged 12–14 a significant effect on glycemic control was observed (p = 0.009 for change from baseline to 24 months; p =0.035 for mixed-effect model across study duration), no effect was found in youth aged 9–11 years. The intervention did not have any significant effect on child or parent reports of adherence.
Conclusions: The low-intensity clinic-integrated behavioral intervention for families of youth with T1D was effective in preventing the deterioration in glycemic control evident during adolescence, and it might represent a model for integrating medical and behavioral sciences in clinical care.

Diabetes management in youth can be challenging, particularly during adolescence. Diabetes treatment is based on the integration of medical therapies, nutrition as well as psychological and behavioral support for children and their families.

Previous studies had already shown the positive effect of behavioral interventions in improving diabetes management. These interventions include greater parental involvement, monitoring responsibility-sharing, lower family conflicts, greater coping and problem-solving skills. However, an important barrier is the translation of behavioral interventions into standard clinical practice. This requires that behavioral interventions are indeed effective, but also simple and feasible.

The present multicenter study was performed on 390 families of youth with T1D and an age range between 9 and 14.9 years. The behavioral intervention, called WE-CAN (Working together, Exploring barriers, Choosing solutions, Acting on our plan, Noting results), was designed to help families improve diabetes management, and its cardinal feature was that it was delivered to both parents and children. The key points on which it was based were: facilitating problem-solving, communication skills, and responsibility sharing. Specially trained personnel were responsible for the different parts of the intervention program, including pre-visit telephone contact, in-person contact during clinic visits, and follow-up telephone calls. Each session lasted about 30 min and feedback about the sessions was collected by phone in the weeks following clinic visits.

This behavioral intervention was successful in improving glycemic control over the study period. The effect was particularly more evident in adolescents than in younger children. This is an important finding given that management of diabetes is particularly complex during adolescence, when dealing with a chronic condition, such as T1D, needs to fit within the complex hormonal, metabolic and psychological changes of this phase of life. In addition, the beneficial effect observed mainly in adolescents suggests that, as previously shown, intervention strategies can be particularly effective when youth start taking greater responsibility for their diabetes management.

The take-home message of this study is the utility of incorporating a low-intensity behavioral intervention into clinical care in order to improve glycemic control, particularly in adolescents.

Clinical trials, new treatments 1
New insulin on the horizon

Insulin degludec, an ultralong-acting basal insulin, versus insulin glargine in basal-bolus treatment with mealtime insulin aspart in type 1 diabetes (BEGIN basal-bolus type 1): a phase 3, randomized, open-label, treat-to-target noninferiority trial

Heller S, Buse J, Fisher M, Garg S, Marre M, Merker L, Renard E, Russell-Jones D, Philotheou A, Francisco AM, Pei H, Bode B
University of Sheffield, Sheffield, UK
s.heller@sheffi eld.ac.uk

Lancet 2012;379:1489–1497

Background: In patients with T1D, intensive basal-bolus insulin therapy can improve glycemic control and reduce the risk of long-term complications. Insulin degludec is a new ultralong-acting basal insulin. The present study aimed to compare the efficacy and safety of insulin degludec and insulin glargine, both administered once daily with mealtime insulin aspart, in basal-bolus therapy for T1D.

Methods: An open-label, treat-to-target, noninferiority trial, was undertaken at 79 sites in six countries, and recruited adults (aged ≥18 years) with T1D (HbA_{1c} ≤10% (86 mmol/mol)) and who had been treated with basal-bolus insulin for at least 1 year. Participants were randomly assigned in a 3:1 ratio, with a computer-generated blocked allocation sequence, to insulin degludec or insulin glargine. The primary outcome was noninferiority of degludec to glargine, assessed as a reduction in HbA_{1c} after 52 weeks, with the intention-to-treat analysis.

Results: Of 629 participants, 472 were randomly assigned to insulin degludec and 157 to insulin glargine; all were analyzed in their respective treatment groups. After 1 year of treatment, HbA_{1c} declined by 0.40% points (SE 0.03) with insulin degludec and 0.39% points (0.07) with insulin glargine (estimated treatment difference −0.01% points (95% CI −0.14 to 0.11); p < 0.0001 for noninferiority testing). A similar number of participants (40 vs. 43%) achieved a target HbA_{1c} below 7% (<53 mmol/mol). Rates of overall confirmed hypoglycemia (plasma glucose <3.1 mmol/l or severe) were similar in insulin degludec and insulin glargine groups (42.54 vs. 40.18 episodes per patient-year of exposure). The rate of nocturnal confirmed hypoglycemia was 25% lower with degludec than with glargine (4.41 vs. 5.86 episodes per patient-year of exposure; 0.75 (0.59–0.96); p = 0.021). Occurrence of serious adverse events (14 vs. 16 events per 100 patient-years of exposure) was similar for insulin degludec and insulin glargine groups.

Conclusions: Insulin degludec appears to be a useful basal insulin for patients with T1D, providing effective glycemic control and reducing the risk of nocturnal hypoglycemia.

Basal-bolus insulin regimen is the standard approach for patients with T1D. However, this approach is far from perfect in mimicking the physiological endogenous insulin pattern.

A new insulin analogue is now on the horizon and phase 2 trials have already shown promising results. Insulin degludec is a new basal insulin with an amino acid sequence identical to human insulin except for removal of threonine at B30. At B29, a glutamic acid spacer is attached that bridges to a 16-carbon diacid. This new insulin forms soluble multihexamer assemblies after subcutaneous injection, resulting in an ultralong action profile, with a reported half-life >25 h and activity >40 h. These characteristics reduce plasma concentrations and variability and create a flat steady-state profile following a once-daily injection.

In this recent phase 3 trial, designed as a 52-week randomized, controlled, open-label, treat-to-target noninferiority trial, insulin degludec, in combination with prandial insulin aspart, led to similar glycemic control as insulin glargine, but the main study finding was a 25% reduction in nocturnal hypoglycemia associated with insulin degludec. This finding is of note and likely reflects the flatter profile of insulin degludec than glargine.

Nocturnal hypoglycemia is associated with poor quality of sleep, decreased sense of wellbeing, reduced productivity and fatigue. Therefore, reducing nocturnal hypoglycemia could significantly improve quality of life. Asymptomatic episodes of hypoglycemia are very common in children and adolescents, in whom they can reduce counterregulation and thereby increase the risk of subsequent prolonged and severe hypoglycemia, associated occasionally with coma. Therefore, there is a great interest in testing insulin degludec in this age group in order to improve their glycemic control while avoiding episodes of hypoglycemia.

GAD65 antigen therapy in recently diagnosed type 1 diabetes mellitus

Ludvigsson J, Krisky D, Casas R, Battelino T, Castano L, Greening J, Kordonouri O, Otonkoski T, Pozzilli P, Robert JJ, Veeze HJ, Palmer J
Division of Pediatrics, Department of Clinical and Experimental Medicine, Linkoping University, Linkoping, Sweden
johnny.ludvigsson@liu.se
N Engl J Med 2012;366:433–442

Background: The 65-kDa isoform of glutamic acid decarboxylase (GAD65) is a major autoantigen in T1D. This study assessed whether treatment with alum-formulated GAD65 (GAD-alum) can preserve β-cell function in patients with recent-onset T1D.
Methods: The study population included 334 patients with T1D aged between 10 and 20 years, with fasting C-peptide levels >0.3 ng/ml (0.1 nmol/l), and detectable serum GAD65 autoantibodies. Within 3 months after diagnosis, patients were randomly assigned to receive one of three study treatments: four doses of GAD-alum, two doses of GAD-alum followed by two doses of placebo, or four doses of placebo. The primary study outcome was the change in the stimulated serum C-peptide level between the baseline and the 15-month visit. Secondary outcomes were HbA_{1c} level, mean daily insulin dose, rate of hypoglycemia, and fasting and maximum stimulated C-peptide levels.
Results: A similar decline in stimulated C-peptide levels occurred in all the study groups and there was no significant difference in the primary outcome at 15 months between the combined active drug groups and the placebo group (p = 0.10). In addition, there were no differences in insulin dose, HbA_{1c}, hypoglycemic rates between patients treated with GAD-alum and those receiving placebo. Infrequent and mild adverse events occurred with similar rates in the three groups.
Conclusions: Treatment with GAD-alum did not significantly reduce the loss of stimulated C peptide or improve clinical outcomes over a 15-month period in newly diagnosed patients with T1D.

Disappointing results have emerged from the first phase 3 immune intervention trials in T1D, which are partly unexpected, given that phase II trials showed promising results [10].

In the study of Ludvigsson et al., GAD-alum treatment failed to preserve β-cell secretion over time as well as to improve glycemic control. These results were completely different from those from a previous phase II study, where treatment with GAD-alum was associated with a preserved C-peptide at 30 months and preserved stimulated C-peptide at 15 months.

The authors suggest that differences in populations or the larger number of clinicians, with potential different approaches to conventional treatments, involved in the phase III trial could explain these discordant results. Another hypothesis is that the differences in age between the treatment groups, including more subjects aged 10–11 years in the GAD-alum group, could have influenced the study results. In fact, it is well known that C-peptide tends to decline faster in younger subjects. Differences in the time of year (seasonal effect) when treatment was implemented might be another confounding factor, as suggested by the finding of better outcomes in those treated during March-April (when all the phase II subjects had been treated). In addition, during the GAD-alum phase III trial, an influenza epidemic occurred, with an extensive vaccination program, and these phenomena could have influenced the trial results. Overall, this study highlights some important factors to be taken into account in future studies: (1) a better patient stratification might be implemented; (2) longer treatment periods might be required, and (3) more needs to be learnt on the mechanisms implicated in the pathogenesis of T1D in order to implement better treatment strategies. In addition, the lack of success of GAD-alum as well as of other immunotherapy suggests that, like in other complex diseases, more than one intervention directed towards different targets might be needed.

New Mechanisms

Huntingtin-interacting protein 14 is a type 1 diabetes candidate protein regulating insulin secretion and β-cell apoptosis

Berchtold LA, Storling ZM, Ortis F, Lage K, Bang-Berthelsen C, Bergholdt R, Hald J, Brorsson CA, Eizirik DL, Pociot F, Brunak S, Storling J
Hagedorn Research Institute, Gentofte, Denmark

Proc Natl Acad Sci USA 2011;108:E681–688

Background: T1D is a complex disease with a strong genetic component, and several loci are known to increase T1D susceptibility risk, although only few causal genes have currently been identified. To identify disease-causing genes in T1D, an in-silico 'phenome-interactome analysis' on a genome-wide linkage scan dataset was performed.

Methods: A phenome-interactome network analysis on a published T1D genome-wide linkage study revealed 11 genomic regions with linkage to T1D.

Results: A total of 11 genes were predicted to be likely disease genes in T1D, including the INS gene. An unexpected top-scoring candidate gene was huntingtin-interacting protein (HIP)-14/ZDHHC17. Immunohistochemical analysis of pancreatic sections showed that HIP14 is almost exclusively expressed in insulin-positive cells in islets of Langerhans. RNAi knockdown experiments established that HIP14 is an antiapoptotic protein required for β-cell survival and glucose-stimulated insulin secretion. Proinflammatory cytokines, such as IL-1β and IFN-γ, downregulated HIP14 expression in insulin-secreting INS-1 cells and in isolated rat and human islets. Overexpression of HIP14 was associated with a decrease in IL-1β-induced NF-κB activity and protection against IL-1β-mediated apoptosis.

Conclusions: This study highlights that network biology is a valid approach to identify important genes for T1D that represent the basis for more specific and targeted therapeutic approaches.

Genome-wide association studies (GWAS) have identified many genetic variants associated with complex diseases. More than 40 genetic regions have been significantly associated with T1D, however it is not clear which are the causative variants and the specific genes in these regions. The study from Berchtold et al. is an example of the 'post-GWAS' era, when GWAS data are being implemented with other techniques in order to understand the role and function of identified loci.

Using integrative bioinformatics, based on an in-silico 'phenome-interactome network analysis' approach, 11 T1D candidate proteins were identified, including insulin. However, the new finding was the identification of the huntingtin-interacting protein (HIP)-14 protein as a new candidate protein for T1D. This protein emerged to be expressed in β-cells and to play a key role for β-cell survival. Reduced levels of HIP-14 or knockout of HIP-14 in animal models was associated with increased apoptosis of β-cells. Downregulation of HIP-14 emerged to be the potential mechanism mediating cytokine-induced β-cell apoptosis in T1D. Overall, this study demonstrates the value and feasibility of a new approach based on the systematic integration of genetic information with protein-protein interaction data to identify proteins which could become targets for preventive and therapeutic interventions.

Identification of novel type 1 diabetes candidate genes by integrating genome-wide association data, protein-protein interactions, and human pancreatic islet gene expression

Bergholdt R, Brorsson C, Palleja A, Berchtold LA, Floyel T, Bang-Berthelsen CH, Frederiksen KS, Jensen LJ, Storling J, Pociot F
Hagedorn Research Institute, Gentofte, Denmark
Diabetes 2012;61:954–962

Background: Genome-wide association studies (GWAS) have allowed the discovery of more than 40 susceptibility loci for T1D. However, GWAS do not lead to identification of the gene or genes in a given locus associated with disease, and they do not typically give any information on the broader context in which the disease genes operate.
Methods: T1D GWAS data were integrated with protein-protein interactions to construct biological networks of relevance for disease. Expressional profiling in human pancreatic islets exposed to proinflammatory cytokines was performed. Confirmation of new candidate genes was then performed in insulin-secreting INS-1 β-cells.
Results: A total of 17 networks were identified. Three networks were significantly enriched for cytokine-regulated genes and thus likely to play an important role for T1D in pancreatic islets. Eight of the regulated genes (CD83, IFNGR1, IL17RD, TRAF3IP2, IL27RA, PLCG2, MYC1B, and CXCR7) in these networks also contained single nucleotide polymorphisms nominally associated with T1D. The expression and cytokine regulation of these new candidate genes were confirmed in insulin-secreting INS-1 β-cells.
Conclusions: These data provide novel insight on the T1D pathogenesis and thus may provide the basis for the design of novel treatment strategies.

In line with the other study by Berchtold et al., which led to the identification of HIP-14 as being associated with T1D, through a combination of genetic data with protein-protein interaction data, this study used extended GWAS data in order to characterize the role of previously identified T1D loci. Network- or pathway-based approaches have been applied to extend GWAS in other diseases, and they are considered as the next step in the process of GWAS data mining. In the present study, GWAS data were integrated with protein-protein interactions and gene expression in β-cells in order to facilitate a systems-based understanding of the mechanisms implicated in the pathogenesis of T1D. This approach led to the identification of an initial number of 17 networks. Among them, 3 were particularly enriched for genes affected by proinflammatory cytokines in the human islets and included 8 genes containing SNPs associated with T1D. Further studies using similar approaches will further clarify mechanisms implicated in the complex pathogenesis of T1D.

Identification of type 1 diabetes-associated DNA methylation variable positions that precede disease diagnosis

Rakyan VK, Beyan H, Down TA, Hawa MI, Maslau S, Aden D, Daunay A, Busato F, Mein CA, Manfras B, Dias KR, Bell CG, Tost J, Boehm BO, Beck S, Leslie RD
Blizard Institute of Cell and Molecular Science, Barts and The London School of Medicine and Dentistry, Queen Mary University of London, London, UK
v.rakyan@qmul.ac.uk
PLoS Genet 2011;7:e1002300

Background: Monozygotic (MZ) twin pair discordance for childhood-onset T1D is approximately 50%, implicating roles for both genetic and nongenetic factors in the etiology of the disease. The study aim was to test whether epigenetic variation could underlie some of the nongenetic components of T1D etiology.
Methods: An epigenome-wide association study (EWAS) for T1D was performed. Genome-wide DNA methylation profiles of purified CD14+ monocytes (an immune effector cell type relevant to T1D pathogenesis) from 15 T1D-discordant MZ twin pairs were generated.
Results: The EWAS identified 132 different CpG sites, at which intra-MZ pair DNA methylation differences significantly, correlated with the diabetic state, i.e. T1D-associated methylation variable positions (T1D-MVPs). An independent set of T1D-discordant MZ pairs was used to confirm that the T1D-MVPs display statistically significant intra-MZ pair DNA methylation differences in the expected direc-

tion (p = 0.035). In order to establish the temporal origins of the T1D-MVPs, two further EWAS datasets were generated and they showed that, when compared with controls, T1D-MVPs are enriched in singletons both before (p = 0.001) and at (p = 0.015) disease diagnosis, and also in singletons positive for diabetes-associated autoantibodies but disease-free even after 12 years of follow-up (p = 0.0023).

Conclusions: T1D-MVPs appear to arise very early in the etiological process that leads to overt T1D. This EWAS of T1D represents an important contribution toward understanding the etiological role of epigenetic variation in T1D.

Epigenetic modifications represent important changes which are implicated in physiological processes, such as regulation of gene transcription and maintenance of genome integrity [11]. A contribution of epigenetic modifications has also been shown in several human diseases, and these changes can occur early in life.

Monozygotic twins represent a valuable model to dissect the relative contributions of the genetic background from environmental influences in human diseases, and thus to assess the potential contribution of epigenetic changes in the pathogenesis of T1D.

In the present study, 15 T1D discordant MZ twin pairs were recruited to perform an epigenome-wide association study, which revealed the presence of T1D-specific methylation positions, defined T1D-MVPs, in the coaffected cotwins. Interestingly, further analysis in other sets of twins highlighted that some of the identified T1D-MVPs are present both before and after the onset of T1D and even in individuals positive for autoantibodies, but who have not developed diabetes yet. These results suggest that these T1D-MVPs could have a role in the pathogenesis of T1D and not only reflect a marker of the disease, due to their temporal appearance before the onset of T1D. Further studies need to assess whether these changes occur even before the appearance of autoantibodies in order to further clarify their pathogenic role in T1D, and the stage when they act. This study represents an important step forwards in understanding the pathogenesis of T1D and it is a good example of a well-designed epigenetic study, which allowed assessment of the temporal origin of T1D-associated epigenetic variations.

Cesarean section and interferon-induced helicase gene polymorphisms combine to increase childhood type 1 diabetes risk

Bonifacio E, Warncke K, Winkler C, Wallner M, Ziegler AG
Center for Regenerative Therapies, Dresden University of Technology, Dresden, Germany
Diabetes 2011;60:3300–3306

Background: The aim of the study was to investigate the association between cesarean delivery, islet autoimmunity and T1D, and genes involved in T1D susceptibility.

Methods: Cesarean section was examined as a risk factor in 1,650 children born to a parent with T1D and followed from birth for the development of islet autoantibodies and T1D.

Results: Children delivered by cesarean section (n = 495) had a more than twofold higher risk for T1D than children born by vaginal delivery (hazard ratio (HR) 2.5 (95% CI 1.4–4.3); p = 0.001, adjusted HR 2.7; 1.5–5.0; p = 0.001). Cesarean section did not increase the risk for islet autoantibodies (p = 0.6) but was associated with a faster progression to diabetes after the appearance of autoimmunity (p = 0.015). The reported association was detected in children with and without high-risk HLA genotypes. In addition, cesarean section appeared to interact with immune response genes, including CD25 and the interferon-induced helicase 1 gene (IFIH1). With regard to IFH1 genotypes, an increased risk for T1D was only seen in children who were delivered by cesarean section and had T1D-susceptible IFIH1 genotypes (12-year risk 9.1 vs. <3% for all other combinations; p < 0.0001).

Conclusions: The present study suggests that T1D risk modification by cesarean section may be linked to viral responses in the preclinical autoantibody-positive disease phase.

The pathogenesis of T1D is well established to be multifactorial with a contribution of genetic and environmental factors along with their interaction.

Several environmental factors have been investigated. Interestingly, cesarean section has been one of these factors, mainly due to the observation that in parallel with the increasing incidence of T1D, there has been an increasing number of children delivered by cesarean section. A recent meta-analysis including 20 retrospective studies highlighted a 20% increased risk of T1D in children delivered by cesarean section [12]. This association has been explained by the finding that children delivered by cesarean section have altered gut microbiotic composition and immune response. In particular, it seems that the types of bacterial found on the newborn skin are different in those delivered by cesarean as compared to those born by vaginal delivery [13]. This in turn could influence immune responses and susceptibility to autoimmune diseases.

This recent study is based on follow-up of children recruited to the BABYDIAB study, a longitudinal prospective study which recruited around 1,650 children born to a parent with T1D between 1989 and 2000, and has been following them since. Autoantibodies have been measured during follow-up and new cases of diabetes recorded. The risk of developing T1D by age 12 in this cohort was higher in children delivered by cesarean section than in those born by vaginal delivery (4.8 vs. 2.8%). A further assessment was the potential interaction between cesarean section, as an environmental determinant, with the genetic background. Genotypes of four genetic regions, known to be associated with T1D and with the immune response, were assessed: IF1H1, CD25. PTPN22 and HLA class II genes. Interaction was found for CD25 and IFIH1. Interestingly for IF1H1, only children with the combination of the risk genotype and delivered by cesarean section were at higher risk of developing T1D. IFIH1 is known to induce the secretion of immune mediators in response to viral infection, mediators which generally block viral replication and can stimulate expression of MHC complex proteins, which can promote destruction of β-cells.

This study sheds more light on the complex pathogenesis of T1D, mainly highlighting the importance of considering the interaction between environmental factors and the individual genetic background when considering disease risk.

New Genes

The human pancreatic islet transcriptome: expression of candidate genes for type 1 diabetes and the impact of proinflammatory cytokines

Eizirik DL, Sammeth M, Bouckenooghe T, Bottu G, Sisino G, Igoillo-Esteve M, Ortis F, Santin I, Colli ML, Barthson J, Bouwens L, Hughes L, Gregory L, Lunter G, Marselli L, Marchetti P, McCarthy MI, Cnop M
Laboratory of Experimental Medicine, Université Libre de Bruxelles (ULB), Brussels, Belgium
deizirik@ulb.ac.be
PLoS Genet 2012;8:e1002552

Background: T1D is an autoimmune disease in which pancreatic β-cells are destroyed by infiltrating immune cells and by cytokines released by these cells. Signaling events occurring in the pancreatic β-cells are decisive for their survival or death in diabetes.

Methods: RNA sequencing was used to identify transcripts, including splice variants, expressed in human islets of Langerhans under control conditions or following exposure to the proinflammatory cytokines interleukin-1β (IL-1β) and interferon-γ (IFN-γ). In addition, it was assessed whether putative candidate genes for T1D, previously identified by GWAS, are expressed in human islets.

Results: A total of 29,776 transcripts were identified as expressed in human islets. Expression of around 20% of these transcripts was modified by proinflammatory cytokines, including apoptosis- and inflammation-related genes. Chemokines were among the transcripts most modified by cytokines. 35% of the genes expressed in human islets undergo alternative splicing, and cytokines caused substantial changes in spliced transcripts. 25/41 of the candidate genes for T1D were expressed in islets, and cytokines modified expression of several of these transcripts.

Conclusions: The present study doubles the number of known genes expressed in human islets and shows that cytokines modify alternative splicing in human islet cells. A large number of cytokines and chemokines are expressed in β-cells exposed to cytokines and 60% of the known T1D candidate genes are expressed in human islets.

The novelty of this study is the application, for the first time, of whole-genome RNA sequencing, to define all transcripts expressed in human pancreatic islets under basal conditions and following exposure to cytokines.

Whole-genome RNA sequencing is a new tool for transcriptomic studies, which does not require a priori knowledge of the targets. Combined with other tools, it also allows detection of splice variants. Sequencing was performed on RNA from human islets obtained from five organ donors, exposed or not to the proinflammatory cytokines IL-1β and IFN-γ.

This approach allowed the identification of up to 15,200 genes expressed in the pancreas, thus doubling the number of previously known genes. Interestingly, 60% of the candidate genes for T1D were found to be expressed in the pancreas. Another interesting finding was that cytokines can modulate the expression of genes in the pancreas and this happens mainly by modifying alternative splicing in human islets. In addition, pancreatic cells themselves expressed cytokines and chemokines. Altogether these data suggest that there should be a close 'talk' between the immune system and pancreatic β-cells early in the natural history of T1D, leading to insulinitis and subsequent progression to diabetes.

The present study supports the value of whole-genome RNA sequencing for the identification of transcripts of specific cells/organs. In addition, this study provides a valuable dataset which could drive future genetic and functional studies in β-cells.

Reviews

The clinical potential of C-peptide replacement in type 1 diabetes

Wahren J, Kallas A, Sima AA
Department of Molecular Medicine and Surgery, Karolinska Institutet, Stockholm, Sweden
john.wahren@ki.se
Diabetes 2012;61:761–772

This review offers a comprehensive overview on what is known on C-peptide physiology and function.

It is well known that C-peptide fulfills an important function in the synthesis of insulin. However, there is now also extensive evidence highlighting that C-peptide is a hormone with its own effects and ability to bind to cell membranes and activate specific intracellular pathways.

Persistence of C-peptide has been associated with better metabolic control in newly diagnosed patients with T1D. In addition, residual C-peptide is also associated with a reduced risk of diabetic vascular complications. Several studies in animal models of diabetes and early clinical trials in patients with T1D have demonstrated that replacement of C-peptide results in beneficial effects on the diabetes-induced functional and structural abnormalities of peripheral nerves, kidneys, and brain. Based on this evidence, preservation or replacement of C-peptide is one of the key targets of new treatment strategies for improving outcomes in patients with diabetes. The development of long-acting C-peptide will facilitate further clinical trials and determine the potential role of C-peptide in the treatment of T1D.

Advanced glycation end products are direct modulators of β-cell function

Coughlan MT, Yap FY, Tong DC, Andrikopoulos S, Gasser A, Thallas-Bonke V, Webster DE, Miyazaki J, Kay TW, Slattery RM, Kaye DM, Drew BG, Kingwell BA, Fourlanos S, Groop PH, Harrison LC, Kn p M, Forbes JM
Division of Diabetes Complications, Diabetes and Metabolism Division, Baker IDI Heart and Diabetes Institute, Melbourne, Vic., Australia
josephine.forbes@bakeridi.edu.au
Diabetes 2011;60:2523–2532

Background: Advanced glycation end products (AGEs) are known to contribute to aging and chronic diseases. The aim of this study was to investigate whether AGEs also have a role in the development of T1D.
Methods: The effect of AGEs on insulin secretion was assessed in MIN6N8 cells and mouse islets and in vivo in three separate rodent models: AGE-injected or high AGE-fed Sprague-Dawley rats and non-obese diabetic (NODLt) mice. Rodents were also treated with the AGE-lowering agent alagebrium.
Results: β-Cell exposure to AGEs showed several abnormalities, including defects in acute glucose-stimulated insulin secretion, mitochondrial dysfunction characterized by increased superoxide generation, a decline in ATP content, loss of manganese superoxide dismutase (MnSOD) activity, reduced calcium flux, and increased glucose uptake. Interestingly, these abnormalities improved following treatment with alagebrium or with MnSOD adenoviral overexpression. Isolated mouse islets exposed to AGEs showed reduced glucose-stimulated insulin secretion, increased mitochondrial superoxide production, and depletion of ATP content. Again, all these abnormalities ameliorated following treatment with alagebrium or with the SOD mimetic, MnTBAP. In rats, transient or chronic exposure to AGEs caused progressive insulin secretory defects, superoxide generation, and β-cell death and these effects were improved by alagebrium. NODLt mice had increased circulating AGEs in association with an increase in islet mitochondrial superoxide generation, which was prevented by alagebrium, which also reduced the incidence of autoimmune diabetes. AGEs levels were also assessed in children, where they were found to be increased in those at risk of developing T1D compared to nonprogressors.
Conclusions: This study shows that AGEs can directly cause insulin secretory defects, most likely by impairing mitochondrial function, and in this way they may contribute to the development of T1D.

In last year's chapter, we commented on a study by Forbes et al., that reported that polymorphisms in the receptor for the AGEs (AGER) contributed to the susceptibility to T1D [14].

More recently the same group published this new study where the direct effect of AGEs on the development of T1D was investigated. Through a series of elegant in-vivo and in-vitro experiments, the authors convincingly showed that exposure to high levels of AGEs could significantly impair insulin secretion, and this effect was reversed by treatment with an AGEs antagonist. Interestingly, mitochondrial dysfunction, leading to increased oxidative stress, appeared to be a main mediator of AGEs effect on β-cells. However, further studies are required to understand whether oxidative stress is the sole mechanism mediating the negative effect of AGEs on β-cells or there are other mechanisms implicated.

Taken together, the results of the present study are in support of AGEs being implicated in the pathogenesis of T1D and thus being a potential target for new intervention strategies aiming at preserving β-cell function.

References
1. Brom M, Andralojc K, Oyen WJ, Boerman OC, Gotthardt M: Development of radiotracers for the determination of the β-cell mass in vivo. Curr Pharm Des 2010;16:1561–1567.
2. Uhlen M, Ponten F: Antibody-based proteomics for human tissue profiling. Mol Cell Proteomics 2005;4:384–393.
3. Uhlen M, Oksvold P, Fagerberg L, Lundberg E, Jonasson K, Forsberg M, Zwahlen M, Kampf C, Wester K, Hober S, Wernerus H, Bjorling L, Ponten F: Towards a knowledge-based Human Protein Atlas. Nat Biotechnol 2010;28:1248–1250.
4. De Kort H, de Koning EJ, Rabelink TJ, Bruijn JA, Bajema IM: Islet transplantation in type 1 diabetes. BMJ 2011;342:d217.
5. Danescu LG, Levy S, Levy J: Vitamin D and diabetes mellitus. Endocrine 2009;35:11–17.

6. Cooper JD, Smyth DJ, Walker NM, Stevens H, Burren OS, Wallace C, Greissl C, Ramos-Lopez E, Hypponen E, Dunger DB, Spector TD, Ouwehand WH, Wang TJ, Badenhoop K, Todd JA: Inherited variation in vitamin d genes is associated with predisposition to autoimmune disease type 1 diabetes. Diabetes 2011;60:1624–1631.
7. Hewison M: Vitamin D and the immune system: new perspectives on an old theme. Endocrinol Metab Clin North Am 2010;39:365–379.
8. Gillespie KM, Bain SC, Barnett AH, Bingley PJ, Christie MR, Gill GV, Gale EA: The rising incidence of childhood type 1 diabetes and reduced contribution of high-risk HLA haplotypes. Lancet 2004;364:1699–1700.
9. Magee GM, Bilous RW, Cardwell CR, Hunter SJ, Kee F, Fogarty DG: Is hyperfiltration associated with the future risk of developing diabetic nephropathy? A meta-analysis. Diabetologia 2009;52:691–697.
10. Ludvigsson J, Faresjo M, Hjorth M, Axelsson S, Cheramy M, Pihl M, Vaarala O, Forsander G, Ivarsson S, Johansson C, Lindh A, Nilsson NO, Aman J, Ortqvist E, Zerhouni P, Casas R: GAD treatment and insulin secretion in recent-onset type 1 diabetes. N Engl J Med 2008;359:1909–1920.
11. Jaenisch R, Bird A: Epigenetic regulation of gene expression: how the genome integrates intrinsic and environmental signals. Nat Genet 2003;33 Suppl:245–254.
12. Cardwell CR, Stene LC, Joner G, Cinek O, Svensson J, Goldacre MJ, Parslow RC, Pozzilli P, Brigis G, Stoyanov D, Urbonaite B, Sipetic S, Schober E, Ionescu-Tirgoviste C, Devoti G, de Beaufort CE, Buschard K, Patterson CC: Caesarean section is associated with an increased risk of childhood-onset type 1 diabetes mellitus: a meta-analysis of observational studies. Diabetologia 2008;51:726–735.
13. Vehik K, Dabelea D: Why are C-section deliveries linked to childhood type 1 diabetes? Diabetes 2012;61:36–37.
14. Forbes JM, Soderlund J, Yap FY, Knip M, Andrikopoulos S, Ilonen J, Simell O, Veijola R, Sourris KC, Coughlan MT, Forsblom C, Slattery R, Grey ST, Wessman M, Yamamoto H, Bierhaus A, Cooper ME, Groop PH: Receptor for advanced glycation end-products (RAGE) provides a link between genetic susceptibility and environmental factors in type 1 diabetes. Diabetologia 2011;54:1032–1042.

M. Loredana Marcovecchio/Francesco Chiarelli

Obesity and Weight Regulation

Martin Wabitsch, Daniel Tews, Christian Denzer, Anja Moss, Belinda Lennerz,
Julia von Schnurbein and Pamela Fischer-Posovszky

Division of Pediatric Endocrinology and Diabetes, and Endocrine Research Laboratory, Department of
Pediatrics and Adolescent Medicine, University of Ulm, Ulm, Germany

We have been very happy to get 1,669 papers out of our established search strategy in PubMed
which have been saved in our 2012 *Yearbook* EndNote database. We then selected 25 papers which
in our mind have been the most exciting ones.

The highlights in this year's chapter are papers about longitudinal studies of body weight changes in
children and new insights into the long-term risk of childhood obesity, reports about a larger group
of patients with congenital leptin deficiency in Pakistan, several papers on remodeling of white adipose tissue and the biology of brown adipose tissue, and two exciting clinical studies published in the
New England Journal of Medicine: Long-term persistence of hormonal adaptions to weight loss, and
Neighborhoods, obesity, and diabetes – a randomized social experiment.

Thus, this *Yearbook* chapter on obesity and weight regulation covers again a broad research area
ranging from genetics and epigenetics to human social environment.

Recent development in childhood obesity prevalence rates

Evidence that the prevalence of childhood overweight is plateauing: data from nine countries

Olds T, Maher C, Zumin S, Péneau S, Lioret S, Castetbon K, Bellisle, De Wilde J, Hohepa M, Maddison R, Lissner L,
Sjöberg A, Zimmermann M, Aeberli I, Ogden C, Flegal K, Summerbell C
Health and Use of Time Group, University of South Australia, Adelaide, SA, Australia
carol.maher@unisa.edu.au
Int J Pediatr Obes 2011;6:342–349

Background: Especially in developed countries, pediatric obesity has been described as the primary health
problem in children. In the past 15 years increasing prevalence rates for overweight and obesity in children were reported in several states of the Western world as well as in developing countries. However,
during the last few years several countries reported a slowing in the rise of childhood obesity, stagna-
tion, or even a decline. This study assembles evidence from nine countries (Australia, China, England,
France, Netherlands, New Zealand, Sweden, Switzerland, and USA).
Methods: Via literature autoalerts and personal contacts, authors who had recently published or presented plateauing data on childhood obesity were identified and asked to contribute to this paper.
Other publications on prevalence data regarding childhood obesity have not been included. For cross-
country comparison, data from all countries were compiled using the International Obesity Task Force
(IOTF) cut-offs. With linear regression the yearly rate of change in the prevalence rates was calculated.
Results: With the exception of the French INCA1 study (n = 1,017 self-reported data), objectively measured weight and height data from 466,277 children aged 2–19 years could be analyzed. Between 1995
and 2008 a mean (SD) change of +0.00 (0.49)% in overweight and obesity prevalence rates across all
age and sex groups and all countries could be calculated per year. Classified in overweight alone and
obesity alone, the change was +0.01 (0.56)% and –0.01 (0.24)%, respectively. The authors could find
differences in the rates of change according to sex, age, socioeconomic status and ethnicity.

This review article shows high-quality data concerning a plateauing of the rate of childhood overweight and obesity from nine countries. Analyzing 112 reports, the mean (SD) change in prevalence
rates of overweight and obesity was +0.00 (0.49)% per year between 1995 and 2008. In 45% of the
reports (n = 50) the authors found even declines. This leveling off in childhood obesity has also been

reported in Germany, Denmark, Scotland, Greece, Greenland and Russia [1–6]. Additionally, more recent data from the USA showed no further change in prevalence of obesity among US children and adolescents in 2009–2010 compared with 2007–2008 [7].

When comparing gender, the flattening was more marked for girls than for boys. Furthermore, the authors described age-related differences whereby declining prevalence rates were found more in preschool children (age 2–5 or 6) compared to primary school-aged children (6–11 or 12 years) or adolescents (12–19 years). Blüher et al. [8] could also show an age-specific stabilization in prevalence rates in German children with an upward trend for overweight and obesity prevalence rates in older children (8–16 years) compared to a downward trend in younger children (4–7.99 years).

There are a number of possible reasons for this declining trend. Factors in the social and physical environment probably play a role. One hypothesis is that these findings are the results of the cumulative effect of programs for preventing the development of childhood overweight and obesity, i.e. focusing on healthy eating and increased physical activity, initiated several years ago. In the last years, the awareness of this health problem has increased in healthcare professionals, schools, community organizations, industry, and governments which decreased environmental factors contributing to inappropriate weight gain. Another explanation is the saturation equilibrium hypothesis which says that overweight and obesity rates have reached a race- and/or country-specific ceiling.

Despite the globally reported stabilization or decline, the prevalence rates of overweight and obesity in children remain on a high level and represent still a significant health issue. It is also not clear whether the reported stabilization represents a long-term change or is only a temporary finding. Because of this lack of clarity, this stagnating trend and possible causal factors should be further analyzed.

Food for thought

Progression from childhood overweight to adolescent obesity in a large contemporary cohort

Reilly JJ, Bonataki M, Leary SD, Wells JC, Davey-Smith G, Emmett P, Steer C, Ness AR, Sherriff A
University of Glasgow, Division of Developmental Medicine, Yorkhill Hospitals Glasgow, UK
jjr2y@clinmed.gla.ac.uk
Int J Pediatr Obes 2011;6:e138–e143

Background: Overweight during childhood is likely to persist or to progress to obesity in adolescence. This assumption is the basis for obesity prevention programs during childhood. However, there is only limited evidence for this assumption with respect to contemporary children.
Methods: Data from the Avon Longitudinal Study of Parents and Children (ALSPAC, children born in 1991 and 1992), which have been obtained longitudinally over a 6-year period, have been analyzed.
Results: The progression of overweight at the age of 7 years to obesity at the age of 13 years showed an adjusted odds ratio of 18.1 (95% CI 12.8–25.6). Approximately one third of the overweight children at age 7 were obese at age 13 years, one third in the healthy weight range at 13, and the remaining third remained overweight using definitions of overweight and obesity with UK BMI reference data.
Conclusions: This study quantifies the progression of overweight to obesity in a large contemporary cohort of children. The study provides a scientific basis to decide whether the overweight state might be a useful target for future obesity prevention programs. It supports recent expert committee guidelines stating that change in BMI should be monitored in children who are overweight.

Longitudinal study of body weight changes in children: who is gaining and who is losing weight?

Williamson DA, Han H, Johnson WD, Stewart TM, Harsha D
Pennington Biomedical Research Center, Baton Rouge, LA, USA
williada@pbrc.edu
Obesity (Silver Spring) 2011;19:667–670

Background: Studies of temporal changes in obesity in general use a cross-sectional design to determine the prevalence of overweight and obesity at different time points. In several countries the well-known rise in the prevalence of childhood obesity has subsided. The aim of this study was to longitudinally assess the changes in body weight and body fat across a period of 28 months in a cohort of children who did not participate in a prevention trial and did not undergo extensive outcome assessment.
Methods: A total of 612 children in the 4th to 6th grades have been enrolled (10 schools, rural communities of Louisiana, USA). The follow-up investigation at month 28 could be performed in 74% of the children. Body fat was estimated by a body impedance analysis. The IOTF classification system was used to define overweight and obesity.
Results: Higher BMI percentile scores and percent body fat at baseline were associated with larger decreases in BMI and percent body fat after 28 months. Children with lower BMI percentiles at baseline tended to gain weight and children with higher BMI percentiles at baseline tended to lose weight. Similar findings were observed for changes in percent body fat. When these data were analyzed as cross-sectional studies, prevalence was found to be stable over the 28-month study period because incidence and remission rates were similar.
Conclusions: The results of this study suggest that children who are not overweight tend to gain weight whereas overweight children tend to lose weight as they grow older.

The effectiveness of childhood obesity prevention programs aimed at overweight children was highlighted in the most recent *Cochrane Review* [9]. There is however a yet insufficient evidence base of well-controlled studies with a meaningful long-term follow-up and there is a lack of studies providing an economic evaluation.

A recent systematic review concluded that overweight in childhood was likely to persist or to progress to obesity [10]. However, the evidence summarized in this review was limited in quantity, and was of limited generalizability to contemporary children. Most of the studies included children born before the 1980s.

On the one side, the study of Reilly et al. showed that the risk of obesity was 18–20 times higher for the overweight child at the age of 7 years compared with a normal weight child at the same age. However, on the other side, the absolute risk of obesity development for overweight children was lower than might have been expected (only one third).

The study of Williamson et al. shows that the prevalence of overweight and obesity might remain stable over time in cross-sectional studies although a significant number of normal weight children became overweight (incidence 13.1%) and a significant number of children became obese (incidence 4.3%). The differences in findings from longitudinal and cross-sectional perspectives illustrate how the two research designs can lead to very different conclusions and reinforce the utility of long-term research designs.

The results of both studies support recent expert committee guidelines [11–13] which strongly support that BMI should be monitored regularly in children over time. Longitudinal studies of weight changes in large nationally representative samples in a variety of countries are needed.

Childhood adiposity, adult adiposity, and cardiovascular risk factors

Juonala M, Magnussen CG, Berenson GS, Venn A, Burns TL, Sabin MA, Srinivasan SR, Daniels SR, Davis PH, Chen W, Sun C, Cheung M, Viikari JSA, Dwyer T, Raitakari OT
Department of Medicine, Turku University Hospital, Turku, Finland
mataju@utu.fi
N Engl J Med 2011;365:1876–1885

Background: There is accumulating evidence that cardiovascular risk factors associated with childhood obesity track into adulthood. Currently, the contribution of childhood overweight and obesity to cardiovascular risk in adulthood independent of adult BMI has not been clearly established.

Methods: Combined analysis of data from four prospective cohort studies (Bogalusa Heart Study, Muscatine Study (both USA), Childhood Determinants of Adult Health (Australia), and the Cardiovascular Risk in Young Finns Study (Finland) that measured childhood and adult BMI. For comparison of outcomes, study participants were categorized in four groups: group I included subjects with normal BMI in childhood and adulthood, group II consisted of subjects who were obese in childhood and nonobese as adults, group III those who were obese in childhood as well as in adulthood, and group IV entailed those who were normal weight in childhood and became obese in adulthood. Defined study outcomes were the presence of type 2 diabetes, hypertension, dyslipidemia, and increased intima media thickness (IMT).

Results: For analysis, data from 6,328 subjects with a mean length of follow-up of 23.1 ± 3.3 years were available. Subjects with persisting high BMI from childhood to adulthood (group III) and subjects who became obese as adults (group IV) had significantly elevated relative risks for type 2 diabetes (RR 5.4 (III), RR 4.5 (IV)), hypertension (RR 2.7 (III), RR 2.1 (IV)), high-risk LDL cholesterol (RR 1.8 (III), RR 1.5 (IV)), high-risk HDL cholesterol (RR 2.1 (III), RR 2.2 (IV)), high-risk triglycerides (RR 3.0 (III), RR 3.2 (IV)), and high-risk IMT (RR 1.7 (III), RR 1.5 (IV)) compared to subjects who had a consistently normal BMI (group I). The relative risks for adverse cardiovascular outcomes in subjects who were obese in childhood and nonobese in adulthood (group II) were comparable to the relative risks in group I.

Conclusions: Decreasing obesity between childhood and adulthood is associated with significant reductions in the relative risk for type 2 diabetes, hypertension, dyslipidemia, and increased intima media thickness in adulthood.

Adolescent BMI trajectory and risk of diabetes versus coronary disease

Tirosh A, Shai I, Afek A, Dubnov-Raz G, Ayalon N, Gordon B, Derazne E, Tzur D, Shamis A, Vinker S, Rudich A
Division of Endocrinology, Diabetes, and Hypertension, Brigham and Women's Hospital, Boston, MA, USA
atirosh@partners.org
N Engl J Med 2011;364:1315–1325

Background: Obesity in adulthood is a major risk factor for the development of type 2 diabetes and coronary heart disease. The impact of BMI trajectory from adolescence to adulthood on obesity-related diseases remains to be elucidated.

Methods: This is a prospective study of 37,674 young men followed from the age of 17 years in regular intervals through the Staff Periodic Examination Center of the Israeli Army Medical Corps. Defined outcomes were the presence of type 2 diabetes, or the diagnosis of coronary heart disease defined as angiography-proven stenosis of more than 50% in at least one coronary artery.

Results: Data from study participants were available of a mean follow-up period of 17.4 ± 7.4 years, representing approximately 650,000 person-years. Adolescent BMI at age 17 predicted type 2 diabetes (hazard ratio 2.76, highest vs. lowest BMI decile) and coronary heart disease (hazard ratio 5.43, highest vs. lowest BMI decile) in midlife adjusted for age, blood pressure, sedentary behavior, smoking, family history and a range of biomarkers for cardiovascular risk. Further adjustment for the confounding effect of adult BMI removed the association of adolescent BMI with type 2 diabetes in adulthood (hazard ratio 1.01), but the increased risk for coronary heart disease still remained significant (hazard ratio 6.85). Furthermore, both BMI in adolescence and BMI in adulthood were independently associated with an increased risk for angiography-proven coronary heart disease.

Conclusions: The risk of coronary heart disease in midlife is associated with an elevated BMI in adolescence. This association holds true even for BMI levels in adolescence considered to be in the normal range.

Long-term impact of overweight and obesity in childhood and adolescence on morbidity and premature mortality in adulthood: systematic review

Reilly JJ, Kelly J
University of Glasgow Faculty of Medicine, Yorkhill Hospital, Glasgow, UK
jjr2y@clinmed.gla.ac.uk
Int J Obes (Lond) 2011;35:891–898

Background: Over the last years a fair number of studies have been conducted examining the associations of obesity in childhood and adolescence with morbidity and premature mortality in adulthood. Lacking was a systematic review of the recent published evidence.

Methods: A systematic review of the literature was carried out comprising studies published between January 2002 and June 2010. Studies were eligible for inclusion in the review if they reported a measure of exposure to overweight or obesity in childhood or adolescence and data on morbidity or mortality as outcomes in adulthood. Studies reporting risk factors or surrogate markers of cardiovascular risk in adulthood were excluded.

Results: From an initial search result of 8,535 papers, 28 were identified reporting data on premature mortality in adulthood (8 papers), cardiovascular or metabolic comorbidities (11 papers), and other adverse outcomes (disability, cancer) associated with childhood obesity. Reported hazard ratios for premature mortality in adulthood ranged from 1.4 to 2.9. Only 1 of 8 studies did not find an increased adult mortality. Childhood obesity was uniformly associated with increased hazard ratios for the risk of diabetes, hypertension, coronary heart disease, and stroke (range 1.1–5.1) across 11 eligible studies. A further 9 studies were identified reporting a variety of outcome measures including increased cancer risk (5 studies), disability (2 studies), asthma and atopy (1 study), and polycystic ovary syndrome (1 study) in adulthood.

Conclusions: Recently published evidence demonstrates a substantial adverse impact of overweight and obesity in childhood and adolescence on long-term morbidity and mortality.

The obesity epidemic has now been a major concern for healthcare service providers and policymakers for almost two decades. Often driven by vast media coverage, the threat of childhood obesity to our healthcare systems has been a major focus of the public perception. Remarkably, the interaction of BMI in childhood and adolescence and BMI in adulthood on the risk of future disease has not been well established. In 2011, two landmark studies published in the *New England Journal of Medicine* by Juonala et al. and Tirosh et al. now further our knowledge on the differential impact of childhood versus adult obesity on established cardiovascular risk factors and cardiovascular endpoints.

First, in a pooled analysis of the datasets of four seminal cohort studies, Juonala et al. find a markedly increased cardiovascular risk associated with childhood overweight and obesity. Except for high-risk triglycerides, subjects with a consistently elevated BMI from childhood to adulthood had the most pronounced risk for adverse cardiovascular outcomes, closely followed by those who had a normal BMI during childhood and became obese as adults. However, the most important result of this analysis is the finding of a complete attenuation of the excess cardiometabolic risk by normalization of weight status between childhood and adulthood.

Second, investigating an impressively large database of the Israeli Armed Forces, Tirosh et al. demonstrate that the risk of type 2 diabetes in adulthood depends mainly on adult BMI but not on adolescent BMI. Contrasting this finding, and warranting interesting insight into the age- and time-dependent evolution of different pathophysiological routes to cardiovascular disease, the same study found independent associations of adolescent BMI and adult BMI with angiography-proven coronary heart disease (CHD). In fact, adjusted for a wide array of potential confounders including adult BMI, the risk for clinical CHD in adulthood was elevated sevenfold for adolescents in the highest BMI decile compared to adolescents in the lowest BMI decile. The average BMI trajectories between ages 17 and 45 years for subjects later affected by diabetes or coronary heart disease ranged between the 50th and 75th percentiles of the entire cohort. These results underscore the importance of BMI for the long-term health consequences and will surely refuel the ongoing debate on 'healthy' BMI ranges.

Third, and completing the picture, Reilly and Kelly provide a comprehensive review of recently published studies on this topic. Compared to the last systematic review in 2003 [14], which only found convincing evidence for the tracking of obesity from childhood into adulthood, the authors now present a considerable body of evidence on the relationships between childhood obesity and morbidity and mortality in later life. Childhood obesity was associated with consistently elevated risks for premature mortality, type 2 diabetes, hypertension, coronary heart disease, stroke, polycystic ovary syndrome, cancer (especially breast cancer), and atopy.

Programming and epigenetics

Epigenetic gene promoter methylation at birth is associated with child's later adiposity

Godfrey KM, Sheppard A, Gluckman PD, Lillycrop KA, Burdge GC, McLean C, Rodford J, Slater-Jefferies JL, Garratt E, Crozier SR, Starling Emerald B, Gale CR, Inskip HM, Cooper C, Hanson MA
Institute of Developmental Sciences, Southampton University Hospitals, MRC Lifecourse Epidemiology Unit, NIHR Nutrition, Diet and Lifestyle Biomedical Research Unit, University of Southampton, Southampton, UK
kmg@mrc.soton.ac.uk

Diabetes 2011;60:1528–1534

Background: Genome-wide association studies suggest that fixed genetic variation makes a relatively small contribution to the risk for obesity development. Animal studies as well as epidemiological data provide evidence that perinatal factors have an important influence on obesity development possibly due to epigenetic changes.

Methods: The methylation status of CpGs in the promotors of candidate genes in DNA extracted from umbilical cord tissue obtained at birth was analyzed using Sequenom MassARRAY.

Results: In cohort 1, retinoid X receptor-α (RXRA) chr9: 136355885+ and endothelial nitric oxide synthase (eNOS) chr7: 150315553+ methylation were independently positively associated with gender-adjusted childhood fat mass at the age of 9 years (measured by DEXA), and explained >25% of the variance in childhood adiposity. Higher methylation of RXRA chr9: 136355885+ was associated with lower maternal carbohydrate intake in early pregnancy. The association between fat mass and methylation status was confirmed for RXRA chr9: 136355885+ in a second cohort.

Conclusions: This study provides novel evidence for the importance of the developmental contribution to the growth of body fat mass. The methylation status of RXRA chr9: 136355885+ measured at birth seems to have a strong influence on fat mass development in later childhood.

These are exciting results in humans showing that the epigenetic gene promoter methylation at birth influences the development of body fat mass during childhood. Evidence for perinatal factors in programming metabolism and also body fat mass development during later life has been established in animal studies and was previously only suggested for humans on the basis of epidemiological findings, e.g. famine during pregnancy is associated with obesity in adult offspring [15]. Epigenetic processes such as DNA methylation and histone modifications allow environmental factors to modulate gene transcription. Many of these changes are then stable throughout the life course [16]. Although epigenetic processes operating in perinatal life have been implicated in the origins of obesity, there is yet no direct evidence for this proposition in humans.

The results of this study also indicate a potential mechanistic pathway involved, because induction of transcription by RXRA is dependent on its binding to ligands including the peroxisome proliferator-activated receptors involved in insulin sensitivity, adipogenesis, and fat metabolism.

The findings of this study raise the possibility that the developmental environment and the resulting epigenetic changes may be equally or even more important than germline genetic variations in their contribution to the risk of obesity.

Leptin deficiency and leptin gene mutations in obese children from Pakistan

Fatima W, Shahid A, Imran M, Manzoor J, Hasnain S, Rana S, Mahmood S
Department of Human Genetics and Molecular Biology, University of Health Sciences, Lahore, Pakistan
Sqb_medgen@yahoo.com
Int J Pediatr Obes 2011;6:419–427

Background: Congenital leptin deficiency is an extremely rare monogenetic cause for infant obesity. Nearly half of the known patients have a Pakistani background and carry the same homozygous mutation ΔG133 in the leptin gene.

Methods: A cohort of 25 extremely obese Pakistani children was screened for leptin levels. In all patients with low levels of leptin, leptin gene sequencing was performed.

Results: Low or undetectable leptin levels were found in 9 children. Seven were homozygous for the ΔG133 mutation. The other 2 children carried novel homozygous mutations (c.481_482delCT and c.104_106delTCA).

Conclusion: The ΔG133 mutation appears to be a founder mutation in Pakistan.

High prevalence of leptin and melanocortin-4 receptor gene mutations in children with severe obesity from Pakistani consanguineous families

Saeed S, Butt TA, Anwer M, Arslan M, Froguel P
Department of Genomics of Common Disease, Imperial College London, London, UK
s.saeed08@imperial.ac.uk
Mol Genet Metab 2012;106:121–126

Background: Since Pakistan has a very high rate of consanguinity, a significantly higher incidence of monogenic obesity is expected in this population.

Methods: 62 unrelated obese Pakistani children of consanguineous parents were screened for mutations in the coding regions of the leptin gene (LEP) and the melanocortin-4 receptor (MC4R) gene

Results: LEP mutations were found in 16.1% of the children. Of these, 9 children were homozygous for the ΔG133 mutation, and 1 child had a novel homozygous mutation involving a deletion of 3 base pairs (I35del). In addition, homozygous MC4R mutations, M161T and I316S, were identified in 2 subjects.

Conclusion: In this consanguineous population, up to 20% of childhood obesity is caused by monogenetic forms of obesity.

These two and the following article by Niard et al. all have in common that they challenge our current beliefs on leptin. The adipocyte-derived hormone leptin is one of the key factors regulating weight both in mammals and in human beings. Apart from gross obesity mainly due to hyperphagia, leptin deficiency and resistance also lead to a number of neuroendocrine and metabolic changes.

Before the two articles above were published, only 15 patients with leptin deficiency had been identified worldwide [17–25]. Since nearly half of these patients have a Pakistani background and carry the ΔG133 mutation, it has been suggested that this might be a founder mutation in Pakistan. Both the articles by Fatima et al. and Saeed et al. prove this assumption to be right. Still it is surprising that within their fairly small samples they found such a high number of affected children (28 and 15% respectively). Even more astonishing though is the fact that each group discovered new homozygous leptin gene mutations. For the two mutations found by Fatima et al., it still has to be proven that they are functionally relevant. Both affected children were morbidly obese and had low leptin levels, but as they were only 7 and 18 months old at the time of the screening, their low leptin levels might still be physiological. However, if all three novel gene changes are true mutations we have to ask ourselves why there is such a high number of leptin gene mutations in Pakistan since, despite massive research efforts, no others have been found in other regions of the world, even within consanguineous populations [26]. It is tempting to speculate that the heterozygous state might confer some advantage in a region with recurrent food shortages.

Pregnancy in a woman with a leptin-receptor mutation

Nizard J, Dommergue M, Clément K
Hôpital Pitié-Salpêtrière, Paris, France
karine.clement@psl.aphp.fr
N Engl J Med 2012;366:1064–1065

Background: Human leptin deficiency and resistance have been shown to lead to a severely delayed puberty with irregular menses in women. So far, no pregnancy has been reported in patients with these rare diseases.
Case Report: A patient with a homozygous leptin receptor gene mutation and morbid obesity showed a delayed puberty with irregular cycles after the age of 17 years. A gastric bypass was performed at 24 years of age, leading to a BMI decrease from 81 to 62 kg/m^2.
Results: Two years after gastric bypass the patient became pregnant. After a normal pregnancy she delivered a healthy normal weight son in the 38th gestational week.
Conclusion: Apparently, in humans leptin function is not essential for reproduction.

The most profound neuroendocrine disturbance in mice with homozygous mutations in the leptin receptor gene (*db/db* mice) or in the leptin gene (*ob/ob* mice) [27] is infertility. Until now, it was also assumed that without leptin action humans are not able to reproduce. This described pregnancy in a woman with a homozygous leptin receptor mutation therefore challenges our current knowledge on leptin action. Three possible explanations can be postulated for this unexpected event.

The first explanation for the patient's fertility might be her weight loss. Here we find a connection to the mouse model since male (but not female) *ob/ob* mice become fertile if kept on a severely restricted diet [28]. Another explanation is more complex yet very interesting. There is some evidence that the main effect of leptin is on the timing of maturation of the hypothalamic-pituitary-gonadal axis, rather than on its subsequent function. Patients with leptin deficiency or resistance show hypogonadotropic hypogonadism during adolescence [25, 26, 29], which normalizes rapidly under leptin substitution in those with leptin deficiency [30]. However, even without leptin substitution, patients with leptin deficiency or leptin resistance develop a spontaneous if severely delayed puberty and show normal LH/FSH secretion in adulthood [21, 26, 29]. That a woman with leptin receptor deficiency can become pregnant is consistent with this overall picture.

Leptin has no direct effect on gonadotropin-releasing hormone (GnRh) neurons since those do not express leptin receptors. Therefore other factors must translate the impact of leptin on GnRH secretion. Immediate downstream mediators of leptin include α-MSH and agouti-related peptide. Leptin increases α-MSH secretion, which stimulates MC4R and lowers agouti-related peptide secretion which inhibits MC4R leptin deficiency or resistance leads to an inhibition of MC4R because agouti-related peptide rises. Two very recent studies in *db/db* [31] and *ob/ob* [32] mice showed that ablation of agouti-related protein [31, 32] or heterozygosity of MC4R [31] restores fertility in these mice. Ablation of agouti-related peptide reverses the MC4R inhibition triggered by leptin deficiency or resistance. Also, heterozygosity of MC4R reduces the influence of an inhibited MC4R. Since homozygous or heterozygous MC4R mutations do not lead to changes in pubertal development or fertility either in mice or in humans, MC4R cannot confer a permissive effect of leptin on pubertal development. However, the experiments show that inhibition of MC4R due to leptin deficiency inhibits pubertal development and fertility and an ablation of this inhibition restores fertility. Therefore, a heterozygous MC4R mutation in the above-described patient could also explain the unexpected pregnancy.

Leptin modulated changes in adipose tissue protein expression in *ob/ob* mice

Zhang W, Ambati S, Della-Fera MA, Choi YH, Baile CA, Andacht TM
Department of Animal and Dairy Science, Department of Foods and Nutrition, Proteomics Resource Facility,
Integrated Biotechnology Laboratories, University of Georgia, Athens, GA, USA
cbaile@uga.edu
Obesity 2011;19:255–261

Background: The satiety hormone leptin is produced from adipocytes. It exerts its functions in the central nervous systems regulating food intake and energy expenditure. Leptin-deficient *ob/ob* mice rapidly lose their body fat upon treatment with recombinant leptin. This effect is mainly due to a decrease in food intake. There is increasing evidence that the loss of adipose tissue is also mediated at least in part by apoptosis of fat cells. The aim of this study was to elucidate how subcutaneous infusion of leptin changes the expression profile of adipose tissue in *ob/ob* mice in order to learn how peripheral actions of the hormone might contribute to weight loss.
Methods: Leptin was administered to *ob/ob* mice by osmotic minipumps (0 vs. 10 µg/day for 14 days). Adipose tissues were subjected to two-dimensional gel electrophoresis, MALDI-TOF MS and real-time RT-PCR.
Results: Leptin-treated mice had significantly lower fat pad weights compared to vehicle-treated control animals. Twelve protein groups were differentially expressed in adipose tissues in both groups including chaperones and redox proteins (e.g. calreticulin, prohibitin, peroxiredoxin-6), and cytoskeleton proteins (β-actin, desmin, α-tubulin). These findings were confirmed on the mRNA level.
Conclusions: The authors conclude that the effects of leptin on adipose tissue might be mediated by changes in expression on chaperones and redox proteins, which regulate endoplasmatic reticulum stress, and cytoskeletal proteins, which regulate mitochondrial morphology.

Patients with congenital leptin deficiency suffer from morbid obesity resulting from severe hyperphagia. Upon treatment with recombinant leptin, their body weight decreases and adipose tissue depots rapidly shrink. Suppression of hyperphagia and normalization of food intake via central nervous mechanisms are mainly responsible for the weight loss, but also increased energy expenditure might play a role here. In *ob/ob* mice leptin treatment led to an increase of lipid mobilization and white adipocytes seem to be converted into lipid-oxidizing cells. Most interestingly, the rapid loss of fat mass led was mediated by apoptosis of fat cells, once more demonstrated in this study.

The important finding of this study is that treatment with leptin targets the expression profile of adipose tissue. However, whether leptin is directly acting on adipocytes, whether its effects are mediated via the central nervous system, or whether its effects are secondary to weight loss remain unanswered.

Remodeling of white adipose tissue

Adipose tissue remodeling in children: the link between collagen deposition and age-related adipocyte growth

Tam CS, Tordjman J, Divoux A, Baur LA, Clément K
Institute of Endocrinology and Diabetes (C.S.T.), The Children's Hospital at Westmead, and Discipline of Paediatrics and Child Health (C.S.T., L.A.B.), The Children's Hospital at Westmead Clinical School, University of Sydney, Westmead, N.S.W., Australia; Institute of Cardiometabolism and Nutrition (C.S.T., J.T., A.D., K.C.), Institut National de la Santé et de la Recherche Médicale, Unité 872, Nutriomique; Université Pierre et Marie Curie-Paris 6 (C.S.T., J.T., A.D., K.C.), Centre de Recherche des Cordeliers, Unité Mixte de Recherche en Santé 872, and Assistance Publique-Hôpitaux de Paris (K.C.), Pitié-Salpêtrière Hospital, Nutrition Division, Paris, France
charmaine.tam@pbrc.edu
J Clin Endocrinol Metab 2011;97:1320–1327

Background: Remodeling of the extracellular matrix (ECM) is important for adipose tissue growth and expansion. The aim of this study was to investigate if ECM remodeling plays a role in adipose tissue of healthy, growing children.

Methods: Subcutaneous adipose tissue biopsies were taken from 65 healthy children. Immunohistochemistry and qPCR was performed to study collagen, macrophages and T cells.

Results: Normal weight children had significantly more total collagen than overweight children. Adipocyte size was negatively correlated with total and pericellular collagen, but positively correlated with the percentage of macrophages. The percentage of total collagen was inversely associated with BMI Z-score and age. Older children (>11 years) in the top BMI Z tertile had less collagen (3.8%) than younger (2–5 years) children in the bottom BMI Z tertile (12.6%). There was no evidence of crown-like structures or T-cell infiltration into adipose tissue in children.

Conclusions: Increased collagen in adipose tissue is associated with decreased fat cell size and BMI Z-score and increased anti-inflammatory M2 macrophages in healthy, growing children. This suggests a dynamic interaction between immune cells and ECM remodeling even at an early age.

Subcutaneous adipose tissue remodeling during the initial phase of weight gain induced by overfeeding in humans

Alligier M, Meugnier E, Debard C, Lambert-Porcheron S, Chanseaume E, Sothier M, Loizon E, Hssain AA, Brozek J, Scoazec JY, Morio B, Vidal H, Laville M

Institut National de la Santé et de la Recherche Médicale Unit 1060, CarMeN Laboratory and Centre Européen Nutrition Santé, Lyon 1 University, Oullins, France
Hubert.vidal@univ-lyon1.fr; Martine.laville@chu-lyon.fr

J Clin Endocrinol Metab 2012;97:E183–192

Background: Adipose tissue remodeling plays an important role during weight gain. The aim of this study was to elucidate molecular pathways involved in adipose tissue remodeling during the initial phase of weight gain.

Methods: 44 healthy men received a lipid-enriched diet (+760 kcal/day) for 2 months. Subcutaneous abdominal adipose tissue biopsies were taken und subjected to histology and transcriptomics at baseline, after 2 weeks and after 2 months.

Results: Significant weight gain occurred on overfeeding. Gene expression patterns in adipose tissue were altered with an upregulation of genes related to lipid metabolism and storage, angiogenesis and matrix remodeling. There was increased microvascular density and connective tissue deposition, but no change in adipose tissue inflammation. Induction of the renin-angiotensin system as well as inhibition of Wnt pathway might be implicated in the observed remodeling processes.

Conclusions: Molecular changes during the early phase of weight gain in humans were identified. The identified pathways might provide potential targets for the treatment of pathological adipose tissue development as seen in obesity.

Adipose tissue represents the major store for energy in the body and as such has an almost unlimited capacity to expand. The cellular response to changes in energy intake involves tightly coordinated remodeling processes.

The paper of Tam et al. demonstrates that remodeling of the extracellular matrix occurs during growth and expansion of healthy children. Several animal models of genetic and diet-induced obesity have demonstrated that increasing fat mass leads to an acceleration of remodeling and subsequently to development of fibrosis. Allgier et al. performed a clinical study in humans to elucidate if diet-induced obesity in fact induces adipose tissue remodeling and fibrosis in humans. As expected, genes involved in ECM remodeling, angiogenesis, inflammation and lipid metabolism were most prominently altered. These pathways and genes represent promising targets to correct the fibrotic/inflammatory orchestration of remodeling processes in obesity.

A PGC1-α-dependent myokine that drives brown-fat-like development of white fat and thermogenesis

Boström P, Wu J, Jedrychowski MP, Korde A, Ye L, Lo JC, Rasbach KA, Boström EA, Choi JH, Long JZ, Kajimura S, Zingaretti MC, Vind BF, Tu H, Cinti S, Højlund K, Gygi SP, Spiegelman BM
Dana-Farber Cancer Institute and Harvard Medical School, Boston, MA, USA
bruce_spiegelman@dfci.harvard.edu
Nature 2012;481:463–468

Introduction: PGC1-α is a transcriptional coactivator which drives many biological pathways related to energy metabolism. Originally described as a modulator of uncoupling protein 1 (UCP-1) expression in brown adipocytes, it has been shown to stimulate mitochondrial biogenesis, angiogenesis and fiber-type switching in exercised muscle. Transgenic mice overexpressing PGC1-α in muscle are resistant to age-related obesity, suggesting the presence of a muscle-secreted factor which affects other tissues.

Methods: The authors used a transgenic mouse model overexpressing PGC1-α in skeletal muscle to investigate PGC1-α effects on energy metabolism and brown adipose tissue recruitment.

Results: Enhanced expression of PGC1-α in muscle stimulates an increase in expression of FNDC5, a membrane protein that is cleaved and secreted as a newly identified hormone, termed irisin. Irisin induces UCP-1 expression and a broad program of brown-fat-like development in white adipocytes in vitro. Furthermore, it is induced with exercise in mice and humans, and the authors could show that mildly increased irisin levels in the blood cause an increase in energy expenditure in mice with no changes in movement or food intake.

Conclusion: The authors conclude that irisin could be therapeutic for human metabolic disease and other disorders that are improved with exercise.

Brown adipose tissue is present and active in adult humans and first evidence has shown that this tissue is involved in cold-induced non-shivering thermogenesis in the human body [33]. In this study, Boström et al. discovered a novel hormone which acts as a chemical messenger between muscle and adipose tissue and has significant impact on brown fat recruitment and energy metabolism. This study elegantly demonstrates the impact of physical exercise on the recruitment of brown adipocytes.

The work group of Paul Spiegelman identified a novel myokine called 'irisin' during a search for genes regulated by PGC1-α. After physical exercise, it is secreted from the muscle into the bloodstream by proteolytic cleavage of its precursor FNDC5 – a type I membrane protein. When irisin levels rise, the hormone acts directly on white adipose tissue by inducing the formation of brown adipocytes. When administered during adipogenic differentiation of primary preadipocytes, FNDC5 induced key molecules of brown adipocytes in vitro. This was accompanied by an increase in oxygen consumption. Overexpression of FNDC5 in mice leads to enhanced irisin plasma levels and the formation of brown adipocyte islets in white adipose tissue. Along with the induction of brown fat recruitment, irisin improved glucose tolerance and reduced fasting insulin in mice fed a high-fat diet.

This discovery might be a first step in understanding the biological mechanisms that translate physical exercise into beneficial changes throughout the body, both in healthy people and in preventing or treating obesity and type 2 diabetes mellitus. This definitely will lead to further attempts to develop strategies to use irisin as an antiobesity drug.

Pediatric brown adipose tissue: detection, epidemiology, and differences from adults

Drubach LA, Palmer EL 3rd, Connolly LP, Baker A, Zurakowski D, Cypess AM
Department of Radiology, Children's Hospital Boston, Boston, MA, USA
laura.drubach@childrens.harvard.edu
J Pediatr 2011;159:939–944

Introduction: Previous histological studies have suggested that brown adipose tissue (BAT) peaks in childhood and declines into adulthood. However, recent studies using PET-CT revealed the existence of active brown fat even in adults with a characteristic anatomical distribution. Moreover, a strong negative correlation between BMI and BAT activity has been shown. The objective of this study was to evaluate the prevalence and factors affecting the detection of active brown adipose tissue (BAT) in children and adolescents using ^{18}F-fluorodeoxyglucose positron emission tomography.

Methods: A retrospective review of 385 PET-CT scans for different oncologic indications of 172 patients aged 5–21 years was performed. BAT activity in the neck, thorax, and abdomen was compared to liver values. Clinical indices were recorded.

Results: There was no significant difference between prevalence of BAT activity in girls vs. boys and highest activities were found in cervical-supraclavicular regions. The highest percentage of patients with detectable BAT and the highest BAT/liver activity were in the 13- to 14.99-year age group in both males and females. BMI percentile correlated negatively with BAT activity, while BAT activity did not show any correlation with outdoor temperature and diagnosis.

Conclusion: BAT is detected more frequently in children than in adults under clinical, temperature uncontrolled conditions. BAT activity correlated inversely with obesity, suggesting that BAT plays a fundamental role in pediatric metabolism.

Despite the relative high number of studies investigating the relationship of BAT and factors which affect its activity status, little was known regarding the demographics of active BAT in children and adolescents.

In this study, 385 scans of pediatric patients undergoing PET-CT for cancer surveillance were investigated. In contrast to adults, there was no sexual dimorphism. BAT activity was negatively correlated with BMI. Interestingly, BAT appearance and BAT/liver activity was highest in the 13- to 14.99-year group, pointing to a potential important role of BAT on metabolism at the time of the adolescent growth spurt. That is even more striking, since it was the dogma for a long time that BAT appearance peaks after birth and declines subsequently afterwards.

This study shows for the first time that BAT activity peaks in adolescents and that BAT activity negatively correlates with BMI in children. However, these data were acquired without controlling for body temperature. As admitted by the authors, this might interfere with measures of active BAT.

Functional brown adipose tissue is related to muscle volume in children and adolescents

Gilsanz V, Chung SA, Jackson H, Dorey FJ, Hu HH
Department of Radiology, Children's Hospital Los Angeles, Los Angeles, CA, USA
vgilsanz@chla.usc.edu
J Pediatr 2011;158:722–726

Introduction: It has been suggested in PET-CT studies that brown adipose tissue (BAT) activity is correlated with anthropometric measures in adults. The aim of this study was to test if BAT activity correlated with anthropometric parameters in children.

Methods: Regression analyses were performed in 71 pediatric patients with or without BAT activity in PET/CT scans to assess the relation between BAT and body mass, obesity and musculature.

Results: 30 patients had detectable BAT in PET-CT scans (10 girls and 20 boys). There were no differences in age, BMI and subcutaneous fat mass between the groups. However, patients with BAT had significantly greater neck and gluteus musculature. With logistic regression analyses, neck and pelvic musculature predicted the presence of BAT independently of age, sex, body size, and season of scan.

Conclusion: The authors conclude that pediatric patients with visualized BAT on PET/CT examinations have significantly greater muscle volume than patients with no visualized BAT.

Unlike white adipocytes, brown adipocytes and myocytes share the same progenitor cell originating from the paraxial mesoderm. Moreover, brown adipocyte progenitors have been found in muscle. In the present study, the correlation between BAT appearance in PET/CT scans with BMI, age and skeletal muscle volume was investigated. Interestingly, they found a correlation between visualized BAT and muscle volume underlining the potential relationship between muscle and BAT development. However, one has to be careful about drawing such conclusions from retrospective PET-CT scans, as the patients were not scanned under controlled temperature conditions. Moreover, it has been shown that PET-CT is not sensitive enough to detect small amounts of BAT [34].

Retinaldehyde dehydrogenase-1 regulates a thermogenic program in white adipose tissue

Kiefer FW, Vernochet C, O'Brien P, Spoerl S, Brown JD, Nallamshetty S, Zeyda M, Stulnig TM, Cohen DE, Kahn CR, Plutzky J

Cardiovascular Division, Department of Medicine, Brigham and Women's Hospital, Harvard Medical School, Boston, MA, USA
jplutzky@rics.bwh.harvard.edu
Nat Med 2012 (E-pub ahead of print)

Introduction: Brown adipose tissue (BAT) may be involved in body weight regulation and recruitment of BAT may prevent obesity. Recent data link retinoids to energy balance, but a specific role for retinoid metabolism in white versus brown fat is unknown. Rate-limiting enzymes in retinol metabolism are retinaldehyde dehydrogenases (Aldhs).

Methods: The authors used an Aldh1a1 knockout mice to investigate the impact of retinol metabolism on energy metabolism and BAT recruitment.

Results: Aldh1a1 is predominately expressed in white adipose tissue (WAT). Deficiency of the Aldh1a1 gene induced genes characteristic for BAT leading to uncoupled mitochondrial respiration and adaptive thermogenesis. WAT-selective Aldh1a1 knockdown resulted in reduced weight gain and improved glucose homeostasis in mice. Rald induced uncoupling protein-1 (Ucp1) mRNA and protein levels in white adipocytes by selectively activating the retinoic acid receptor (RAR), recruiting the coactivator PGC-1α and inducing Ucp1 promoter activity

Conclusion: Aldh1a1 and its substrate Rald are regulators of thermogenesis in white adipocytes. These findings may have potential therapeutic implications.

Metabolites of vitamin A – retinoids – have been linked to diverse biological functions including adipogenesis and energy homeostasis. The rate-limiting step of retinol metabolism is the conversion of retinaldehyde (Rald) to retinoic acids by aldehyde dehydrogenases (Aldh). This study nicely shows the impact of Rald on brown adipocyte formation in white adipose tissue.

First, the authors found a high expression of Aldh1a1 in mouse WAT compared to BAT. Moreover, the expression of this enzyme was found to be increased in obese humans and in mice on a high-fat diet, pointing to its role in regulating fat mass. They further investigated the phenotype of Aldh1a1$^{-/-}$ mice. Interestingly, these animals had higher energy expenditure and body temperature compared to wild-type mice, which was accompanied by the formation of brown adipocytes in visceral adipose tissue. The authors then further investigated this effect on white adipocyte in vitro. Treating the cells with either Rald or with antisense oligonucleotides directed against Aldh1a1 induced brown adipocyte marker genes in white adipocytes. Moreover, Rald treatment induced the recruitment of PGC1- via a RAR-dependent mechanism and induced UCP-1 promoter activation.

Dissipating energy stores by promoting thermogenesis in WAT has been proposed to be an approach to combat overweight and obesity. Disruption of Aldh1a1 in white adipose tissue might lead to new therapeutic strategies in obesity treatment.

Orexin is required for brown adipose tissue development, differentiation, and function

Sellayah D, Bharaj P, Sikder D
Metabolic Signaling and Disease Program, Diabetes and Obesity Research Center, Sanford-Burnham Medical Research Institute, Orlando, FL, USA
dev@sanfordburnham.org
Cell Metab 2011;14:478–490

Background: Orexin (OX) neuropeptides play a role in regulating food intake and wakefulness. Deficiency of orexin has been linked to narcolepsy, a disease which is associated with obesity.
Methods: Orexin-deficient mice were metabolically characterized. The effect of orexin-A on brown adipose tissue (BAT) development was investigated.
Results: Obesity in orexin knockout mice is associated with impaired BAT thermogenesis due to a defect in differentiation of brown adipocyte precursor cells. This defect was circumvented by orexin injection to orexin-null dams. In vitro, orexin was able to induce the full differentiation program into brown adipocytes of mesenchymal progenitor stem cells, embryonic fibroblasts and brown preadipocytes dependent on p38, bone morphogenetic protein receptor-1a (BMPR1A) and Smad 1/5 signaling.
Conclusion: The authors conclude that orexin plays an important role in brown adipose tissue differentiation and function with effects on adaptive thermogenesis and body weight regulation.

Several transcription factors which promote brown adipocyte differentiation have been identified. However, much less is known about factors which initiate these transcriptional events. In this study, Sellayah et al. provide surprising data connecting orexin neuropeptides with brown adipocyte formation.

Orexins are neuropeptides which regulate wakefulness and also food intake. Interestingly, they have been mentioned also in context of obesity. The authors found that orexin knockout mice became obese while eating less compared to wild-type animals. They showed also that this effect was due to an increased metabolic efficiency, which led them to investigate brown adipose tissue plasticity in these animals. In orexin-deficient mice, BAT was delipidated which was accompanied by reduction in the expression of brown adipocyte marker genes. In an elegant experiment, this effect could be circumvented in the offspring of orexin-null dams by injecting orexin in the dams during pregnancy. Interestingly, the effects of orexin on BAT development are mediated directly, as shown in in vitro experiments using mouse embryonic stem cells or primary brown preadipocytes.

This study provides evidence that orexin plays a significant role in the development of brown adipose tissue. Investigating the signaling pathways activated by orexin might lead to new and promising strategies to develop therapies against obesity and its related comorbidities.

New mechanisms

Dysfunction of lipid sensor GPR120 leads to obesity in both mouse and human

Ichimura A, Hirasawa A, Poulain-Godefroy O, Bonnefond A, Hara T, Yengo L, Kimura I, Leloire A, Liu N, Iida K, Choquet H, Besnard P, Lecoeur C, Vivequin S, Ayukawa K, Takeuchi M, Ozawa K, Tauber M, Maffeis C, Morandi A, Buzzetti R, Elliott P, Pouta A, Jarvelin MR, Körner A, Kiess W, Pigeyre M, Caiazzo R, Van Hul W, Van Gaal L, Horber F, Balkau B, Lévy-Marchal C, Rouskas K, Kouvatsi A, Hebebrand J, Hinney A, Scherag A, Pattou F, Meyre D, Koshimizu TA, Wolowczuk I, Tsujimoto G, Froguel P
Department of Genomic Drug Discovery Science, Graduate School of Pharmaceutical Sciences, Kyoto University, Sakyo-ku, Kyoto, Japan
p.froguel@imperial.co.uk; gtsuji@pharm.kyoto-u.ac.jp
Nature 2012;483:350–354

Background: Free fatty acids (FFA) serve as important energy source and signaling molecules at the same time. Several G-protein-coupled receptors for FFA have been identified so far, among them GPR120.

GPR120 is a receptor for unsaturated long-chain FA and is not only important for regulation of appetite and food preference, but also adipogenesis.

Methods: GPR120 knockout mice were generated and metabolically characterized. ~7,000 obese patients and ~7,000 controls were genotyped for variants in the GPR120 gene.

Results: GPR120-deficient mice develop obesity, glucose intolerance and fatty liver on a high-fat diet. Adipocyte differentiation and lipogenesis were impaired in these mice, while hepatic lipogenesis was enhanced. Mice were characterized by insulin resistance with reduced insulin signaling and increased adipose tissue inflammation. The expression of GPR120 in adipose tissue was significantly higher in obese humans compared to lean controls. A deleterious non-synonymous mutation (p.R270H), which inhibited GPR120 signaling, was discovered by exon sequencing. This variant was associated with increased obesity risk in Europeans.

Conclusions: The authors demonstrate that GPR120 is an important lipid sensor, which plays an important role in controlling energy balance in both humans and rodents.

GPR120 is highly abundant in the digestive tract. When food enters the gut, fatty acids bind to and activate GPR120 leading to secretion of gastrointestinal peptides such as cholecystokinin, glucagon-like peptide-1 and peptide YY. This informs the central nervous system about the availability of fatty acids and allows an adaptive response. Therefore, activation of GPR120 is one of the first steps in sending a satiety signal from the periphery to the brain.

The study from Ichimura et al. underlines the importance of GPR120 for the development of overweight and obesity. Mice deficient in GPR120 are more prone to diet-induced obesity and hepatic steatosis. Certain mutations in the GPR120 gene, which lead to inactivation of the receptor, seem to increase a person's risk of obesity by 60%.

Modulating the function of receptors involved in nutrient signaling, among them GPR120, might be a new pharmacological option for the treatment of obesity and its comorbidities.

Long-term persistence of hormonal adaptations to weight loss

Sumithran P, Prendergast LA, Delbridge E, Purcell K, Shulkes A, Krikrtos, A, Proietto A
Department of Medicine (Austin and Northern Health), University of Melbourne, Melbourne, Vic., Australia
jproietto@unimelb.edu.au
N Engl J Med 2011;365:1597–1604

Background: Weight loss alters the circulating levels of several peripheral hormones involved in body weight regulation and increases subjective appetite. Whether these changes are transient or persistent over time will further the understanding of the widely observed challenges in maintaining the lowered body weight.

Methods: 50 overweight and obese subjects were enrolled in an 8-week weight loss program, followed by a 1-year weight maintenance period. Circulating levels of leptin, ghrelin, peptide YY (pYY), gastric inhibitory polypeptide (GIP), glucagon-like peptide 1 (GLP-1), amylin, pancreatic polypeptide (PP), cholecystokinin (CCK), and insulin were measured along with subjective ratings of hunger proxies at baseline, 2 weeks, and 1 year after completion of the weight loss period. At each time point, samples were obtained before and 30, 60, 120, 180 and 240 min after a standardized breakfast to shed light on changes in fasting values as well as modifications in postprandial hormone excursions.

Results: 36 subjects completed the study and were included in the analyses. Subjects lost 13.5 ± 0.5 kg (SE) on average, weight after 1 year remained 7.9 ± 1.1 kg below baseline. Weight loss produced significant reductions in leptin (p < 0.001), leptin/fat mass (p < 0.001), pYY (p < 0.001), CCK (p < 0.001), insulin (p < 0.001), and amylin (p = 0.002), and increases in ghrelin (p < 0.001), GIP (p = 0.004), PP (p = 0.008), and subjective appetite (p < 0.001). One year after the initial weight loss, these changes persisted for leptin (p < 0.001), pYY (p < 0.001), CCK (p = 0.04), insulin (p = 0.01), ghrelin (p < 0.001), GIP (p < 0.001), PP (p = 0.002), and subjective hunger (p < 0.001).

Conclusions: The authors conclude that weight loss-induced changes in peripheral hormones persist after 1 year. Thereby, they may contribute to the observed propensity to regain weight, and long-term strategies to counteract these changes may prevent obesity relapse.

It is known from previous studies that leptin, an adipocyte hormone, acts in the hypothalamus to reduce food intake and increase energy expenditure. The gastrointestinal hormones PYY, GLP-1, CCK, PP and amylin are released postprandially and inhibit hunger and further food intake [35–39]. To an opposite effect, ghrelin stimulates hunger [40] and GIP promotes energy storage [41, 42]. Thus, the hormonal changes found in this study can be expected to promote increased food intake, and thereby contribute to weight gain. This is substantiated by the reported increase in hunger and appetite ratings.

However, no comparison was made with a BMI-matched control group that did not undergo weight loss. Thus, some of the reported changes might be physiological at the lower BMI. Analogous to the reduction in insulin levels that go along with increased insulin sensitivity, as illustrated by the HOMA-IR reported in the supplemental materials, other hormonal alterations might be an effect of altered end-organ sensitivity and have no immediate consequences on intake regulation.

Despite these limitations, the study sheds light on possible physiological factors that contribute to the widely observed rebound phenomenon after weight reduction diets, and will certainly inform further investigations to clarify the underlying mechanisms.

Clinical review

Regulation of food intake, energy balance, and body fat mass: implications for the pathogenesis and treatment of obesity

Guyenet SJ, Schwartz MW
Diabetes and Obesity Center of Excellence and Division of Metabolism, Endocrinology, and Nutrition, Department of Medicine, University of Washington School of Medicine, Seattle, WA, USA
mschwart@u.washington.edu
J Clin Endocrinol Metab 2012;97:745–755

Background: Although substantial progress has identified neurohumoral mechanisms underlying obesity, current nonsurgical treatment approaches are insufficient to help most obese individuals in achieving and maintaining a meaningful reduction in body weight. This review provides a synthesis of research articles providing insight into the mechanisms controlling food intake in the context of energy homeostasis with a focus on obesity pathogenesis, the dramatic recent increase in obesity prevalence, and the insufficient effectiveness of current nonsurgical treatment programs.
Methods: Research articles with highest quality evidence were included in the review.
Results: The authors summarized research findings in a structured way under six headlines: short-term, meal-related determinants of food intake, long-term regulation of food intake and energy balance, food reward and palatability, obesity and energy homeostasis, genetic factors, and leptin resistance: cause or effect of obesity? Interventions that reduce body fat stores elicit compensatory responses that promote the recovery of lost fat and are difficult to consciously override. Obesity involves the biological defense of an elevated level of body fat.
Conclusion: Essential breakthroughs are needed in understanding the biological defense of elevated body fat mass required to enable the development of effective new obesity prevention and treatment strategies.

This clinical review summarizes the current scientific knowledge about the regulation of food intake, energy balance, and body fat mass in a comprehensive manner. It explains why obesity is resistant to effective, long-term treatment when classical non-surgical approaches are applied. Body fat stores are subject to homeostatic regulation in obese individuals, just as in lean individuals. We are still waiting for essential breakthroughs in understanding the biological mechanisms that 'defend' against any reductions in our high levels of body fat mass.

Ghrelin levels increase after pictures showing food

Schüssler P, Kluge M, Yassouridis A, Dresler M, Uhr M, Steiger A
Max Planck Institute of Psychiatry, Munich, Germany
steiger@mpipsykl.mpg.de
Obesity 2012;385:1–6

Background: The neuropeptide ghrelin is mainly secreted by the stomach and small intestine. It represents a potent orexigenic stimulus, as it increases self-rated appetite, caloric intake, and the propensity to initiate a meal. Ghrelin levels physiologically increase before meals, but to date the interplay of intrinsic and external factors that modulate this rise is incompletely understood. If external factors such as visual food cues play a role, this might be one of the mechanisms through which environmental factors potentiate obesity risk.
Methods: The influence of viewing pictures of food on circulating levels of ghrelin, leptin and insulin was assessed in comparison to neutral pictures with non-food contents. In two sessions, food vs. non-food pictures were shown to 8 healthy male volunteers in a cross-over design. Subjects were provided a standard breakfast at 08:00 h and lunch at 12:00 h. 50 pictures were repeatedly presented for 30 min starting at 10:30 h. Pictures displayed food contents during the first and non-food contents during the second session. Serial blood sampling of ghrelin, leptin, and insulin was performed every 10–15 min throughout the test sessions.
Results: As expected, ghrelin levels increased before each meal, independent of the picture contents. In addition, ghrelin levels during the 30-min interval following the food picture presentation increased significantly compared to the 30-min interval prior to the visual stimulation (AUC 188 vs. 155%, p < 0.05). There was no rise in ghrelin after the non-food pictures. The difference between the two picture conditions was significant (p < 0.05). Neither picture session affected levels of leptin or insulin.
Conclusion: The authors conclude that food pictures elevate ghrelin levels, while insulin and leptin levels are not affected. Thus, the ubiquitous food cues displayed in today's environment may contribute to increased hunger, food intake and obesity rates via elevations in ghrelin levels.

Visual food cues have been used in multiple studies investing the central regulation of food intake using functional MRI (fMRI). The implementation of this method in the investigation of peripheral processes is more innovative and represents an elegant way of investigating changes of the cephalic phase of food intake. From fMRI studies, it is known that viewing food pictures activates brain areas involved in food anticipation and reward calculation [43]. It has been shown that ghrelin release is regulated by the central nervous system via sympathic efferences [44, 45]. Vice versa, ghrelin's orexigenic effect is mediated by vagal afferences to the brainstem and hypothalamus [46], and ghrelin is actively transported through the blood-brain barrier [47]. Ghrelin administration increases the neural response to food pictures in areas of appetite control [48]. Through these pathways, ghrelin may represent a link between regulatory brain areas and gut mechanisms when it comes to food anticipation and intake initiation. Its rise in response to visual food cues may denote one of the mechanisms linking environmental factors to eating behavior and increased obesity rates.

Ghrelin mediates food-reward behavior in mice

Chuang J, Perello M, Sakata I, Osborne-Lawrence S, Savitt J, Lutter M, Zigman J
Division of Hypothalamic Research, Department of Internal Medicine, The University of Texas Southwestern Medical Center, Dallas, TX, USA
jeffrey.zigman@utsouthwestern.edu
J Clin Invest 2011;121:2684–2692

Background: Increased appetite and food intake has been observed in individuals suffering from chronic stress or depression and may contribute to the increased prevalence of obesity in these individuals. There is evidence from animal models and human data that ghrelin might play a role in stress-related eating. However, the underlying mechanisms are incompletely understood.
Methods: In a mouse system, food-reward behavior was assessed using a conditioned place preference (CPP) task after prolonged exposure to chronic social defeat stress (CSDS), a model of psychosocial

stress featuring aspects of major depression and posttraumatic stress disorder. Three different mice were examined: wild-type (WT) mice, ghrelin receptor (GSHR) knockout (GSHR-null) mice, and mice with isolated GSHR expression in catecholaminergic, thyrosine hydroxylase (TH) expressing neurons in the brain (GSHR-null/TH).

Results: WT mice, but not GSHR-null mice, responded to ghrelin injections by increasing their intake of chow. This effect could be restored in the GSHR-null/TH mice. During the CSDS exposure, GSHR-null mice showed increased social isolation compared to the WT and GSHR-null/TH mice. WT and GSHR-null/TH mice, but not GSHR-null mice, demonstrated increased weight gain and CPP for intake of the high-intake diet.

Conclusion: The authors conclude that increased intake and preference for a high-fat diet during social stress is ghrelin-dependent and mediated by signaling in catecholaminergic neurons in the brain.

By crossing GHSR-null mice, which contain a loxP-flanked transcriptional blocking cassette inserted into the GHSR gene, with mice in which Cre recombinase expression is driven by the TH promoter (TH-Cre mice) [49, 50], the authors developed an elegant mouse model to study ghrelin-mediated central nervous and peripheral processes.

With the limitation in mind that mice experiments cannot be directly transferred to humans, the authors provide a possible mechanism linking chronic stress and depression to eating behavior. Psychosocial stress leads to elevations in circulating levels of acyl-ghrelin. As sympathoadrenal tone is increased in stress, speculatively, this stress-induced elevation may involve stimulation of β_1-adrenergic receptors on ghrelin cells, a pathway that has been implicated in ghrelin release in response to fasting [44, 51]. Ghrelin, in turn, interacts with its receptor, GHSR, which is distributed throughout the brain and periphery [52]. The data in this report suggest that direct ghrelin signaling, specifically on GHSR-TH-coexpressing neurons, is sufficient to decrease social avoidance and induce hedonic eating behavior in mice. The effects on eating behavior led to increased intake of calorically dense foods and increased body weight, a correlate of the observed increased prevalence of obesity in humans with chronic stress or depression.

Food for thought

Neighborhoods, obesity, and diabetes – a randomized social experiment

Ludwig J, Sanbonmatsu L, Gennetian L, Adam E, Duncan GJ, Katz LF, Kessler RC, Kling JR, Tessler Lindau S, Whitaker RC, McDade TW
University of Chicago, Chicago, IL, USA
jludwig@uchicago.edu
N Engl J Med 2011;365:1509–1519

Background: There is observational evidence that neighborhood environments may contribute to the development of obesity and diabetes. The association of obesity and diabetes with social environment was studied in a large-scale social experiment by randomly assigning different neighborhood conditions.

Methods: During the timeframe from 1994 to 1998, 4,498 women with children living in public developments in high-poverty areas of Baltimore, Boston, Chicago, or New York were randomly assigned to one of three groups. Families in the intervention group received short-term counseling on housing search plus housing vouchers which had to be used in a low-poverty census tract (n = 1,788); a second group received conventional, unrestricted housing vouchers and no additional counseling (n = 1,312), and the control group received neither counseling nor vouchers (n = 1,398). A long-term follow-up survey was carried out from 2008 through 2010 including measurement of weight status, HbA_{1c}, and health outcomes.

Results: Compared with the control group, participants receiving a low-poverty voucher had lower prevalences of BMI >35 kg/m^2 (–4.61 percentage points) and BMI >40 kg/m^2 (–3.38 percentage points) at 10–15 years of follow-up. Furthermore, the prevalence of HbA_{1c} levels >6.5% was reduced in the intervention group compared to controls (–4.31 percentage points), corresponding to a relative reduction of 21.6%. Observed differences in health outcomes between the low-poverty and conventional voucher group did not reach statistical significance.

Conclusions: Moving from high-level to lower-level poverty neighborhoods was associated with moderate but significant reductions in the prevalence of different degrees of obesity and in the prevalence of diabetes. Although the underlying mechanisms remain unclear, it is reasonable to assume that community level interventions have the potential to improve health.

Obesity research taught us that obesity is a multifaceted, multiorgan disease mainly originating from complex gene-environment interactions. The present study by Ludwig et al. now vividly illustrates that the 'environmental' determinants of obesity are not limited to individual-level factors (e.g. diet and physical activity) but also includes important area-level factors: poverty, segregation, impaired collective efficacy, poor infrastructure, and limited access to higher education. In a large-scale 'social experiment' (which undoubtedly could not have been carried out at least in most Western European countries due to ethical concerns), the authors demonstrate that giving mainly Black and Hispanic families the opportunity of moving from high- to low-poverty neighborhoods ameliorates the prevalence of marked obesity and type 2 diabetes during long-term follow-up. Moving to lower poverty neighborhoods not only improved health outcomes, but also increased the reported collective efficacy as a measure of solidarity as well as the subjective feeling of safety, and furthermore changed the structure of social contacts and friendship. Although the mechanisms responsible for the association of local socioeconomic structures and health outcomes remain to be elucidated, the present study clearly shows that any public health intervention targeted at obesity and diabetes should consider effective social policy measures.

Important for clinical practice

Effects of metformin on body weight and body composition in obese insulin-resistant children – a randomized clinical trial

Yanovski JA, Krakoff J, Salaita CG, McDuffie JR, Kozlosky M, Sebring NG, Reynolds JC, Brady SM, Calis KA
Unit on Growth and Obesity, Program in Developmental Endocrinology and Genetics, Eunice Kennedy Shriver National Institute of Child Health and Human Development (NICHD), Bethesda, MD, USA
jy15i@nih.gov
Diabetes 2011;60:477–485

Background: Metformin suppresses hepatic glucose production, improves peripheral insulin sensitivity and can induce weight stabilization or moderate weight loss in obese adults. Although small trials reported similar positive effects of metformin in obese adolescents, data on the efficacy of metformin in younger children are missing.

Methods: In a randomized double-blind placebo-controlled trial, 100 markedly obese children and adolescents (mean BMI 34.6 ±6.6 kg/m^2, age range 6–12 years) with fasting hyperinsulinemia (insulin ≥15 µU/ml) were randomized to either 1,000 mg metformin or placebo twice daily for 6 months followed by 6 months of open-label metformin treatment. All participating families underwent an accompanying clinic-based lifestyle intervention.

Results: After completion of the 6-month randomized phase, mean BMI (–1.09 kg/m^2), mean body weight (–3.38 kg), mean BMI Z-score (–0.07), and mean fat mass (–1.40 kg) were significantly reduced in the metformin group compared to the placebo group. Fasting plasma glucose slightly decreased in the metformin group (–0.88 mg/dl) and increased in the placebo group. Concordantly, HOMA-IR index significantly improved under metformin treatment, whereas first-phase insulin secretion and whole-body insulin sensitivity measured by hyperglycemic clamp remained unchanged between the groups. No serious adverse events occurred, however dose reductions due to side effects of metformin had to be applied in 17% of the children in the intervention group. Continued metformin treatment during the open-label phase did not result in further weight reduction in the metformin group, but subjects who previously received placebo significantly decreased their BMI Z-score.

Conclusions: In the setting of a low-intensity lifestyle intervention program, metformin facilitated a moderate reduction in BMI Z-score and fat mass and improved fasting glucose and HOMA-IR in severely obese, insulin-resistant children.

Metformin was first synthesized in the early 1920s and developed – after a changeful history – into one of the most widely prescribed antidiabetic drugs in the world today. Given the limited short- and long-term efficacy of lifestyle interventions in achieving persistent weight loss in severely obese children and adolescents, there is a continuing interest in developing alternative treatment approaches. Currently – in most countries – there are no approved pharmacologic treatment options available for obese children in the prepubertal age range. As onset and course of pubertal development and associated metabolic changes, e.g. in whole-body insulin sensitivity, may represent an important event in the evolution of cardiovascular disease risk in later life, tailoring interventions for obese prepubertal children could be a rewarding aim. In the present study by Yanovski et al., adding metformin to a basic, low-level lifestyle intervention was proven to be a safe and moderately favorable treatment option for at least a duration of up to 1 year in severely obese children aged 6–12 years. Although the reported changes in BMI Z-score induced by metformin seem to be unimpressive, more importantly metformin stabilized levels of fasting glycemia in contrast to the further increasing fasting glucose levels in the placebo group. This finding may provide a rationale for further investigations exploring the potential preventive effect of early-onset metformin treatment on the risk for developing type 2 diabetes.

References

1. Moss A, Klenk J, Simon K, Thaiss H, Reinehr T, Wabitsch M: Declining prevalence rates for overweight and obesity in German children starting school. Eur J Pediatr 2012;171:289–299.
2. Matthiessen J, Velsing Groth M, Fagt S, Biltoft-Jensen A, Stockmarr A, Andersen JS, et al: Prevalence and trends in overweight and obesity among children and adolescents in Denmark. Scand J Public Health 2008;36:153–160.
3. Mitchell RT, McDougall CM, Crum JE: Decreasing prevalence of obesity in primary schoolchildren. Arch Dis Child 2007;92:153–154.
4. Tambalis KD, Panagiotakos DB, Kavouras SA, Kallistratos AA, Moraiti IP, Douvis SJ, et al: Eleven-year prevalence trends of obesity in Greek children: first evidence that prevalence of obesity is leveling off. Obesity (Silver Spring) 2010;18:161–166.
5. Schnohr C, Sorensen TI, Niclasen BV: Changes since 1980 in body mass index and the prevalence of overweight among in schooling children in Nuuk, Greenland. Int J Circumpolar Health 2005;64:157–162.
6. Popkin BM, Conde W, Hou N, Monteiro C: Is there a lag globally in overweight trends for children compared with adults? Obesity (Silver Spring) 2006;14:1846–1853.
7. Ogden CL, Carroll MD, Kit BK, Flegal KM: Prevalence of obesity and trends in body mass index among US children and adolescents, 1999–2010. JAMA 2012;307:483–490.
8. Blüher S, Meigen C, Gausche R, Keller E, Pfaffle R, Sabin M, et al: Age-specific stabilization in obesity prevalence in German children: a cross-sectional study from 1999 to 2008. Int J Pediatr Obes 2011;6:e199–e206.
9. Summerbell CD, Waters E, Edmunds LD, Kelly S, Brown T, Campbell KJ: Interventions for preventing obesity in children. Cochrane Database Syst Rev 2005;3:CD001871.
10. Singh AS, Mulder C, Twisk JW, van Mechelen W, Chinapaw MJ: Tracking of childhood overweight into adulthood: a systematic review of the literature. Obes Rev 2008;9:474–488.
11. Barlow SE: Expert committee recommendations regarding the prevention, assessment, and treatment of child and adolescent overweight and obesity: summary report. Pediatrics 2007;120(suppl 4):S164–S192.
12. August GP, Caprio S, Fennoy I, Freemark M, Kaufman FR, Lustig RH, et al: Prevention and treatment of pediatric obesity: an Endocrine Society clinical practice guideline based on expert opinion. J Clin Endocrinol Metab 2008;93:4576–4599.
13. National Institute for Health: Obesity: the prevention, identification, assessment, and management of overweight and obesity in adults and children. National Institute for Health and Clinical Excellence Guideline, December 2006, No 43 (www.nice.org.uk/guidance/CG43).
14. Reilly JJ, Methven E, McDowell ZC, Hacking B, Alexander D, Stewart L, et al: Health consequences of obesity. Arch Dis Child 2003;88:748–752.
15. Ravelli GP, Stein ZA, Susser MW: Obesity in young men after famine exposure in utero and early infancy. N Engl J Med 1976;295:349–353.
16. Godfrey KM, Lillycrop KA, Burdge GC, Gluckman PD, Hanson MA: Epigenetic mechanisms and the mismatch concept of the developmental origins of health and disease. Pediatr Res 2007;61:5R–10R.
17. Montague CT, Farooqi IS, Whitehead JP, Soos MA, Rau H, Wareham NJ, et al: Congenital leptin deficiency is associated with severe early-onset obesity in humans. Nature 1997;387:903–908.
18. Strobel A, Issad T, Camoin L, Ozata M, Strosberg AD: A leptin missense mutation associated with hypogonadism and morbid obesity. Nat Genet 1998;18:213–215.
19. Farooqi IS, Matarese G, Lord GM, Keogh JM, Lawrence E, Agwu C, et al: Beneficial effects of leptin on obesity, T-cell hyporesponsiveness, and neuroendocrine/metabolic dysfunction of human congenital leptin deficiency. J Clin Invest 2002;110:1093–1103.
20. Gibson WT, Farooqi IS, Moreau M, DePaoli AM, Lawrence E, O'Rahilly S, et al: Congenital leptin deficiency due to homozygosity for the Δ133G mutation: report of another case and evaluation of response to four years of leptin therapy. J Clin Endocrinol Metab 2004;89:4821–4826.
21. Ozata M, Ozdemir IC, Licinio J: Human leptin deficiency caused by a missense mutation: multiple endocrine defects, decreased sympathetic tone, and immune system dysfunction indicate new targets for leptin action, greater central than peripheral resistance to the effects of leptin, and spontaneous correction of leptin-mediated defects. J Clin Endocrinol Metab 1999;84:3686–3695.

22. Paz-Filho GJ, Babikian T, Asarnow R, Delibasi T, Esposito K, Erol HK, et al: Leptin replacement improves cognitive development. PloS One 2008;3:e3098.
23. Mazen I, El-Gammal M, Abdel-Hamid M, Amr K: A novel homozygous missense mutation of the leptin gene (N103K) in an obese Egyptian patient. Mol Genet Metab 2009;97:305–308.
24. Farooqi IS: Monogenic human obesity. Front Horm Res 2008;36:1–11.
25. Fischer-Posovszky P, von Schnurbein J, Moepps B, Lahr G, Strauss G, Barth TF, et al: A new missense mutation in the leptin gene causes mild obesity and hypogonadism without affecting T-cell responsiveness. J Clin Endocrinol Metab 2010;95:2836–2840.
26. Farooqi IS, Wangensteen T, Collins S, Kimber W, Matarese G, Keogh JM, et al: Clinical and molecular genetic spectrum of congenital deficiency of the leptin receptor. N Engl J Med 2007;356:237–247.
27. Ingalls AM, Dickie MM, Snell GD: Obese, a new mutation in the house mouse. J Hered 1950;41:317–318.
28. Lane P, Dickie MM: Relative sterility in obese males corrected by dietary restriction. J Hered 1954;54:56–58.
29. Clement K, Vaisse C, Lahlou N, Cabrol S, Pelloux V, Cassuto D, et al: A mutation in the human leptin receptor gene causes obesity and pituitary dysfunction. Nature 1998;392:398–401.
30. Von Schnurbein J, Moss A, Nagel SA, Muehleder H, Debatin KM, Farooqi IS, et al: Leptin substitution results in the induction of menstrual cycles in an adolescent with leptin deficiency and hypogonadotropic hypogonadism. Horm Res Paediatr 2012;77:127–133.
31. Israel DD, Sheffer-Babila S, de Luca C, Jo YH, Liu SM, Xia Q, et al: Effects of leptin and melanocortin signaling interactions on pubertal development and reproduction. Endocrinology 2012;153 2408–2419.
32. Wu Q, Whiddon BB, Palmiter RD: Ablation of neurons expressing agouti-related protein, but not melanin concentrating hormone, in leptin-deficient mice restores metabolic functions and fertility. Proc Natl Acad Sci USA 2012;109:3155–3160.
33. Ouellet V, Labbe SM, Blondin DP, Phoenix S, Guerin B, Haman F, et al: Brown adipose tissue oxidative metabolism contributes to energy expenditure during acute cold exposure in humans. J Clin Invest 2012;122:545–552.
34. Lee P, Zhao JT, Swarbrick MM, Gracie G, Bova R, Greenfield JR, et al: High prevalence of brown adipose tissue in adult humans. J Clin Endocrinol Metab 2011;96:2450–2455.
35. Batterham RL, Cowley MA, Small CJ, Herzog H, Cohen MA, Dakin CL, et al: Gut hormone PYY(3-36) physiologically inhibits food intake. Nature 2002;418:650–654.
36. Batterham RL, Le Roux CW, Cohen MA, Park AJ, Ellis SM, Patterson M, et al Pancreatic polypeptide reduces appetite and food intake in humans. J Clin Endocrinol Metab 2003;88:3989–3992.
37. Flint A, Raben A, Astrup A, Holst JJ: Glucagon-like peptide-1 promotes satiety and suppresses energy intake in humans. J Clin Invest 1998;101:515–520.
38. Morley JE, Flood JF: Amylin decreases food intake in mice. Peptides 1991;12:865–869.
39. Gibbs J, Young RC, Smith GP: Cholecystokinin decreases food intake in rats. J Comp Physiol Psychol 1973;84:488–495.
40. Wren AM, Seal LJ, Cohen MA, Brynes AE, Frost GS, Murphy KG, et al: Ghrelin enhances appetite and increases food intake in humans. J Clin Endocrinol Metab 2001;86:5992.
41. Hauner H, Glatting G, Kaminska D, Pfeiffer EF: Effects of gastric inhibitory polypeptide on glucose and lipid metabolism of isolated rat adipocytes. Ann Nutr Metab 1988;32:282–288.
42. Knapper JM, Puddicombe SM, Morgan LM, Fletcher JM: Investigations into the actions of glucose-dependent insulinotropic polypeptide and glucagon-like peptide-1(7-36)amide on lipoprotein lipase activity in explants of rat adipose tissue. J Nutr 1995;125:183–188.
43. Carnell S, Gibson C, Benson L, Ochner CN, Geliebter A: Neuroimaging and obesity: current knowledge and future directions. Obes Rev 2012;13:43–56.
44. Mundinger TO, Cummings DE, Taborsky GJ Jr: Direct stimulation of ghrelin secretion by sympathetic nerves. Endocrinology 2006;147:2893–2901.
45. Cummings DE, Overduin J: Gastrointestinal regulation of food intake. J Clin Invest 2007;117:13–23.
46. Murphy KG, Dhillo WS, Bloom SR: Gut peptides in the regulation of food intake and energy homeostasis. Endocr Rev 2006;27:719–727.
47. Banks WA, Tschop M, Robinson SM, Heiman ML: Extent and direction of ghrelin transport across the blood-brain barrier is determined by its unique primary structure. J Pharmacol Exp Ther 2002;302:822–827.
48. Malik S, McGlone F, Bedrossian D, Dagher A: Ghrelin modulates brain activity in areas that control appetitive behavior. Cell Metab 2008;7:400–409.
49. Zigman JM, Nakano Y, Coppari R, Balthasar N, Marcus JN, Lee CE, et al: Mice lacking ghrelin receptors resist the development of diet-induced obesity. J Clin Invest 2005;115:3564–3572.
50. Savitt JM, Jang SS, Mu W, Dawson VL, Dawson TM: Bcl-x is required for proper development of the mouse substantia nigra. J Neurosci 2005;25:6721–6728.
51. Zhao TJ, Sakata I, Li RL, Liang G, Richardson JA, Brown MS, et al: Ghrelin secretion stimulated by β_1-adrenergic receptors in cultured ghrelinoma cells and in fasted mice. Proc Natl Acad Sci USA 2010;107:15868–15873.
52. Zigman JM, Jones JE, Lee CE, Saper CB, Elmquist JK: Expression of ghrelin receptor mRNA in the rat and the mouse brain. J Comp Neurol 2006;494:528–548.

Type 2 Diabetes, Metabolic Syndrome and Lipids

Orit Pinhas-Hamiel

Pediatric Endocrinology and Diabetes Unit, Edmond and Lily Safra Children's Hospital, Sheba Medical Center, Tel-Hashomer, Ramat-Gan and Maccabi Juvenile Diabetes Center, Raanana, Sackler School of Medicine, Tel-Aviv University, Israel

The complexity of the development of type 2 diabetes mellitus (T2DM) is exhibited in the story of the Oji-Cree people. Long-term surveillance of the offspring of mothers who were diagnosed with T2DM in their own childhood demonstrates the interaction between the changing environment, genetics, and antenatal factors.

This year we learnt of yet another group at risk for early-onset T2DM: children treated with growth hormone (GH). The results of the first long-term clinical trial to maintain glycemic control among adolescents with T2DM are worrisome. Even more worrisome are the findings of a computer model calculating the risk of morbidity and mortality for youngsters with T2DM. We learnt that the development of the metabolic syndrome (MetS) during adolescence can be predicted by natal and parental profiles. This is important since children with MetS are at risk for developing kidney stones. The hours of sleep and the quality of sleep contribute to the development of MetS.

New guidelines for universal screening for dyslipidemia in children were published this year. Studies in adults show that intensive statin treatment is associated with an increased risk of new-onset T2DM. It is comforting to know that there are new drugs to reduce LDL levels in the pipeline.

Type 2 diabetes
New paradigms

Obesity and type 2 diabetes mellitus in a birth cohort of First Nation children born to mothers with pediatric-onset type 2 diabetes

Mendelson M, Cloutier J, Spence L, Sellers E, Taback S, Dean H
Section of Endocrinology and Metabolism, Department of Pediatrics, University of Manitoba, Winnipeg, Man., Canada
Pediatr Diabetes 2011;12:219–228

Background: Children who are born to mothers with pediatric-onset type 2 diabetes mellitus (T2DM) are exposed to a hyperglycemic intrauterine environment throughout pregnancy. The growth patterns and risk of T2DM in these offspring may be influenced by unique gene-environment interactions during intrauterine and postnatal life.

Methods: A cohort of offspring of First Nation mothers with onset of T2DM before age 18 years in Manitoba, Canada, was established. Height or length and weight at study entry and annually thereafter with fasting blood glucose in offspring aged ≥7 years were measured. Birth and breastfeeding history were collected, as well as specific hepatic nuclear factor-1α (HNF-1α) G319S genotype of offspring at age 7 years.

Results: From July 2003 to April 2008, 76 offspring of 37 mothers were enrolled. 64% (23/36) of the offspring aged 2–19 years were obese at initial assessment. The rates of obesity remained constant throughout the 5 years. As of April 2008, 7/28 (25%) of the offspring aged 7–19 years have diabetes including 6/14 (43%) aged 10–19 years. Most offspring with diabetes (5/7, 71%) were obese at diagnosis. All of the 7 offspring with diabetes have one or two copies of the G319S polymorphism.

Conclusions: The prevalence of T2DM in this cohort of offspring of First Nation women with pediatric-T2DM is the highest ever reported in children. Obesity is an important postnatal risk factor for T2DM in this population and may result from a unique gene-environment interaction.

This report, which tells us the story of the Oji-Cree people, is a result of 'The Next Generation Project' that began in 2003. The project has established long-term surveillance of the offspring of Aboriginal mothers who were diagnosed with T2DM during their own childhood or adolescence. The prevalence of T2DM in the Canadian Oji-Cree population ranks among the highest in the world. They were the first population to experience T2DM in a pediatric age group. Subjects from the Oji-Cree population were found to have a private polymorphism of the hepatic nuclear factor-1α (HNF-1α) [1]. HNF-1 α is a transcriptional activator of many genes including insulin, albumin, α_1-antitrypsin, and fibrinogen; it is expressed predominantly in the liver and the kidney, but also in the pancreas. Rare deleterious mutations in HNF-1α occur in maturity-onset diabetes of the young type 3 (MODY-3). The Oji-Cree polymorphism in the HNF-1α gene leads to an amino acid substitution of glycine to serine at codon 319 (G319 to S319). Carriers of a single copy of the S319 allele have about 3-fold higher risk of T2DM, whereas S319/S319 homozygotes have a 120-fold higher risk. Moreover, the age of onset of T2DM is earlier with an increased number of the S319 alleles. This polymorphism occurs in about 8% of the general Oji-Cree population but it is present in about 40% of those who developed T2DM. Two generations ago the diagnosis of diabetes was virtually unknown among the Oji-Cree people, though the S319 mutation must have been present, thus HNF-1α appears to be a susceptibility gene in subjects exposed to an abundance of food and limited physical activity.

In the current study, because of the high rates and the early onset of T2DM among the offspring, the authors suggest that the intrauterine exposure to maternal obesity and diabetes may have accelerated the progression of T2DM. Alteration of β-cell mass through prenatal programming of the fetus by epigenetic influences might possibly explain the high rate of early-onset diabetes in this cohort [2].

Type 2 diabetes
New concerns

Prevalence and incidence of diabetes mellitus in GH-treated children and adolescents: analysis from the GeNeSIS observational research program

Child CJ, Zimmermann AG, Scott RS, Cutler GB Jr, Battelino T, Blum WF
Lilly Research Laboratories, Erl Wood Manor, Windlesham, UK
cjc@lilly.com
J Clin Endocrinol Metab 2011;96:E1025–1034

Background: GH has an insulin antagonist effect, and GH treatment has therefore been suggested to impair glucose metabolism and increase risk of diabetes mellitus.
Methods: Data from 11,686 GH-treated patients in the Genetics and Neuroendocrinology of Short Stature International Study (GeNeSIS), a multinational observational study of children with growth disorders, were analyzed for diabetes incidence. Baseline diabetes prevalence was determined from a GH-naive subgroup. Prevalence and incidence (by standardized incidence ratio) were compared with results from patients aged less than 20 years in the US SEARCH for Diabetes in Youth study.
Results: Baseline type 1 diabetes (T1DM) prevalence per 1,000 persons was 4.92 (95% CI 1.91–12.58) in GeNeSIS and 1.03 (0.97–1.10) in SEARCH for 0- to 9 year-olds, and 7.33 (4.20–12.77) and 2.99 (2.78–2.98), respectively, for 10- to 19-year-olds. There were no GeNeSIS cases of T2DM before GH initiation. During a median 1.8 years of GH treatment, diabetes standardized incidence ratios for US patients were 1.4 (0.5–3.1) for T1DM and 8.5 (2.8–19.5) for T2DM, and for all patients was 1.4 (0.7–2.4) for T1DM and 6.5 (3.3–11.7) for T2DM. Among the 11 patients with incident T2DM, preexisting risk factors for diabetes were identified in 10. Glucose concentrations normalized in 7 of 9 patients for whom glycemic status could be determined, 3 of whom continued GH therapy and 4 who discontinued.
Conclusion: The incidence of T2DM was higher in GH-treated children than the general population. Monitoring of glucose, before and periodically during GH treatment, is recommended for those with preexisting T2DM risk factors.

Besides regulating growth, GH has a major function in maintaining carbohydrate and lipid homeostasis which may have important relevance in conditions in which GH activity is high. When GH is secreted in excess, it acts directly to block insulin signaling, which then causes an elevation of glucose and insulin concentrations. Indeed impaired glucose intolerance, relative hyperinsulinemia, and overt T2DM are common features in acromegaly. Similarly, an increased incidence for T2DM in GH-treated children and adolescents was reported a decade ago [3]. In light of the rising prevalence of obesity in the general pediatric population and the trend toward higher GH doses, the objective of the study was to reevaluate the impact of GH treatment.

The Genetics and Neuroendocrinology of Short Stature International Study (GeNeSIS) is an open-label multinational observational safety study. The findings show that children who received growth hormone treatment had more than 8-fold increased risk of developing T2DM compared with unselected children. Children with organic growth hormone deficiency had a higher incidence of T2DM than children with idiopathic growth hormone deficiency. The majority of patients who developed T2DM had preexisting risk factors for diabetes such as Turner syndrome, Prader-Willi syndrome, and obesity, as well as small for gestational age and growth hormone deficiency due to leukemia and irradiation. Among the 11 patients who developed T2DM, hyperglycemia resolved in 7 patients. It is noteworthy that an additional 13 children had abnormal glucose tolerance.

This is an observational study and the value of the analysis depends on the accurate reporting of all events by the participating physicians, thus the rates might be biased. However, it seems that clinicians need to notify parents about the risk of T2DM, especially those with high-risk factors. Attention to glucose metabolism, both before and during GH treatment, is warranted.

Type 2 diabetes
Important for clinical practice

A clinical trial to maintain glycemic control in youth with type 2 diabetes

TODAY Study Group, Zeitler P, Hirst K, Pyle L, Linder B, Copeland K, Arslanian S, Cuttler L, Nathan DM, Tollefsen S, Wilfley D, Kaufman F
N Engl J Med 2012;366:2247–2256

Background: Despite the increasing prevalence of T2DM in youth, there are few data to guide treatment. The efficacies of three treatment regimens to achieve durable glycemic control in children and adolescents with recent-onset T2DM were compared.
Methods: All eligible patients 10–17 years of age were treated with metformin (1,000 mg twice daily) during the run-in phase to attain a glycated hemoglobin level of less than 8%, and were then randomly assigned to continued metformin alone, or metformin plus rosiglitazone (4 mg twice daily) or metformin plus a lifestyle-intervention program focusing on weight loss through eating and activity behaviors. The primary outcome was loss of glycemic control, defined as a glycated hemoglobin level of at least 8% for 6 months or sustained metabolic decompensation requiring insulin.
Results: Of the 699 randomized participants (mean duration of T2DM, 7.8 months), 319 (45.6%) reached the primary outcome over an average follow-up of 3.86 years. Rates of treatment failure were 51.7% (120/232), 38.6% (90/233), and 46.6% (109/234) for metformin alone, metformin plus rosiglitazone, and metformin plus lifestyle intervention, respectively. Metformin plus rosiglitazone was superior to metformin alone (p = 0.006); metformin plus lifestyle intervention was intermediate but not significantly different to the other groups. Prespecified subgroup analyses showed differences in sustained effectiveness, with metformin alone least effective in non-Hispanic black participants and metformin plus rosiglitazone most effective in girls. Serious adverse events were reported in 19.2%.
Conclusions: Monotherapy with metformin was associated with durable glycemic control in approximately half of children and adolescents with T2DM. The addition of rosiglitazone, but not an intensive lifestyle intervention, was superior to metformin alone.

The findings of this report are highly disappointing. Regardless of the therapy, about half of adolescents with T2DM failed to achieve adequate metabolic control of HbA_{1c} <8%. The American Diabetes Association recommends target HbA_{1c} values <7.5% for adolescents with T1DM aged 13–18 years. There is no reason to assume that a different target should be set for those with T2DM; on the contrary, youth with T2DM have additional risk factors that put them at increased risk for morbidity. T2DM is becoming increasingly common among youth in parallel with rates of childhood obesity. Despite this trend, there have been only a limited number of clinical trials investigating pharmacotherapy for T2DM in youth. Therapeutic modalities remain extremely limited and there are insufficient data on their effectiveness in children and adolescents. Most of the recommendations for treating T2DM in childhood are extrapolated from adults [4]. This is why this study is so important. Although the addition of rosiglitazone improved primary outcomes, this group showed increased weight gain. In contrast, metformin plus lifestyle intervention decreased the percentage of overweight adolescents. Two more noteworthy findings were: serious adverse effects were reported in 19.2% of adolescents, and there was no difference in rate of loss of glycemic control between participants who adhered to their medication regimen and those who did not. If metformin monotherapy at maximal tolerated dose is insufficient, additional treatment must be sought. In adults, intensive treatment with insulin in newly diagnosed T2DM can result in sustained remission. Studies on the efficacy and safety of long-acting glucagon-like peptide-1 (GLP-1) analog in combination with metformin and a selective dipeptidyl peptidase IV (DPP-4) inhibitor are currently ongoing. Long-term clinical studies with insulin treatment for youth with T2DM are needed.

Type 2 diabetes
Food for thought

Estimated morbidity and mortality in adolescents and young adults diagnosed with type 2 diabetes mellitus

Rhodes ET, Prosser LA, Hoerger TJ, Lieu T, Ludwig DS, Laffel LM
Division of Endocrinology, Children's Hospital Boston, Boston, MA, USA
erinn.rhodes@childrens.harvard.edu

Diabet Med 2012;29:453–463

Background: To estimate remaining life expectancy (RLE), quality-adjusted life years (QALY), causes of death and lifetime cumulative incidence of microvascular/macrovascular complications of diabetes for youths diagnosed with T2DM.

Methods: A Markov-like computer model simulated the life course for a hypothetical cohort of adolescents/young adults in the USA, aged 15–24 years, newly diagnosed with T2DM following either conventional or intensive treatment based on the UK Prospective Diabetes Study. Outcomes included RLE, QALYs, cumulative incidence of microvascular/macrovascular complications and causes of death.

Results: Compared with a mean RLE of 58.6 years for a 20-year-old in the USA without diabetes, those with T2DM on conventional treatment had an average RLE of 43.09 years and 22.44 discounted QALYs. Intensive treatment increased RLE by 0.98 years and QALYs by 0.44 years, and lowered lifetime cumulative incidence of microvascular complications and mortality from microvascular complications (e.g. end-stage renal disease (ESRD) death 19.4 vs. 25.2%). Approximately 5% with both treatments had ESRD within 25 years. Lifetime cumulative incidence of coronary heart disease (CHD) increased with longer RLE and greater severity of CHD risk factors. When incorporating disutility (loss in health-related quality of life), intensive treatment resulted in net loss of QALYs.

Conclusions: Adolescents/young adults with T2DM lose approximately 15 years from RLE and will experience severe, chronic complications of T2DM by their 40s. The net benefit of intensive treatment may be sensitive to preferences for treatment. A comprehensive management plan that includes early and aggressive control of cardiovascular risk factors is likely needed to reduce lifetime risk of CHD.

The onset of T2DM in adolescence appears to place the individual at very high risk for later major morbidity. The rate of progression of complications in adolescents with T2DM may be more rapid than in adolescents with T1DM. Understanding the true risks of early-onset T2DM on life expectancy may take decades. These authors used an alternative computer model to simulate a hypothetical course in adolescents with T2DM.

The authors estimated that an adolescent with T2DM on conventional treatment would be expected to survive until their early 60s, compared the late 70s in a healthy 20-year-old in the USA. Moreover, QALYs were reduced to only 22 years, suggesting that they may experience severe complications of T2DM by their 40s. The concept of quality-adjusted life-years (QALYs) is key to understanding this report. QALY is a measure for survival that accounts for the suboptimal quality of life due to poor health. One year of life lived in perfect health equals 1 QALY, while 1 year of life lived in poor health equals less than 1, ranging in number down to zero for death. The computer model relied on several assumptions about rates of complications and the impact of intervention. Risks were calculated from existing studies in adolescents with T2DM, and the effects of intervention (intensive vs. conventional) were based on the United Kingdom Prospective Diabetes Study (UKPDS) of adults with T2DM. One can only hope that the reality is more encouraging than these estimates.

Metabolic syndrome
New concerns

Metabolic syndrome in obese adolescents is associated with risk for nephrolithiasis

Tiwari R, Campfield T, Wittcopp C, Braden G, Visintainer P, Reiter EO, Allen HF
Department of Pediatrics, Baystate Medical Center/Tufts University School of Medicine, Boston, MA, USA

J Pediatr 2012;160:615–620 e2

Background: To examine the relationship between urinary pH and metabolic syndrome risk factors along with insulin resistance in obese adolescents, and to evaluate the relationship between other urinary stone-forming and -inhibiting markers and MetS.
Methods: 46 obese adolescents (mean age 14.6 ± 2.0 years; mean BMI 36 ± 6.3 kg/m^2) were enrolled. 24-Hour and random urine samples were analyzed for urinary pH, promoters of stone formation (uric acid, oxalate, and relative saturation ratio of calcium oxalate (RSR-CaOx)), and inhibitors of stone formation (citrate and osteopontin). Height, weight, blood pressure, and fasting lipid, insulin, and glucose levels were also collected.
Results: Random urine pH was inversely related to the number of MetS risk factors (r = –0.34; p = 0.02). RSR-CaOx was positively related to both the insulin resistance score (r = 0.38; p < 0.01) and number of MetS risk factors (r = 0.47; p = 0.001).
Conclusion: Decreased urinary pH and increased RSR-CaOx were associated with MetS risk factors in obese adolescents.

Among adults the prevalence of nephrolithiasis is increasing in parallel with the rising prevalence of obesity, and the risk of nephrolithiasis is increased in adults with obesity, MetS, and T2DM [5]. Insulin resistance plays a key role in the development of renal stones, being associated with low urinary pH, a potential cause of uric acid nephrolithiasis.

An increase in the number of children with nephrolithiasis has been documented in the last decade as well. In the current study, urine pH was unrelated to BMI Z-score, but pH declined with an increasing number of MetS traits in obese adolescents. The mean fresh urine pH was 5.23 in obese adolescents with 3 or more metabolic risk factors, compared with 6.12 in those with no risk factors. In addition, the relative saturation of calcium oxalate, a measure of the likelihood of precipitation of minerals in renal stones, was elevated in obese adolescents with more metabolic syndrome risk factors. These findings again show that the pathophysiological process of adult disease begins in childhood.

Michelangelo (1475–1564) suffered from recurrent urinary stones throughout his life and possibly died of fluid overload due to obstructive nephropathy. This may account for his interest in kidney function, evident in his poetry and drawings [6]. Most impressive is the mantle of the Creator in his painting of the Separation of Land and Water on the ceiling of the Sistine Chapel, which is in the shape of a bisected right kidney. His use of the renal outline in a scene representing the separation of solids (Land) from liquid (Water) suggests that Michelangelo was likely familiar with the anatomy and function of the kidney.

Metabolic syndrome in adolescence: can it be predicted from natal and parental profile? The Prediction of Metabolic Syndrome in Adolescence (PREMA) study

Efstathiou SP, Skeva II, Zorbala E, Georgiou E, Mountokalakis TD
Center for Cardiovascular Disease Prevention, Hygeias Melathron Infirmary, Athens, Greece
stamatise@gmail.com
Circulation 2012;125:902–910

Background: There are well-established predisposing factors for the metabolic syndrome (MetS) in childhood or adolescence, but no specific risk profile has yet been identified. The Prediction of Metabolic Syndrome in Adolescence (PREMA) study was conducted (1) to construct a classification score to detect children at high risk for MetS in adolescence and (2) to test its predictive ability.
Methods: In the derivation cohort (1,270 children), data from natal and parental profiles and from initial laboratory assessment at 6–8 years of age were used to select independent predictors of MetS at 13–15 years of age, as defined by the International Diabetes Federation criteria. In the independent validation cohort (1,091 adolescents), the discriminatory capacity of the derived prediction score was tested.
Results. MetS was diagnosed in 105 adolescents in the derivation cohort (8%). Independently, predictors of adolescent MetS were: low birth weight <10th percentile (odds ratio 6.02; 95% CI 2.53–10.12, p < 0.001), small birth head circumference <10th percentile (4.15; 2.04–7.14, p < 0.001), and at least one parent overweight or obese (3.22; 1.30–5.29, p < 0.01). In the validation cohort, 86 developed MetS (8%). These three factors predicted MetS with a sensitivity of 91% and a specificity of 98%.
Conclusions: The coexistence of low birth weight, small birth head circumference, and parental history of overweight or obesity predicts infants at risk of developing MetS in adolescence.

Metabolic syndrome (MetS) is a cluster of interconnected factors that increases the risk of cardiovascular atherosclerotic diseases and T2DM. Its main components are dyslipidemia (elevated triglycerides and low high-density lipoproteins (HDL), elevation of arterial blood pressure (BP) and dysregulated glucose homeostasis, abdominal obesity and insulin resistance. The International Diabetes Federation criteria are: abdominal obesity (waist circumference ≥90th percentile) combined with at least two of the following characteristics: hypertension (systolic pressure ≥130 mm Hg or diastolic pressure ≥85 mm Hg), fasting plasma glucose ≥100 mg/dl, triglycerides ≥150 mg/dl, and HDL cholesterol <40 mg/dl. Known risk factors for MetS include family history, poor diet, and inadequate exercise. The value of early recognition of risk factors of the MetS is clear.

After assessment of 2,361 white children and adolescents over a 10-year period, the present study showed that birth measurements and family history of obesity proved to be good predictors of future MetS. Prevalence of MetS increased with the number of risk factors, from 0% for those with no risk factors to 81% for those with all three risk factors. Combining all three predictors provided high sensitivity and specificity with a positive predictive value over 75% and a negative predictive value of 99%. These findings allow the very early identification of high-risk individuals for future targeted early life interventions.

 Orit Pinhas-Hamiel

Chemerin as a mediator between obesity and vascular inflammation in children

Landgraf K, Friebe D, Ullrich T, Kratzsch J, Dittrich K, Herberth G, Adams V, Kiess W, Erbs S, Korner A
Pediatric Research Center, Department of Women's and Child Health, University of Leipzig, Leipzig, Germany
Antje.Koerner@medizin.uni-leipzig.de
J Clin Endocrinol Metab 2012;97:E556–564

Background: The chemoattractant protein chemerin is expressed in adipose tissue. This study aimed to evaluate the association of chemerin with obesity and early-onset metabolic and vascular sequelae in children.

Methods: Serum chemerin concentrations were measured in 69 lean and 105 obese children and were related to their metabolic and cardiovascular parameters. In addition, a potential direct effect of chemerin on the expression of endothelial adhesion molecules and cell viability was assessed in human coronary artery endothelial cells in vitro.

Results: Chemerin concentrations were significantly higher in obese compared to lean children and were positively correlated with BMI SD score, leptin, and skinfold thickness. Moreover, significant associations were identified with the inflammatory markers: high-sensitive C-reactive protein and white blood cell count, and with markers of endothelial activation: intercellular adhesion molecule-1 (ICAM-1) and E-selectin. Multiple regression analyses confirmed chemerin as the strongest predictor of ICAM-1 and E-selectin, independent of BMI SD score. Chemerin induced ICAM-1 and E-selectin expression in endothelial cells in vitro, whereas VCAM-1 and eNOS expression and endothelial cell viability were unaffected.

Conclusion: These findings support a role for chemerin as a molecular link between fat mass and an early atherogenic risk profile in obese children.

The chemerin gene, also known as retinoic acid receptor responder 2 (RARRES2), was originally identified to be associated with psoriatic skin lesions. It is a secreted ligand of the orphan G-protein-coupled receptor chemokine-like receptor (CMKLR) [7]. The chemerin protein is a chemoattractant that promotes the recruitment of various cell types involved in innate and adaptive immunity to lymphoid organs and sites of tissue injury. In parallel, chemerin expression and secretion was found to increase dramatically with adipogenesis, while reduced chemerin expression in preadipocytes severely impairs differentiation into mature adipocytes. Beyond this autocrine function in adipocytes, chemerin/CMKLR1 signaling might have paracrine functions with in adipose tissue by contributing to obesity-related inflammation.

Among adults, plasma chemerin levels have been shown to correlate positively with body mass index (BMI), fasting glucose, fasting serum insulin, plasma triglycerides, and total serum cholesterol, and to correlate negatively with high-density lipoprotein (HDL) cholesterol. Unlike the findings in adult studies, the current study shows that in children, the correlation of chemerin with parameters of glucose and insulin metabolism, as well as with HDL-C and triglycerides and blood pressure, were due to underlying obesity. This suggests that the children in this study represent an earlier stage of secondary morbidity of obesity. Separate from BMI, chemerin levels in children correspond directly to CRP, the number of white blood cells. This suggests that chemerin levels play a role in low-grade systemic inflammation. To investigate a direct link between chemerin and vascular inflammation, chemerin levels were analyzed in association with measures of endothelial activation. Endothelial inflammatory markers such as intracellular adhesion molecule-1 (ICAM-1) and E-selectin were found to be associated with chemerin levels independent from the degree of obesity. This finding suggests that chemerin plays a role in early vascular inflammation.

In recent years, it has become clear that obesity is commonly associated with chronic low-grade systemic inflammation. The chemerin protein may be one of the mediators between the accumulation of fat mass and the induction of early atherogenesis in obese children.

Sleep architecture and glucose and insulin homeostasis in obese adolescents

Koren D, Levitt Katz LE, Brar PC, Gallagher PR, Berkowitz RI, Brooks LJ
Division of Pediatric Endocrinology and Diabetes, The Children's Hospital of Philadelphia, PA, USA
koren@email.chop.edu
Diabetes Care 2011;34:2442–2447

Background: Sleep deprivation is associated with increased risk of adult T2DM. It is uncertain whether sleep deprivation and/or altered sleep architecture affects glycemic regulation or insulin sensitivity or secretion.

Methods: In a cross-sectional observational study, 62 obese adolescents underwent oral glucose tolerance test (OGTT), anthropometric measurements, overnight polysomnography, and frequently sampled intravenous glucose tolerance test (FSIGT). HbA_{1c} and serial insulin and glucose levels were obtained, indices of insulin sensitivity and secretion were calculated, and sleep architecture was assessed. Correlation and regression analyses were performed to assess the association of total sleep and sleep stages with measures of insulin and glucose homeostasis, adjusted for confounding variables.

Results: There were significant U-shaped (quadratic) associations between sleep duration and both HbA_{1c} and serial glucose levels on OGTT and positive associations between slow-wave sleep (N3) duration and insulin secretory measures, independent of degree of obesity, pubertal stage, sex, and obstructive sleep apnea measures.

Conclusions: Both insufficient and excessive sleep were associated with short-term and long-term hyperglycemia in obese adolescents. Decreased N3 was associated with decreased insulin secretion. These effects may be interrelated, with reduced insulin secretory capacity leading to hyperglycemia. Optimizing sleep may prevent the development of T2DM in obese adolescents.

In addition to reduced physical activity and increased calorie intake, other putative causes have been suggested for the increased prevalence of obesity in recent decades [8]. These include endocrine disruptors, decreased smoking, reduction in variability of ambient temperature, pharmaceutical iatrogenesis, and a reduction in hours of sleep. The average hours of sleep have steadily decreased among US adults and children during the past several decades. Moreover, for children and adults, hours of sleep per night is inversely related to BMI, and sleep deprivation is associated with insulin resistance, increased risk of T2DM, and higher fasting glucose among adults with preexisting diabetes.

The metabolic consequences of insufficient sleep may be the result of a lack of total sleep hours or insufficiency in a certain sleep component. We therefore need to understand the four different sleep components as defined by the American Academy of Sleep Medicine. N sleep (non-rapid eye movement sleep) is made up of three stages. *Stage N1* is an initial very brief stage when one first falls asleep and again after awakenings during the night. Each episode lasts <10 min. Stage N2 makes up about 50% of total sleep time in normal adult sleep. *Stage N3*, which is known as 'deep sleep', makes up about 20% of total sleep time in normal adult sleep. The fourth component, REM (rapid eye movement sleep), typically occupies 20–25% of total sleep. During REM, the activity of the brain is similar to activity during waking hours. The current study suggests that glucose metabolism is optimal when sleep duration is 7.5–8.5 h. The authors encourage teenagers to get more sleep and to adopt good sleep habits by avoiding caffeine and dark chocolate late in the day, and by avoiding bright lights from TV monitors or computer monitors for a few hours before they go to sleep.

Polycystic ovary-like syndrome in adolescent competitive swimmers

Coste O, Paris F, Galtier F, Letois F, Maimoun L, Sultan C
Département d'Hormonologie, Hôpital Lapeyronie, Centre Hospitalo Universitaire Montpellier, Université Montpellier I, Montpellier, France
Fertil Steril 2011;96:1037–1042

Background: To investigate the potential effects of intensive swimming on clinical and hormonal pubertal development in adolescent girls and to determine whether hyperandrogenism contributes to menstrual disorders.
Methods: In a cross-sectional study, 18 competitive swimmers and 18 age-matched control subjects with breast stages IV or V. Clinical, biologic, and ultrasonographic investigations were done.
Results: A high number of cases of hyperandrogenism was seen in swimmers compared with control subjects (11 vs. 5 with T level >0.5 ng/ml), as well as a higher LH/FSH ratio (1.5 vs. 0.9) and SHBG level (58.4 vs. 39.5 nmol/l) and more oligomenorrhea (9 vs. 4). Half of the swimmers with hyperandrogenism presented pauci- or multifollicular ovaries determined by pelvic ultrasound. Free T was not significantly different between the two groups.
Conclusions: Hyperandrogenism and oligomenorrhea may be part of the spectrum of polycystic ovary syndrome in elite swimmers. These findings suggest that hyperandrogenism may have preceded the intensive training of these swimmers and may have predisposed the choice of sport for these girls. Intensive swimming may in turn have attenuated the clinical expression of their hyperandrogenism. Follow-up after the cessation of intensive activity would be helpful to evaluate the endocrine and metabolic profiles of these swimmers.

How many times has a parent asked you 'if my son plays basketball will he be taller'? Studies in gymnasts have shown that short stature in active gymnasts is partly due to a priori selection of individuals with shorter legs rather than being the result of vigorous exercise [9]. In the current study the authors aimed to understand the reasons for menstrual dysfunction among swimmers.

Young female athletes in a wide spectrum of sports activities suffer from menstrual dysfunction. Females with athletic amenorrhea have energy imbalance due to a combination of (1) increased energy expenditure, (2) low caloric intake as a result of body dissatisfaction and increased incidence of eating disorders, and (3) psychogenic stressors due to intense training and the rigors of competition. It is not surprising that the highest prevalence of menstrual dysfunction is observed in sports that emphasize low body weight, such as running and gymnastics. The hormonal profile in these cases is characterized by dysfunction of the hypothalamic-pituitary-ovarian axis with reduced GnRH pulsatility and low estrogen levels. The prevalence of menstrual disorders among swimmers has been reported to range from 15 to 82%.

In the current study, swimmers had lower fat mass and 50% had menstrual disorders, compared to 22% of the control group. 72% of the swimmers had a T level >0.5 ng/ml, defined as hyperandrogenism. The study concluded that the cause for menstrual disorders was not due to dysfunction of the hypothalamic-pituitary-ovarian axis, but was rather secondary to hyperandrogenism. The authors suggest that the PCO-like syndrome in these female athletes is not a coincidence. A predisposition to hyperandrogenism might orient girls toward sports such as swimming, where strength is a performance criterion. Moreover, the authors even speculate that swimming may have attenuated the clinical expression of the hyperandrogenism and decreased the risk of developing MetS.

Expert panel on integrated guidelines for cardiovascular health and risk reduction in children and adolescents: summary report

Expert panel on integrated guidelines for cardiovascular health and risk reduction in children and adolescents
Pediatrics 2011;128(suppl 5):S213–256

Pediatric screening for hypercholesterolemia in Europe

Kusters DM, de Beaufort C, Widhalm K, Guardamagna O, Bratina N, Ose L, Wiegman A
Department of Pediatrics, Academic Medical Center, Amsterdam, The Netherlands
Arch Dis Child 2012;97:272–276

Background: Different screening strategies are currently recommended to identify children with (familial) hypercholesterolemia in order to initiate early lipid management. However, these strategies are characterized to date by low adherence by the medical community and limited compliance by parents and children.
Methods: In a literature review, the authors assessed which children should undergo screening and which children are identified through current recommended strategies. Different screening tools and strategies currently used in Europe and what is known about the negative aspects of screening are discussed.
Results and Conclusions: The authors conclude that currently recommended selective screening strategies, which are mainly based on family history, lack precision and that a large percentage of children at high risk of future coronary artery disease are not being identified. They suggest that universal screening of children between 1 and 9 years of age is likely to be most effective in terms of sensitivity and specificity to identify children with familial hypercholesterolemia. However, this concept has yet to be proven in clinical practice.

The National Heart, Lung and blood Institute (NHLB) expert panel published guidelines for pediatric care providers to reduce cardiovascular disease risks in children. These guidelines were endorsed by the American Academy of Pediatrics (AAP). The recommendations address two different goals: to prevent risk-factor development (primordial prevention), and to prevent cardiovascular disease (primary prevention). These are integrated guidelines regarding nutrition, physical activity, smoking, blood pressure, obesity and the metabolic syndrome management.

Focusing on lipid management these guidelines differ from those published by the US Preventive Services Task Force (USPSTF) 4 years ago. The current guidelines suggest the following actions be carried out: (1) universal lipid screening on all children at 9–11 years of age; (2) selective screening of children aged 2–8 years who have a family history of cardiovascular disease or dyslipidemia or risk factors such as diabetes, hypertension or medical conditions; (3) no routine screening for children aged 12–16 years of age; screen only if there is new family history or at-risk medical condition; (4) universal screening once between age 17 and 21 years, and (5) the cut-off points used to consider use of drug therapy did not change.

These recommendations were supported by level B evidence, i.e. randomized control trials or diagnostic studies with minor limitations, genetic natural history studies, and overwhelmingly consistent evidence from observational studies. However, they have been much criticized because there are no long-term trials of treatment on cardiovascular outcomes and there are no data on the safety of lipid-lowering drugs in children. The proponents of universal screening suggest that children with moderate hyperlipidemia may benefit from lifestyle intervention and children with severe hyperlipidemia would benefit from decreased morbidity.

In light of disagreements in the USA, it is interesting to read the European recommendations published in the same year by Kusters et al. The authors reviewed current practices in Europe. In the Netherlands, Norway and the UK there is an ongoing cascade-screening program for children with positive index cases with familial hyperlipidemia. In Slovenia, there is general cholesterol screening in preschool children at the age of 5 years, and in Italy a selective screening program for children with a positive family history. The authors propose a strategy of universal screening when children have routine vaccinations between 1 and 9 years of age. Yet they admit that this concept has yet to be tested. Clinicians are advised that guidelines are based on the best available information and it is up to them whether or not to follow them. Personally, I believe that children should be tested for high cholesterol levels, which may uncover not only their own FH but also the possible risk heart disease for their parents.

New concerns

Risk of incident diabetes with intensive-dose compared with moderate-dose statin therapy: a meta-analysis

Preiss D, Seshasai SR, Welsh P, Murphy SA, Ho JE, Waters DD, DeMicco DA, Barter P, Cannon CP, Sabatine MS, Braunwald E, Kastelein JJ, de Lemos JA, Blazing MA, Pedersen TR, Tikkanen MJ, Sattar N, Ray KK
BHF Glasgow Cardiovascular Research Centre, University of Glasgow, Glasgow, UK
david.preiss@glasgow.ac.uk

JAMA 2011;305:2556–2564

Background: A recent meta-analysis demonstrated that statin therapy is associated with excess risk of developing diabetes mellitus. This study aimed to investigate whether intensive-dose statin therapy increases the risk of incident diabetes compared with moderate-dose statin therapy.

Methods: Relevant trials in a literature search of MEDLINE, EMBASE, and the Cochrane Central Register of Controlled Trials (January 1, 1996, through March 31, 2011) were identified. Unpublished data were obtained from investigators. Randomized controlled endpoint trials that compared intensive-dose versus moderate-dose statin therapy and included more than 1,000 participants who were followed up for more than 1 year were included. Trial-specific odds ratios (ORs) for incident diabetes and major cardiovascular events were calculated using random-effects model meta-analysis.

Results: In 5 statin trials with 32,752 participants without diabetes at baseline, 2,749 developed diabetes (1,449 assigned intensive-dose therapy, 1,300 assigned moderate-dose therapy, representing 2.0 additional cases in the intensive-dose group per 1,000 patient-years) and 6,684 experienced cardiovascular events (3,134 and 3,550, respectively, representing 6.5 fewer cases in the intensive-dose group per 1,000 patient-years) over a weighted mean ± SD follow-up of 4.9 ± 1.9 years. Odds ratios were 1.12 (95% CI 1.04–1.22; I^2 = 0%) for incident diabetes and 0.84 (95% CI 0.75–0.94; I^2 = 74%) for cardiovascular events for intensive- versus moderate-dose therapy. As compared with moderate-dose statin therapy, the number needed to harm per year for intensive-dose statin therapy was 498 for incident diabetes while the number needed to treat per year for intensive-dose statin therapy was 155 for cardiovascular events.

Conclusion: In a pooled analysis of data from 5 statin trials, intensive- versus moderate-dose statin therapy increased the risk of incident diabetes but reduced the risk of cardiovascular events.

Statins effectively improve survival in subjects with acute coronary syndrome or other risk factors for atherosclerotic coronary artery disease. A decrease in LDL-C levels of 40 mg/dl translates to a 13% lower risk of death. However, studies variably report that statins increase the risk for diabetes [10]. JUPITER (Justification for the Use of Statins in Primary Prevention: An Intervention Trial Evaluating Rosuvastatin) showed that statins increased the risk of newly diagnosed diabetes by 25%; on the other hand, a meta-analysis of 13 randomized trials involving 91,140 patients concluded that the risk of diabetes was only 9% higher [11]. It is interesting that there was no relationship between the degree of lowering of LDL-C levels and risk of new-onset diabetes. Risk factors for diabetes include older age, higher baseline fasting glucose levels, and higher dose of statins.

The current study now shows that intensive- versus moderate-dose statin therapy increases the risk of new-onset diabetes by 12%, but reduced the risk of cardiovascular events by16%. One additional patient develops diabetes for every 3 patients protected from a major cardiovascular event. How statins increase the incidence of diabetes is still unknown. These findings shed a warning for the use of statins in children, who may require statin therapy for many decades; the risk:benefit ratio of long-term statin therapy in children should be monitored.

Effect of a monoclonal antibody to PCSK9 on LDL cholesterol

Stein EA, Mellis S, Yancopoulos GD, Stahl N, Logan D, Smith WB, Lisbon E, Gutierrez M, Webb C, Wu R, Du Y, Kranz T, Gasparino E, Swergold GD
Metabolic and Atherosclerosis Research Center, Cincinnati, OH, USA
esteirmrl@aol.com
N Engl J Med 2012;366:1108–1118

Background: Proprotein convertase subtilisin/kexin 9 (PCSK9), one of the serine proteases, binds to low-density lipoprotein (LDL) receptors, leading to their accelerated degradation and to increased LDL-C levels. Three phase 1 studies of a monoclonal antibody to PCSK9 designated as REGN727/SAR236553 (REGN727) are reported.
Methods: Two randomized, single ascending-dose studies of REGN727 administered either intravenously (40 subjects) or subcutaneously (32 subjects), as compared with placebo, were performed in healthy volunteers. In addition, a randomized, placebo-controlled, multiple-dose trial in adults with heterozygous familial hypercholesterolemia who were receiving atorvastatin (21 subjects) and those with nonfamilial hypercholesterolemia who were receiving atorvastatin (30 subjects) (baseline LDL-C, >100 mg/dl (2.6 mmol/l)) or a modified diet alone (10 subjects) (baseline LDL-C, >130 mg/dl (3.4 mmol/l)). REGN727 doses of 50, 100, or 150 mg were administered subcutaneously on days 1, 29, and 43. The primary outcome for all studies was the occurrence of adverse events. The principal secondary outcome was the effect of REGN727 on the lipid profile.
Results: There were no discontinuations of REGN727 due to adverse events. REGN727 significantly lowered LDL-C levels in all the studies. In the multiple-dose study, REGN727 doses of 50, 100, and 150 mg reduced measured LDL-C levels in the combined atorvastatin-treated populations to 77.5 mg/dl (2.00 mmol/l), 61.3 mg/dl (1.59 mmol/l), and 53.8 mg/dl (1.39 mmol/l); differences in the change from baseline were −39.2, −53.7, and −61.0 percentage points, respectively, as compared with placebo (p < 0.001 for all comparisons).
Conclusions: In three phase 1 trials, a monoclonal antibody to PCSK9 reduced LDL-C levels in healthy volunteers and in subjects with familial or nonfamilial hypercholesterolemia.

Safety and efficacy of a monoclonal antibody to proprotein convertase subtilisin/kexin type 9 serine protease, SAR236553/REGN727, in patients with primary hypercholesterolemia receiving ongoing stable atorvastatin therapy

McKenney JM, Koren MJ, Kereiakes DJ, Hanotin C, Ferrand AC, Stein EA
Virginia Commonwealth University and National Clinical Research, Inc., Richmond, VA, USA
J Am Coll Cardiol 2012;59:2344–2353

Background: The primary objective of this study was to evaluate the LDL-C-lowering efficacy of 5 SAR236553/REGN727 (REGN727) dosing regimens versus placebo at week 12 in patients with LDL-C ≥100 mg/dl on stable atorvastatin therapy. Secondary objectives included other lipid parameters and the attainment of LDL-C treatment goals of <100 mg/dl (2.59 mmol/l) and <70 mg/dl (1.81 mmol/l).
Methods: This double-blind, parallel-group, placebo-controlled trial randomized 183 patients with LDL-C ≥100 mg/dl (2.59 mmol/l) on stable-dose atorvastatin 10, 20, or 40 mg for ≥6 weeks to: subcutaneous placebo every 2 weeks (Q2W); REGN727 at 50, 100, or 150 mg (Q2W), or REGN727 at 200 or 300 mg every 4 weeks (Q4W), alternating with placebo for a total treatment period of 12 weeks.
Results: REGN727 demonstrated a clear dose-response effect on percentage LDL-C lowering for both Q2W and Q4W administration: 40, 64, and 72% with 50, 100, and 150 mg Q2W, respectively, and 43 and 48% with 200 and 300 mg Q4W, compared to 5% with placebo. REGN727 also substantially reduced non-HDL cholesterol, apolipoprotein B, and lipoprotein(a). REGN727 was generally well tolerated. One patient on REGN727 experienced a serious adverse event of leukocytoclastic vasculitis.

Conclusions: When added to atorvastatin, PCSK9 inhibition with REGN727 further reduces LDL-C by 40–72%. These additional reductions are both dose- and dosing frequency-dependent.

Familial hypercholesterolemia (FH) is an autosomal dominant disorder that causes extreme elevations in total cholesterol and LDL-C, and occurs in approximately 1 per 500 persons worldwide. It is most often associated with loss-of-function mutations in the gene encoding the LDL receptor (LDLR), and familial defective Apo-B100 (FDB) caused by mutations in ApoB-100 (APOB) that disrupt the binding of LDL to its receptor. In 2003, proprotein convertase subtilisin kexin type 9 (PCSK9) was discovered as the third class of mutations involved in autosomal dominant FH [12]. PCSK9 is synthesized primarily in the liver, and enters the circulatory system, where it binds to and accelerates the degradation of hepatic LDL receptors. This process reduces the capacity of the liver to remove LDL-C from the circulation. Patients with PCSK9 gain-of-function mutations have high LDL-C levels whereas patients with PCSK9 loss-of-function mutations have low levels of LDL-C and low incidence of coronary heart disease. Based on this knowledge, pharmacologic inhibition of PCSK9 is sought either by blocking its action or preventing its formation.

Stein et al. report phase 1 data on REGN727, a monoclonal antibody specific to PCSK9 which reduced LDL-C levels by 73% compared to a placebo in healthy volunteers and in statin-treated subjects with familial and nonfamilial forms of hypercholesterolemia. The short duration of this trial limited the ability to evaluate its safety profile. McKenney et al. confirm in a phase 2 trial that REGN727 reduced LDL cholesterol levels by 39.6% with the 50-mg dose to 72% on 150 mg. The biweekly injection was more potent than four weekly. At week 12, 100% of the patients treated with a 150-mg injection of REGN727 had LDL-C levels <70 mg/dl. One patient developed diarrhea and a rash, which was diagnosed as leukocytoclastic vasculitis and was considered to be a significant medical event. Six other patients discontinued the drug owing to adverse events such as neutropenia, fatigue, rash, headache, and nausea.

Although concerns have been raised regarding the cost of PCSK9-directed antibodies, it is clear that this new drug is a landmark in the treatment for FH.

Important for clinical practice

Pregnancy outcomes in familial hypercholesterolemia: a registry-based study

Toleikyte I, Retterstol K, Leren TP, Iversen PO
Department of Nutrition, Institute of Basic Medical Sciences, University of Oslo, Oslo, Norway
Circulation 2011;124:1606–1614

Background: Women with familial hypercholesterolemia (FH) are prone to early cardiovascular disease and death. It is unknown whether FH adversely affects pregnancy and birth outcomes. This study aimed to determine whether heterozygous FH women are at higher risk of premature birth (<37 gestational weeks), delivering infants with low birth weight (<2,500 g) and/or congenital malformations.
Methods: Information from the Medical Genetics Laboratory was linked to the Medical Birth Registry of Norway. 1,869 FH women (≥14 years) from the Medical Genetics Laboratory and about 2 million (general population) from the Medical Birth Registry of Norway during the period 1967–2006 were included. The registry match allowed analysis of 2,319 births in 1,093 women with heterozygous FH.
Results: The mean ± SD prepregnancy total cholesterol concentration was 9.59 ± 2.06 mmol/l (370 ± 80 mg/dl). The frequencies of prematurity, low birth weight, and congenital malformations in the FH population were 6.8, 5.0, and 3.3%, respectively, compared to 6.2, 5.2, and 3.2% in the general population. The corresponding odds ratios were 1.11 (95 CI 0.94–1.31; p = 0.23), 0.96 (0.79–1.15; p = 0.64), and 1.09 (0.87–1.37; p = 0.45).
Conclusions: Women with FH do not have higher risks of adverse pregnancy outcomes.

During pregnancy, plasma cholesterol may increase by 25–50% and plasma triglycerides by 50–300%. Women with heterozygous familial hypercholesterolemia (FH) show similar relative changes, but higher absolute changes, in plasma lipid levels than in healthy women. Moreover, lipid-lowering drugs are not recommended during preconception, pregnancy and lactation. Hyperlipidemia during pregnancy may induce atherosis in the uteroplacental spiral arteries that, combined with hypercoagulation, may result in thrombosis and placental infarctions, leading to placental insufficiency and thereby fetal compromise.

In this retrospective study, no maternal cardiovascular deaths were observed. Also, children of mothers with FH were no more likely than the general population to be born prematurely, have low birth weight, or have congenital malformations. The accompanying editorial [13] emphasized that high LDL-C levels during childbearing years may have long-term implications for women with FH.

While no congenital malformations were observed in the 19 pregnancies associated with the use of lipid-lowering drugs, statins are classified as category X in pregnancy, which means they have been linked to fetal abnormalities in animal and human studies, and their benefits do not outweigh their potential risks. Statin exposure during the first trimester is associated with defects of the central nervous system and unilateral limb deficiencies. The Food and Drug Administration classifies ezetimibe and niacin as category C in pregnancy, which means 'animal reproduction studies have shown an adverse effect on the fetus and there are no adequate and well-controlled studies in humans, but potential benefits may warrant use of the drug in pregnant women despite potential risks'.

Food for thought

Improbable research: the German beer belly is misunderstood

Abrahams M

Mini-Annals of Improbable Research 'mini-AIR' April 2012

I encourage you to check the mini-AIR website: http://www.improbable.com/airchives/miniair/. It is the simplest way to keep informed about Improbable and Ig Nobel news and events. It is advertised as 'the magazine about research that makes people laugh and then think, and it will bring a smile to your face'.

The above review cites work by scientists who questioned whether beer is the main cause of beer bellies in Germans [14]. The weight, waist and hip circumferences of 19,941 men and women were recorded related to self-reported surveys of beer consumption. Their estimates were based on the size of a typical bottle of beer in Germany. Women were placed in four categories from 'no beer' to 'moderate drinkers'. Men were placed in five categories from 'no beer' to 'heavy drinkers'. For women, 'moderate' meant consuming at least 250 ml of beer a day. For men, 'moderate' meant 500–1,000 ml/day. The authors conclude that their study 'does not support the common belief of a site-specific effect of beer on the abdomen, the beer belly'. So now, enjoy Gose, a top-fermented beer characteristic of Leipzig. Cheers. . .!

References
1. Hegele RA, Zinman B, Hanley AJ, Harris SB, Barrett PH, Cao H: Genes, environment and Oji-Cree type 2 diabetes. Clin Biochem 2003;36:163–170.
2. Millar K, Dean HJ: Developmental origins of type 2 diabetes in aboriginal youth in Canada: it is more than diet and exercise? J Nutr Metab 2012;2012:127452.
3. Cutfield WS, Wilton P, Bennmarker H, et al: Incidence of diabetes mellitus and impaired glucose tolerance in children and adolescents receiving growth-hormone treatment. Lancet 2000;355:610–613.
4. Flint A, Arslanian S: Treatment of type 2 diabetes in youth. Diabetes Care 2011;34(suppl 2):S177–183.
5. Sakhaee K, Maalouf NM, Sinnott B: Kidney stones 2012: pathogenesis, diagnosis, and management. J Clin Endocrinol Metab 2012.
6. Eknoyan G: Michelangelo: art, anatomy, and the kidney. Kidney Int 2000;57:1190–1201.
7. Ernst MC, Sinal CJ: Chemerin: at the crossroads of inflammation and obesity. Trends Endocrinol Metab 2010;21:660–667.
8. Keith SW, Redden DT, Katzmarzyk PT, et al: Putative contributors to the secular increase in obesity: exploring the roads less traveled. Int J Obes (Lond) 2006;30:1585–1594.

9. Bass S, Bradney M, Pearce G, et al: Short stature and delayed puberty in gymnasts: influence of selection bias on leg length and the duration of training on trunk length. J Pediatr 2000;136:149–155.
10. Goldfine AB: Statins: is it really time to reassess benefits and risks? N Engl J Med 2012;366:1752–1755.
11. Sattar N, Preiss D, Murray HM, et al: Statins and risk of incident diabetes: a collaborative meta-analysis of randomised statin trials. Lancet 2010;375:735–742.
12. Abifadel M, Varret M, Rabes JP, et al: Mutations in PCSK9 cause autosomal dominant hypercholesterolemia. Nat Genet 2003;34:154–156.
13. Rutherford JD: Maternal heterozygous familial hypercholesterolemia and its consequences for mother and child. Circulation 2011;124:1599–1601.
14. Schutze M, Schulz M, Steffen A, et al: Beer consumption and the 'beer belly': scientific basis or common belief? Eur J Clin Nutr 2009;63:1143–1149.

Evidence-Based Medicine in Pediatric Endocrinology and Diabetes

Gary Butler[a,b], Carrie Williams[a,b], Lee Hudson[a,b] and Stephen O'Riordan[c]

[a]University College London Hospital, London, UK
[b]Institute of Child Health, University College London, UK
[c]Cork University Hospital, Cork, Ireland

The principal themes in this year's chapter are hypoglycemia, its problems and prevention, strategies to improve bone health and growth, and hyperandrogenism, new insights into the diagnosis and treatment together with reports of novel uses of growth hormone. Although the studies selected are among the best we identified, the challenges of obtaining high quality clinical evidence are there to see. Important consensus documents released include the American Diabetes Association statement about transitional care [1] and continuous glucose monitoring [2]. New information about the longer term safety of growth hormone treatment is gradually emerging albeit piecemeal at the present time (see chapter on Growth and Growth Factors) [3, 4], but as yet there is not enough high quality evidence to make it into this *Yearbook* chapter. However, when concerns are raised, we need to be reminded of why we use such a treatment to improve short stature [5]. As ever, what is presented is a small selection from an outstandingly good publication year, selected principally to inform and guide your everyday clinical practice.

Mechanism of the year
Keeping the β cell going

Teplizumab for the treatment of type 1 diabetes (Protégé Study): 1-year results from a randomized placebo-controlled trial

Sherry N, Hagopian W, Ludvigsson J, Jain SM, Wahlen J, Ferry RJ Jr, Bode B, Aronoff S, Holland S, Carlin D, King KL, Wilder RL, Pillemer S, Bonvini E, Johnson S, Stein KE, Koenig S, Herold KC, Daifotis AG
General Hospital for Children, Boston, MA, USA
nsherry@partners.org
Lancet 2011;378:487–497

Background: Small studies have suggested that short treatments with anti-CD3 monoclonal antibodies (mutated to reduce Fc receptor binding) may preserve β-cell function and decrease insulin needs in patients with recent-onset type 1 diabetes. This phase 3 trial aims to assess the safety and efficacy of teplizumab, one such anti-CD3 monoclonal antibody.

Methods: The paper describes interim data from the first year of this 2-year trial. Patients, aged 8–35 years, who had been diagnosed with type 1 diabetes for 12 weeks or fewer were enrolled and treated at 83 clinical centers in North America, Europe, Israel, and India. Participants were allocated (2:1:1:1 ratio) by an interactive telephone system, according to computer-generated block randomization, to receive one of three regimens of teplizumab infusions (14-day full dose, 14-day low dose, or 6-day full dose) or placebo at baseline and at 26 weeks. The primary composite outcome was the percentage of patients with insulin use of <0.5 U/kg/day and glycated hemoglobin A_{1c} (HbA_{1c}) of <6.5% at 1 year. Analyses included all patients who received at least one dose of study drug. As this study is still underway, patients and study staff remain masked through to study closure.

Results: 513 of 763 patients screened were randomized to receive 14-day full-dose teplizumab (n = 209), 14-day low-dose teplizumab (n = 102), 6-day full-dose teplizumab (n = 106), or placebo (n = 99). Two patients in the 14-day full-dose group and 1 patient in the placebo group did not start treatment, leaving 513 patients eligible for efficacy analyses. The primary outcome did not differ between groups at 1 year: 19.8% (41/207) in the 14-day full-dose group, 13.7% (14/102) in the 14-day low-dose group, 20.8% (22/106) in the 6-day full-dose group, and 20.4% (20/98) in the placebo group. 5% (19/415) of patients in the teplizumab groups were not taking insulin at 1 year, compared with no patients in the placebo group at 1 year (p = 0.03). Similar proportions of patients had adverse events across the four study groups (99% in the teplizumab groups vs. 99% in the placebo group) and serious adverse events (10 vs. 9%). The most common clinical adverse event in the teplizumab groups was rash (53 vs. 20% in the placebo group).

Conclusion: Findings of exploratory analyses suggest that future studies of immunotherapeutic intervention with teplizumab might have increased success in prevention of a decline in β-cell function (measured by C-peptide) and provision of glycemic control at reduced doses of insulin if they target patients early after diagnosis of diabetes and especially children aged 8–11 years.

> The Protégé Study is a very impressive well-designed, large, multicenter (83 centers), randomized, double-blind, placebo-controlled trial. Although the interim primary outcome, presented above, does not differ between treatment and placebo groups, it is definitely worth taking the time to delve a little deeper into this study as the post-hoc analysis has some interesting findings. At any given HbA$_{1c}$ threshold, the authors found a greater percentage of patients in the 14-day full-dose group achieved that threshold at lower insulin doses than in the placebo group at all stages of the study. This was particularly the case for children and for adults recently diagnosed with type 1 diabetes. This study is pushing the frontiers of diabetes care both at clinical and experimental levels. It highlights the importance of including children in large, multicenter, randomized, double-blind, placebo-controlled trials and the importance of translational research linking bench to bedside. This study not only supports the need for further studies investigating this fascinating and promising mechanism, it also serves as a reminder of the importance of choosing the most appropriate primary outcome for any study.

New paradigms
Building bones

Influence of a 3-year exercise intervention program on fracture risk, bone mass, and bone size in prepubertal children

Lofgren B, Detter F, Dencker M, Stenevi-Lundgren S, Nilsson JA, Karlsson MK
Clinical and Molecular Osteoporosis Research Unit, Department of Orthopaedics, Lund University, Skane University Hospital, Malmo, Sweden
bjarne.lofgren@med.lu.se

J Bone Miner Res 2011;26:1740–1747

Background: Previous publications showing that exercise during childhood can improve bone mineral density have tended to follow up after short periods (<12 months) and have reported other endpoints than actual fracture rates. There has been debate as to whether an increased risk of fracture from moderate exercise regimes outweighs the benefits of bone mineral density accrual.

Methods: Fractures were registered prospectively in 446 boys and 362 girls in an intervention group of an additional 40 min exercise per day over the 3-year study period, and 807 boys and 780 girls in a control group following a standardized national program of 60 min per week. A subgroup of 76 male and 48 female cases aged 7–9 years and 55 males and 44 female controls in the same age range had serial measurements of lumbar and hip bone mineral content as well as bone size using DEXA prospectively over 3 years. Presence of a fracture was also collected prospectively for all children from local hospital data.

Results. There were 108 fractures during the study period. Rate ratio of fractures between cases and controls was 1.08 (95% CI 0.71, 1.62) with no gender differences. There were no differences at baseline in age, anthropometrics, or bone traits between cases and controls. The mean annual gain in the intervention group in lumbar spine BMC was 0.9 SD higher in girls and 0.8 SD higher in boys (both p < 0.001) and in the third lumbar vertebra width 0.4 SD higher in girls and 0.3 SD higher in boys (both p < 0.05) than in control children.

Conclusion: A moderately intense 3-year exercise program compared with standard school ones can increase bone mineral content and possibly bone size without increasing short-term fracture risk.

This paper and the one below share the theme of the importance of childhood and adolescence in the acquisition of longer-term bone health but look separately at an intervention to promote bone strength in childhood and a potential treatment for those with anorexia nervosa-related osteopenia.

In the study of Lofgren et al., both controls and cases received the same type of physical education, but for more regular and frequent periods than usual. The consistency of duration of physical education ensured was measured with accelerometers in both groups. Differences in extracurricular physical activity were ascertained and accounted for through questionnaires. Important baseline and follow-up analysis was made looking at changes in pubertal stage and body composition with control for the impact of both as they could potentially be confounders on evaluation of bone mineral density and bone size between groups. Furthermore, in addition to the increases in bone mineral content associated with greater physica activity, in both males and females, vertebral size was increased in those who received higher levels of regular physical education. The authors argue that this may provide additional benefits to bone strength alongside greater bone mineral content. This might be especially important in the vertebral region where crush fractures are a difficult, aged-related later-life pathology [6]. The lack of difference in fracture rates between those in a more intensive level of physical act vity regimen reassures concerns over short-term negative effects of more intensive activity regimens Interestingly, girls in with higher level of activities saw significantly bigger yearly increases in body fat. A limitation of this paper is the small number of children finally recruited into the detailed study from a larger proportion of children receiving the intervention and control across the four schools, but most likely reflects the multitude of difficulties facing all researchers when recruiting children into studies. Ultimately this paper adds to a number of health benefits associated with adequate and regular exercise for all children [7–9] and perhaps particularly highlights the importance of school-based physical education.

Physiologic estrogen replacement increases bone density in adolescent girls with anorexia nervosa

Misra M, Katzman D, Miller KK, Mendes N, Snelgrove D, Russell M, Goldstein MA, Ebrahimi S, Clauss L, Weigel T, Mickley D, Schoenfeld DA, Herzog DB, Klibanski A
Neuroendocrine Unit, Massachusetts General Hospital and Harvard Medical School, Boston, MA, USA
mmisra@partners.org

J Bone Miner Res 2011;26:2430–2438

Background: Underweight and amenorrhea are associated with reduced bone mineral density (BMD) and accrual of BMD in anorexia nervosa, as a result of nutritional and hormonal abnormalities. Previous studies of oral estrogen supplementation had not shown improvements in BMD.

Methods: 110 girls with a diagnosis of anorexia nervosa were recruited with 40 normal-weight controls. Mature girls with bone age ≥15 years (96) were randomized to either transdermal 100 µg of 17β-estradiol (with cyclic progesterone) or transdermal placebo for 18 months. Immature girls with bone age ≤15 years were randomized to low-dose incremental oral ethinylestradiol (3.75 mg daily from 0 to 6 months, 7.5 mg from 6 to 12 months, 11.25 mg from 12 to 18 months) or placebo for 18 months. Participants were assessed by dual-energy X-ray absorptiometry (DEXA) at 6, 12 and 18 months. Participants and assessors were blind to intervention or control status (double-blind).

Results: At baseline, in both immature and mature participants, spine and hip BMD did not differ between cases provided with estrogen compared to those with placebo. Spine and hip BMI Z-scores increased over time in those treated with estrogen compared with placebo.

Conclusion: Physiological estradiol replacement increases spine and hip BMD in girls with anorexia nervosa.

The authors report a double-blind RCT which brings some hope for treatment of adolescent females with prolonged periods of underweight and persistent amenorrhea secondary to anorexia nervosa. Although weight restoration is the best treatment for improving (or least preventing deterioration in) bone mineral density consequent to underweight [10], a significant number of patients fail to achieve this, or if it happens it is very delayed [11]. Results from previous RCTs using oral estrogen have been disappointing, showing no benefit [12–14]. The authors hypothesize that the physiological doses of oral estrogen given in this study avoid suppression of IGF-1 secretion and the consequent reduced impact on bone formation which may occur with higher doses of estrogen therapy. The study found no effect on body mass or composition, an important finding when prescribing for patients with anorexia. The authors did not report incidence of side effects of sudden administration of estrogen to postmenarchal patients (such as mood disturbances). The study had a high attrition rate (of 150 cases and controls originally recruited, only 90 completed the trial). The long-term safety profile of estrogen in this context also remains unknown, especially in the immature group. The authors used oral progesterone to counter the possible late effects of unopposed estrogen activity in those with higher doses by transdermal route.

Finally, as with so many studies of bone mineral density in children and adolescence, this study and the one above provide detailed analysis of measured bone density which can only be used as a proxy for future fracture risk. It is important to note that neither of them are currently able to provide differences in actual long-term fracture rates between controls and cases. Thus longer-term studies are indeed essential to defend the relative costs and risks of both implementing public interventions to promote bone health and prescribing hormonal treatments for those viewed most at risk, such as those with anorexia nervosa.

New hope
Getting better at preventing hypos

Sensor-augmented pump therapy for HbA$_{1c}$ reduction (STAR 3) study: results from the 6-month continuation phase

Bergenstal RM, Tamborlane WV, Ahmann A, Buse JB, Dailey G, Davis SN, Joyce C, Perkins BA, Welsh JB, Willi SM, Wood MA, STAR 3 Study Group
International Diabetes Center at Park Nicollet, Minneapolis, MN, USA
richard.bergenstal@parknicollet.com
Diabetes Care 2011;34:2403–2405

Background: This study examined the effects of crossing over from optimized multiple daily injection (MDI) therapy to sensor-augmented pump (SAP) therapy for 6 months, and the sustained effects of 18 months' of SAP usage.

Methods: This study was a 6-month, single-crossover continuation phase of the Sensor-Augmented Pump Therapy for HbA$_{1c}$ Reduction (STAR 3) trial which provided SAP therapy to 420 patients after completing the 1-year randomized study. Change in HbA$_{1c}$ was the primary outcome in the crossover group.

Results: The HbA$_{1c}$ values were initially lower in the continuing-SAP group than in the crossover group (7.4 vs. 8.0%, p < 0.001). HbA$_{1c}$ values remained lower in the SAP group. After 3 months on the SAP system, HbA$_{1c}$ decreased to 7.6% in the crossover group (p < 0.001) and there was a sustained and significant decrease in both adult and pediatric groups (p < 0.05).

Conclusions: Converting from optimized MDI to SAP therapy allowed for rapid and safe HbA$_{1c}$ reductions. Glycemic benefits of SAP therapy were sustained at 18 months in children and adults.

Prevention of hypoglycemia by using low glucose suspend function in sensor-augmented pump therapy

Danne T, Kordonouri O, Holder M, Haberland H, Golembowski S, Remus K, Blasig S, Wadien T, Zierow S, Hartmann R, Thomas A
Children's Hospital on the Bult, Hannover, Germany
danne@hka.de
Diabetes Technol Ther 2011;13:1129–1134

Background: This study reports on the severe hypoglycemic episodes as a barrier for achieving optimal glycemic control. Sensor-augmented pump (SAP) therapy with insulin in combination with a novel mechanism of automatic insulin shutoff (low glucose suspend (LGS)) can be used to prevent and reduce hypoglycemia. This prospective study investigated the effect of the LGS on the frequency of hypoglycemia in children and adolescents with type 1 diabetes in routine clinical practice.

Methods: 21 patients with type 1 diabetes (10.8 ± 3.8 years old, duration of diabetes 5.9 ± 3.0 years, pump therapy for 3.7 ± 1.7 years, glycated hemoglobin level 7.8 ± 1.1%) from three pediatric centers used the Paradigm Veo system during two subsequent time periods: SAP without LGS for 2 weeks and then SAP with LGS activated for 6 weeks. The primary aim was to assess the frequency of hypoglycemic episodes when using the LGS feature with an insulin delivery shutoff of a maximum of 2 h at a sensor glucose level <70 mg/dl (3.9 mmol/l).

Results: In total, 1,298 LGS alerts occurred (853 <5 min). 42% of LGS activations (>5 min) lasted <30 min, whereas 24% had a duration of 2 h. The number of hypoglycemic excursions (average/day) was reduced during SAP + LGS (<70 mg/l, 1.27 ± 0.75 vs. 0.95 ± 0.49, p = 0.010; ≤40 mg/dl, 0.28 ± 0.18 vs. 0.13 ± 0.14, p = 0.005) as was the time spent in hypoglycemia (average minutes/day, 101 ± 68 vs. 58 ± 33, p = 0.002) without significant difference in the mean glucose level (145 ± 23 vs. 148 ± 19 mg/dl). While LGS was activated, no episodes of diabetic ketoacidosis or severe hyperglycemia were observed.

Conclusions: This study provides evidence that SAP with LGS reduces the frequency of hypoglycemia without compromising safety.

Continuous glucose monitoring (CGM) has been an exciting evolving theme through the EBM chapter over the last 3 years [15]. Both of these new studies focus on the utility of continuous glucose monitoring (CGM) in children and adults with type 1 diabetes. Both studies have a good study design and sound evidence-based methodology. Bergenstal's study is a single-crossover continuation phase of 420 subjects who completed the 1-year randomized STAR 3 study [16, 17]. The trial results of STAR 3 showed a 1% reduction in HbA$_{1c}$ in adults and 0.5% reduction in children over 1 year on the SAP compared with MDI. This 6-month follow-up study reports the effects of crossing over from optimized MDI to SAP. Bergenstal et al. report safe, rapid and sustained reductions in HbA$_{1c}$ in both adults and children. This study highlights the importance of translating clinical trials to clinical practice and allows us to provide good evidence to guide our day-to-day management of all adults and children with type 1 diabetes.

The second study by Danne et al. is a multicenter prospective study, assessing 21 children with type 1 diabetes using SAP for 2 weeks with the LGS feature turned off followed by 6 weeks with the LGS feature activated. The Paradigm Veo is the first insulin pump equipped with a low glucose suspend (LGS) feature which leads to an interruption in the supply of insulin for a period of up to 120 min. This occurs when the glucose value falls below an adjustable hypoglycemia threshold (set by the patient and/or healthcare professional). If the patient does not respond to the alert and the insulin is automatically suspended. After the LGS is triggered, if the patient fails to respond by resuming insulin delivery, insulin suspension will last for 120 min, after which insulin delivery will be automatically resumed for 4 h. Danne et al. report that the LGS feature reduces the frequency of hypos without compromising pump safety. This is a major finding in pediatric diabetes and a very useful tool in management of nocturnal hypoglycemia and hypoglycemia unawareness, particularly in young children (<5 years). Both studies highlight the importance of larger multicenter trials with realistic outcomes, which include children so this important evidence is also available for pediatric endocrinologists around the globe.

The effect of recurrent severe hypoglycemia on cognitive performance in children with type 1 diabetes: a meta-analysis

Blasetti A, Chiuri RM, Tocco AM, Di Giulio C, Mattei PA, Ballone E, Chiarelli F, Verrotti A
Department of Pediatrics, University of Chieti, Chieti, Italy
ablasetti@tiscalinet.it
J Child Neurol 2011;26:1383–1391

Background: The aim of this study was to investigate the extent of cognitive impairment in children with type 1 diabetes with recurrent severe hypoglycemia, using meta-analysis to synthesize data across studies.
Methods: 441 children with diabetes and recurrent severe hypoglycemia and 560 children with diabetes and without recurrent severe hypoglycemia were included in this meta-analysis.
Results: Children with type 1 diabetes and recurrent severe hypoglycemia had lower performance than type 1 diabetes children without severe hypoglycemia only in some cognitive domains: learning, memory, intelligence and verbal fluency/language. Greater impairment was found in memory and learning. Motor speed was not impaired.
Conclusions: This study confirms the hypothesis that recurrent severe hypoglycemia has a selective negative effect on the children's cognitive functions.

Effective treatment of hypoglycemia in children with type 1 diabetes: a randomized controlled clinical trial

McTavish L, Wiltshire E
Department of Diabetes and Endocrinology, Capital and Coast District Health Board, Wellington, New Zealand
Pediatr Diabetes 2011;12:381–387

Background: This study aimed to identify the most effective of four oral treatments for hypoglycemia in children with type 1 diabetes using a weight-based protocol during a diabetes camp.
Methods: At children's diabetes camp, the treatment of hypoglycemia was randomized to one of the four treatments, randomly assigned for each episode using a sealed envelope: glucose tablets, jellybeans, orange juice, and sugar mints. The appropriate carbohydrate dose was calculated for each child for each treatment (0.3 g carbohydrate/kg) and provided to camp leaders. Blood glucose was measured at 0, 2, 5, 10, and 15 min and symptoms recorded.
Results: 191 hypoglycemia episodes were recorded in 39 children (1–12 episodes per child), with 2 episodes excluded because of protocol violations. 52 episodes were treated with glucose tablets, 45 with jellybeans, 44 with juice, and 48 with sugar mints. Change in glucose at 10 (p = 0.034) and 15 min (p = 0.005) and glucose at 15 min (p = 0.026) were significantly different between treatment groups, with jellybeans produced the lowest and slowest response. Glucose tablets did not differ significantly from juice or sugar mints. Symptoms occurred in 112 episodes, with a median time to symptom resolution of 12 min (interquartile range 8–15 min).
Conclusions: Jellybeans are less effective treatment for hypoglycemia than the other three treatments. Glucose tablets, sugar mints and orange juice are equally effective. Treatment with 0.3 g/kg of carbohydrate (excluding jellybeans) effectively resolved hypoglycemia in most children, with 15 min often required to normalize blood glucose.

These two studies report good evidence on a well-recognized theme: hypoglycemia in children with type 1 diabetes. The first study is a meta-analysis and the second a randomized control trial.

Blasetti et al. use a meta-analysis to generate these data, however these results must be considered with caution taking into account factors such as small sample sizes, the different definitions of severe hypoglycemia, and the variety of neuropsychological tests used. On the other hand, the overall hypothesis is confirmed that in type 1 diabetes recurrent severe hypoglycemia has a selective negative effect on the children's cognitive functions.

 Gary Butler/Carrie Williams/Lee Hudson/Stephen O'Riordan

McTavish et al. report four treatment options that were used randomly at children's diabetes camps: glucose tablets, jellybeans, orange juice, and sugar mints. All were effective and rapid using a 0.3-g/kg equivalent carbohydrate dose protocol. Jellybeans were least effective and there was a trend towards the need for repeat treatments with jellybeans to correct hypogycemia, which was not present with the other treatments.

Both these studies provide practical data on everyday events in the lives of children with type 1 diabetes: diabetes camps and treatment of hypoglycemia. These important but perhaps small studies are warranted to lead our clinical practice with sound evidence.

Concepts revised
Metformin in PCOS: angel or demon?

Effects of metformin in adolescents with polycystic ovary syndrome undertaking lifestyle therapy: a pilot randomized double-blind study

Ladson G, Dodson WC, Sweet SD, Archibong AE, Kunselman AR, Demers LM, Lee PA, Williams NI, Coney P, Legro RS
Department of Obstetrics and Gynecology, Meharry Medical College, Nashville, TN, USA
Fertil Steril 2011;95:2595–2598 e1–6

Background: A good evidence base for metformin in obese adolescents with PCOS is lacking.

Methods: 22 females (13–18 years) meeting an agreed (NIH/NICHD) PCOS definition were randomized to treatment with 500 mg metformin four times per day (stepped up over 5 days) or placebo. Treatment regimen was double blinded. Both groups received a combined diet and exercise lifestyle intervention over 6 months. Participants were assessed monthly over a 6-month period.

Results: Baseline ages and BMI were similar in intervention and control groups. A significant decrease in serum testosterone, free androgen index was seen at 3 and 6 months in the metformin group compared with baseline. There was significant ($p < 0.05$) improvement of acne at each month over the 6 months in the metformin groups compared with baseline using a standardized scoring system. Adverse gastrointestinal effects in the metformin arm were greater: abdominal pain (RR = 3.6, 95% CI 1–12.8) and diarrhea (RR = 4.5, 95% CI 1.5–13.2).

Conclusions: This study could not defend the use of metformin for the management of PCOS in the light of side effects found.

The first comment to make is an important caveat: this study failed to recruit sufficient participants to meet power calculations. The researchers initially powered their RCT to detect a 25% absolute difference in serum testosterone levels based on a log-normal distribution and also for a 15% dropout rate, requiring 50 participants in each arm. Final numbers were only 11 participants in each arm. Thus the small numbers in this study significantly limited power, so much so that in the mean differences after 6 months (metformin-placebo) for over 50 measured outcomes in the trial, only the AUC glucose reached statistical significance. Despite this, the authors used a rigorous definition of PCOS a robust double-blind placebo-controlled RCT design. The results presented graphically in the paper show greater decreases in serum testosterone, free androgen index compared with placebo. They discuss that lack of interest and the burden of the study were the key reasons for the failed recruitment, an important insight into the difficulties faced in research in young people with obesity [18]. The paper reminds us of the importance of side effects of metformin use, which lead the authors to conclude that use of metformin may not be justifiable – although they did not report on adherence during the trial. The authors did not indicate whether or not the metformin formulation used in the trial was slow-release which may balance side effects and increase compliance. The reduction in acne (measured using standardized pro forma for assessment of number of open and closed comedones) at each month might be an important benefit for young people that potentially could improve compliance in the clinical setting. Both cases and controls also received a lifestyle intervention, a context that may be difficult to provide in clinical practice.

Final adult height in children with congenital adrenal hyperplasia treated with growth hormone

Lin-Su K, Harbison MD, Lekarev O, Vogiatzi MG, New MI
Department of Pediatric Endocrinology, Weill Medical College of Cornell University, New York, NY, USA
J Clin Endocrinol Metab 2011;96:1710–1717

Background: This study aimed to examine whether GH alone or in combination with an GnRH analogue (LHRH analogue) improved adult height in patients with congenital adrenal hyperplasia (CAH) due to 21-hydroxylase deficiency as adult height is usually well below midparental/target height.
Methods: This nonrandomized, prospective study included 34 patients (19 males, 15 females) with CAH, treated with GH as they were predicted to be >2 SD below their midparental target height or >2 SD below the population mean. GnRH analogue was also given to 27 patients (16 males, 11 females) for precocious puberty, mean duration was 3.7 ± 1.7 years. The mean duration of GH treatment was 5.6 ± 1.8 years in males and 4.5 ± 1.6 years in females.
Results: Males achieved a significantly taller adult height (172.0 ± 4.8 cm) than predicted (162.8 ± 7.7 cm) (p < 0.00001). Females also became significantly taller (162.2 ± 5.3 cm) than predicted (151.7 ± 5.2 cm) (p < 0.00001). The mean height gain was 9.2 ± 6.7 cm in males and 10.5 ± 3.7 cm in females.
Conclusions: This study demonstrates the possible height gains that can be achieved with GH alone or in combination with GnRH analogue in patients with CAH.

The degree of reduction in adult height in patients with CAH and its causes are well described in this paper, including the tendency to develop central precocious puberty as a result of the chronic hyperandrogenism. This paper presents an important comprehensive extension of the only study that addresses the long-term use of GH in the CAH population, and hence the inclusion in this chapter, despite the study not using a randomized control design. Inclusion criteria were typical to those encountered in routine practice: bone age of at least 6 years and >1 SD ahead of chronological age; adult height prediction by the Bayley-Pinneau method of at least 2 SD below midparental target height or at least 2 SD below the population mean (males 177 ± 7 cm, females 163 ± 6 cm), and with open epiphyses (bone age under 13 years in girls and 15 years in boys), and hence on that count, a very useful exposition of an attempt to rescue growth in these children we often see with difficult CAH. The greater height gain in females over males was explained by the worse initial height prognosis in this group of males. It is important to note that GnRH analogue did not appear to add any clear height gain benefit to GH therapy, so the authors stress that the decision to treat with GnRH analogue should be based on the age of the patient and the social impact of precocious puberty rather than for the sole purpose of increasing the gain in height. This very positive report now gives grounds for further exploration of this treatment approach.

This paper and the RCT of GH in short children with X-linked hypophosphatemic rickets by Zivicnjak et al. (see chapter by Cianfarani) each present evidence of GH efficacy with differing evidence bases, neither perfect. Both are relatively small, one long-term to adult height, and one a medium-term RCT, and both are for clinical indications not currently bearing a license for GH treatment. However, they both provide the necessary groundwork to take trials forward to the next stage.

Prospective study on the prevalence and associated risk factors of cryptorchidism in 6,246 newborn boys from Nice area, France

Wagner-Mahler K, Kurzenne JY, Delattre I, Berard E, Mas JC, Bornebush L, Tommasi C, Boda-Buccino M, Ducot B, Boulle C, Ferrari P, Azuar P, Bongain A, Fenichel P, Brucker- Davis F
Pediatrics Department, CHU, Nice, France
Wagner.k@pediatrie-chulenval-nice.fr; wagner@chu-nice.fr
Int J Androl 2011;34:e499–510

Background: Cryptorchidism is the most common congenital malformation in boys. The incidence appears to vary markedly between studies, and it remains unclear whether the incidence is rising, largely due to methodological limitations in previous studies. Therefore this study aimed to assess the incidence and risk factors of cryptorchidism in the Nice area.

Methods: A prospective study was conducted at two maternity wards over a 3-year period. All boys born ≥34weeks after the last menstrual period during the study period were screened. The methodology was strict with examination at birth, 3 and 12 months by the same pediatrician. Two carefully matched controls were included for each case. Information on child and parents (including lifestyle, medical history and pregnancy) was recorded using medical chart information and self-administered questionnaires.

Results: Of the 6,246 boys born within the duration of the study, a total of 102 were born with cryptorchidism (prevalence 1.6%, 95 included in the study). Half were still cryptorchid at 3 and 12 months with 10% recurrence of cryptorchidism at 12 months, justifying long-term follow-up. Instrumental delivery, inguinal hernia and urogenital malformations, particularly micropenis and paternal history of cryptorchidism, were associated with cryptorchidism at birth. Results suggested that maternal exposure to antirust or phthalates could be a risk factor, whereas eating fruits daily seemed somewhat protective.

Conclusions: The prevalence of cryptorchidism in this study is on the lower side compared with estimates from other countries. Cryptorchidism was found to be associated with both familial and environmental risk factors.

Cryptorchidism is the most common congenital malformation in boys, with estimated incidence varying between 0.9 and 9%. Various authors have suggested a variety of environmental exposures as risk factors for cryptorchidism, and previous studies have attempted to quantify the influence of these exposures. This population-based case-control study is well designed and conducted to overcome limitations of previous studies including those relating to definition and diagnosis. The assessment of children was highly standardized, both between centres and between examinations at different ages. Follow-up rates were very good, between 90 and 96% throughout the study.

At 12 months of age, 41% had spontaneously resolved, the overwhelming majority of these before 3 months (1 case resolved after 3 months but before 12 months). In addition, this paper demonstrates well the need for follow-up of children who have had apparent resolution at 3 months as they reported a 10% recurrence rate between 3 and 12 months of age.

This paper also reports a number of apparent risk factors for cryptorchidism some already well described including a paternal history of cryptorchidism, prematurity, and some less well described including maternal exposure to antirust products and phthalates, living in a rural setting and instrumental delivery. When interpreting these findings, as indeed for all research, authors and readers alike must be cautious. Whilst some association may be true risk factors, other apparent risk factors may be serving as 'proxies' for other factors. For example, this paper found that eating fruit daily appeared to act as a protective factor for the cryptorchidism. The authors point out that this is unlikely to be a true effect, but rather may be due to 'confounding' by some other socioeconomic status-related exposure.

Treatment of androgen excess in adolescent girls: ethinylestradiol-cyproterone acetate versus low-dose pioglitazone-flutamide-metformin

Ibanez L, Diaz M, Sebastiani G, Sanchez-Infantes D, Salvador C, Lopez-Bermejo A, de Zegher F
Endocrinology Unit, Hospital Sant Joan de Déu, University of Barcelona, Esplugues, Barcelona, Spain
libanez@hsjdbcn.org
J Clin Endocrinol Metab 2011;96:3361–3366

Background: Traditional management of the androgen excess in PCOS in postmenarchal females has been by ovarian-focused treatment using combined estrogen and progesterone medication. This study aimed to compare use of such a therapy with a regimen directed towards systemic abnormalities in metabolism and body fat storage.
Methods: An open-labeled, randomized study in postmenarchal girls of ethinylestradiol-cyproterone acetate (EE-CA) or low-dose combination of pioglitazone, flutamide, and metformin (PioFluMet) with comparison of clinical and endocrine-metabolic outcomes at 6 months.
Results: EE-CA and PioFluMet were equally as effective in reducing laboratory and clinical measures of androgen excess. Effects on fasting insulinemia; circulating cholesterol, triglycerides, C-reactive protein, high-molecular-weight adiponectin, leptin, and follistatin; carotid intima-media thickness; lean mass, and on abdominal, visceral, and hepatic fat, were significantly healthier with low-dose PioFluMet compared to EE-CA.
Conclusions: Low-dose PioFluMet compared favorably with EE-CA in adolescents with androgen excess and with no pregnancy risk. The efficacy and safety of low-dose PioFluMet remain to be studied over a longer term and in larger cohorts.

This study challenges the traditional thinking of PCOS as a disorder primarily of the ovary and the associated treatment model of ovarian suppression as route to decreasing androgen excess [19]. Ibáñez et al. propose an alternative way of thinking about PCOS which links hyperandrogenism with abnormalities of body fat storage, in particular visceral adiposity. This they argue would bring together the multiple metabolic and endocrine abnormalities associated with the condition, for example insulin resistance, as well as the chronological pathway from visceral adiposity to PCOS in postmenarche. They tested this proposal in an open-labelled randomized trial comparing traditional estrogen-progesterone therapy (EE-CA) with a combination of two metabolic antidiabetes medications (pioglitazone and metformin) with the antiandrogen flutamide (PioFluMet). Although both regimens produced comparable antiandrogen effects, the more systemic effects on metabolic risk such as fasting insulin, lipids and fat distribution were much more evident with PioFluMet. This trial was not blinded, but this seems appropriate when considering the potential dangers associated with pregnancy whilst on the PioFluMet regimen, a consideration which may also have implications for its clinical application in a postmenarchal group of women. The study does not seem to have been formally powered and numbers were small, though importantly no patients were lost to follow-up. Further study of the PioFluMet is warranted to identify longer term clinical effects in this age group.

Effect of intensive insulin therapy on the somatotropic axis of critically ill children

Gielen M, Mesotten D, Brugts M, Coopmans W, Van Herck E, Vanhorebeek I, Baxter R, Lamberts S, Janssen JAMJL, Van den Berghe G
Department of Intensive Care Medicine, Katholieke Universiteit Leuven, Belgium
Dieter.Mesotten@med.kuleuven.be
J Clin Endocrinol Metab 2011;96:2558–2566

Background: Intensive insulin therapy (IIT) is known to improve outcomes in the adult and pediatric intensive care unit (PICU) compared with conventional insulin therapy (CIT). IIT does not increase the anabolic hormone IGF-I in critically ill adults, but feeding in critically ill children and pediatric hormonal responses may differ. This study hypothesized that IIT reactivates the somatotropic axis and anabolism in PICU patients.
Methods: The authors performed a preplanned subanalysis of a randomized controlled trial of IIT. 369 patients who stayed in PICU for at least 3 days were included in the main analysis (study 1). 126 of these 369 patients were also included in a nested case-control study (study 2). Circulating insulin, C-peptide, GH, IGF-I, bioavailable IGF-I, IGF-binding protein (IGFBP)-1, IGFBP-3, and acid-labile subunit were analyzed upon admission and day 3. In the nested case-control study, the somatotropic axis, cortisol, and glucagon were analyzed before and after hypoglycemia.
Results: On day 3, C-peptide was 10-fold lower (p < 0.0001) in the IIT group than in the CIT group. IIT lowered bioavailable IGF-I (p = 0.002) and increased circulating GH (p = 0.04) and. IIT also decreased IGFBP-3 (p = 0.0005) and acid-labile subunit (p = 0.007), while increasing IGFBP-1 (p = 0.04) and the urea/creatinine ratio, a marker of catabolism (p = 0.03). In the nested case-control study, IGFBP-1 was increased after hypoglycemia. No change was noted in either the somatotropic axis or the counterregulatory hormones cortisol and glucagon.
Conclusion: Despite improved PICU outcome, IIT was not shown to counteract the catabolic state of critical illness. Lower bioavailable IGF-I may have been the result of suppression of portal insulin.

This group's previous study showed that IIT improved both mortality and morbidity in both infants and children admitted to PICU regardless of the cause or severity of illness [20]. In this preplanned analysis of the same RCT, they attempted to investigate the underlying mechanism. Contrary to the a priori hypothesis, this analysis found no evidence that the benefits of IIT are related to counteraction of the catabolic state by reactivation of the GH/IGF-1 axis. In contrast to expected results, this group actually found lowered levels of bioavailable IGF-1. The authors consider a number of possible mechanisms to explain their findings including (1) aggravated GH resistance, (2) induction of a counter-regulatory response by hypoglycemia, and (3) suppression of portal insulin. This last possibility is supported by the low C-peptide levels found in the IIT group. So, if it is not through the reversal of catabolism, what *is* the mechanism by which IIT results in improved outcomes for PICU patients? The authors postulate that IIT is likely to improve outcomes by improving insulin sensitivity. This conclusion is supported by other studies, including a similar study in children with burns reviewed in last year's edition of this chapter [15, 21].

Responsiveness to metformin in girls with androgen excess: collective influence of genetic polymorphisms

Diaz M, Lopez-Bermejo A, Sanchez-Infantes D, Bassols J, de Zegher F, Ibanez L
Endocrinology Unit, Hospital Sant Joan de Déu, University of Barcelona, Barcelona, Spain
Fertil Steril 2011;96:208–213 e2

Background: Metformin exerts metabolic effects at different tissue types and its effect can potentially be modified by a number of regulating genes. This study investigated the relationship between the efficacy of metformin use in girls with known androgen excess and combinations of genetic variants.
Methods: Adolescent girls with known hyperandrogenism and who were treated with metformin were recruited from a university hospital. A polymorphism score was calculated in each participant based on single nucleotide polymorphisms in the OCT1, STK11 and FTO genes, and number of repeats in the SHBG and AR genes. Participants were followed after 1 year of metformin use.
Results: 104 adolescent girls were enrolled. Mean BMI at baseline was 21.8 ± 0.2. All girls were postmenarchal. Both OCT1 and FTO showed no major associations at baseline or follow-up. Polymorphism scores had no association at baseline, however an increasing polymorphism score was associated with more favorable endocrine-metabolic outcomes of metformin use at the 1-year follow-up.
Conclusion: Collectively, genetic polymorphisms appear to have a positive impact on the outcomes of metformin use in postmenarchal girls with androgen excess.

As part of the evidence base for metformin in PCOS in children and adolescence, Diaz et al. examine the important question as to whether varying outcomes within young women receiving metformin is mediated by genetic differences. Metformin acts at a number of sites, and therefore a number of genes may modify its effects at the cellular level [22]. OCT1 encodes the organic cation transporter 1, a regulator of hepatic gluconeogenesis, which metformin is known to decrease [23]. Metformin also influences catalysis of AMP-activated protein kinase by serine-threonine kinase 11 (STK11) [24]. The fat mass and obesity-associated gene (FTO) is associated with degree of fat mass and insulin resistance in PCOS [25]. Variability in the number of repeats in both the sex hormone-binding globulin (SHBG) gene and in the androgen receptor (AR) gene have been hypothesized to alter the phenotype of PCOS and also the response to metformin [26, 27].

Diaz et al. demonstrated that these variants, either in isolation or in combination, showed little associations with baseline endocrine and metabolic features. However, more favorable metabolic responses to metformin (e.g. lower fasting insulin and body fat mass) were seen in participants with certain combinations of variants. A highly specific definition was used to identify this patient group, girls with a sequence of low birth weight, precious puberty and androgen excess. None was obese and all had the same ethnic background. Thus the findings may not be generalizable to other girls with PCOS, in other locations. However it may explain the variable effects of metformin in PCOS in the clinical setting as well as in research studies. Genetic categorization is however unlikely to be readily accessible in the clinical setting in the near future to assist clinical decision-making.

Efficacy and harms of nasal calcitonin in improving bone density in young patients with inflammatory bowel disease: a randomized, placebo-controlled, double-blind trial

Pappa HM, Saslowsky TM, Filip-Dhima R, DiFabio D, Lahsinoui HH, Akkad A, Grand RJ, Gordon CM
Center for Inflammatory Bowel Disease, Children's Hospital Boston, MA, USA
Helen.pappa@childrens.harvard.edu
Am J Gastroenterol 2011;106:1527–1543

Background: Very few published studies have investigated therapies to improve bone health in children with inflammatory bowel disease (IBD). This study aimed to establish the safety and efficacy of intranasal calcitonin in improving bone mineral density (BMD) in young patients with IBD. In addition, the study aimed to identify additional factors that impact bone mineral accrual.

Methods: In a randomized, placebo-controlled, double-blind trial, 63 patients, aged 8–21 years, with IBD and a spinal BMD Z-score ≤–1.0 SD (measured by dual energy X-ray absorptiometry) were randomized to 200 IU intranasal calcitonin (n = 31) or placebo (n = 32) daily. All received age-appropriate calcium and vitamin D supplementation. At 9 and 18 months, BMD was measured.

Results: Intranasal calcitonin was well tolerated. Adverse event frequency was similar in both groups and largely reversible, minor, and limited to the upper respiratory tract. The change in BMD Z-score between 0 and 9 months and 0 and 18 months did not differ between the two trial groups. In the subgroup with Crohn's disease, the spinal BMD Z-score improved between screening and 9 months in the calcitonin group 0.21 (0.37) over the placebo group 0.15 (0.5), p = 0.02. Factors associated with lower bone mineral accrual rate were: IBD severity (indicated by elevated inflammatory markers, need for surgery, hospitalization, and the use of immunomodulators) and higher daily caffeine intake. Factors favoring higher bone mineral accrual rate were: lower baseline BMD and higher baseline body mass index Z-score, improvement in height Z-score, higher serum albumin, hematocrit and iron concentration, and more hours of weekly weight-bearing activity.

Conclusions: Intranasal calcitonin is well tolerated. However, it does not offer a long-term advantage in adolescents with IBD and decreased BMD. Bone mineral accrual rate remains compromised in adolescents with IBD. Improvement in nutritional status, catch-up linear growth, control of inflammation, increase in weight-bearing activity, and lower daily caffeine intake may be helpful in restoring bone density in children with IBD.

This well-designed double-blind, placebo-controlled RCT is the first to investigate the effect of intranasal calcitonin on BMD in children with IBD. Unfortunately, it did not find any evidence to support this treatment. Only one positive finding within the subgroup of children with Crohn's disease was seen out of 32 p value calculations. As the authors do not include a Bonferroni correction for multiple comparisons, carrying out this number of significance tests would mean that it is entirely plausible to find one significant result by chance alone. This could also be the logical explanation, given the lack of a biologically plausible reason for an effect solely in this subgroup. Despite the negative results, the robust design of this study gives directions for future studies. In order to adequately control for confounding factors, the authors have very accurately measured other factors which they found to be affecting BMD, some of which have not been adequately quantified before including the effect of weight-bearing activity, the effect of good disease control (measured via inflammation markers), and the effect of caffeine. The evidence suggests that it is these factors which may hold the key to improved BMD in such patients and indeed, perhaps where future studies should concentrate.

Testosterone and the child (0–12 years) with Klinefelter syndrome (47,XXY): a review

Fennoy I
Department of Pediatrics, Columbia University Medical Center, New York, NY, USA
if1@columbia.edu
Acta Paediatr 2011;100:846–850

Background: This review aimed to explore the evidence base for considering testosterone therapy in infant and prepubertal boys with Klinefelter syndrome (KS).
Methods: The author searched major databases for articles that addressed the role of testosterone in the development of the male fetus with and without KS characterizing testicular function in KS during prepuberty.
Results: There may be an increased frequency of clinical features consistent with deficient testosterone production in infants with KS. However, results are conflicting as to whether testosterone levels are low or normal. There are no complete studies addressing the outcome of therapy in prepubertal boys.
Conclusions: Currently, the only documented benefit for testosterone therapy in these children is for the management of microphallus. There is an absence of data that directly address the risks and benefits of testosterone therapy in prepubertal boys with KS for any other parameter.

It is a great paradox that we know so little about the commonest human chromosome variation, 47,XXY. This review was one of several published in this supplement of *Acta Paediatrica* addressing what is currently known about Klinefelter syndrome, and what the evidence base for clinical practice is or should be [28]. The evidence for androgen deficiency in late puberty and adulthood is better known, but what about in the pre- and peripubertal boy, and indeed what about during infancy? Are variations in gonadal function during mini-puberty responsible for microphallus, or indeed cryptorchidism? The evidence placed before us is mixed, and very dependent upon the source of the subjects. Those where ascertainment is less biased (newborn population screening or antenatal diagnosis) may provide a more realistic prediction of gonadal function. So, infantile testosterone levels are probably within normal or low normal limits, as are those during childhood. In contrast, testosterone concentrations climb to upper normal in the peripubertal age range and can even be high in early puberty. This review also considers the reasons for benefits and potential disadvantages of giving exogenous testosterone to the prepubertal boy and on his testes. Theoretically, due to a possible increased sensitivity of the testis to intratesticular testosterone during this time period, testosterone treatment could even enhance the damage and limit even further the already reduced fertility prospects. So there is much work to do. This series of reviews, although primarily clinical reviews and not truly systematic reviews, significantly enhances our understanding of this condition and should be read by any pediatrician or endocrinologist working in this field.

Milk protein intake, the metabolic-endocrine response, and growth in infancy: data from a randomized clinical trial

Socha P, Grote V, Gruszfeld D, Janas R, Demmelmair H, Closa-Monasterolo R, Subias JE, Scaglioni S, Verduci E, Dain E, Langhendries JP, Perrin E, Koletzko B
Children's Memorial Health Institute, Warsaw, Poland
p.socha@czd.pl
Am J Clin Nutr 2011;94:1776S–1784S

Background: This study examined the influence of protein intake in infancy on serum amino acids, insulin, and the insulin-like growth factor I (IGF-I) axis and its possible relation to growth in the first 2 years of

Gary Butler/Carrie Williams/Lee Hudson/Stephen O'Riordan

life as it has been suggested protein intake in early infancy is an important risk factor for later obesity. Information on potential mechanisms is very limited.

Methods: In a multicenter European double-blind randomized trial, 1,138 healthy, formula-fed infants were randomized to receive cows' milk-based infant and follow-on formulas with lower protein (1.77 and 2.2 g protein/100 kcal) or higher protein (2.9 and 4.4 g protein/100 kcal) contents over the first year. Biochemical variables were measured at age 6 months in 339 infants receiving the lower protein formula and 333 infants receiving the higher protein formula and in a parallel group of 237 breast-fed infants.

Results: Essential amino acids, especially branched-chain amino acids, IGF-I, and urinary C-peptide:creatinine ratio, were significantly (p < 0.001) higher in the higher protein group than in the lower protein group, and more so compared with the breast-fed group, whereas IGF-binding protein (IGF-BP) 2 was lower and IGF-BP3 did not differ significantly. Total IGF-I was significantly associated with growth until 6 months of age but not thereafter. The median IGF-I total serum concentration was 48.4 ng/ml (25th, 75th percentile: 27.2; 81.8 ng/ml) in the higher protein group and 34.7 ng/ml (17.7; 57.5 ng/ml) in the lower protein group.

Conclusions: Higher protein intake stimulates the IGF-I axis and insulin release in infancy. The higher IGF-I may be associated with enhanced growth during the first 6 months of life.

This large European double-blind randomized trial was conceived to further explore mechanisms behind the development of infant obesity, higher protein intake already known to be associated with faster infant growth. The design randomized bottle-fed infants to the variable protein level intake, the comparator being a separate group of breast-fed infants. The size of this trial, despite the high dropout rate, provided sufficient power and the international element avoided the influence of local determinants on the outcome. The endocrine and metabolic parameters studied allowed for a more detailed insight to be gained into the mechanism of faster growth. Key findings include the protein induced drive of IGF-1 production, apparently separate from the GH axis (IGFBP-3 being unchanged between the groups). Insulin secretion increased too with the higher protein intake as deduced from elevated urinary C-peptide:creatinine ratios. Conversely at this age, glucose levels fell in the higher protein group, with insulin sensitivity being retained, again possibly a consequence of unchanged IGFBP-3 concentrations. The observed greater weight-for-length and BMI gains are likely to have been determined by the protein content of the infant feeds, but as the authors discuss, the opportunities for an even more detailed study, especially on amino acid metabolism were not possible, so many questions on the exact mechanism of the faster growth remain unanswered.

Effect of camel milk on glycemic control and insulin requirement in patients with type 1 diabetes: 2-years randomized controlled trial

Agrawal RP, Jain S, Shah S, Chopra A, Agarwal V
Department of Medicine, Diabetes Care & Research Centre, SP Medical College, Bikaner, Rajasthan, India
drrpagrawal@yahoo.co.in

Eur J Clin Nutr 2011;65:1048–1052

Background: Camel milk supplementation has been shown to exert a hypoglycemic effect both in an experimental rat model and previous studies from this group had shown a significant reduction in doses of insulin in type 1 diabetic patients. This was a 2-year randomized open clinical, parallel-design study and was undertaken to assess the efficacy, safety and acceptability of camel milk jointly with insulin therapy in adolescents and young adults with type 1 diabetes.

Methods: 24 patients were selected at random then randomized into two groups. Group I (n = 12; ages 14.5 ± 8.4 years) received usual care comprising of diet, exercise and insulin and group II (n = 12; ages 16.7 ± 8.9 years) additionally received 500 ml camel milk daily. Insulin dosage was titrated weekly following blood glucose estimation.

Results: In the intervention group, the mean blood glucose decreased from 6.6 ± 1.1 to 5.2 ± 0.9 mmol/l, as did HbA$_{1c}$ levels (7.8 ± 1.4 to 5.5 ± 0.8%). There was a fall in and insulin requirement from 32.5 ± 10.0 to 17.5 ± 12.1 U/day (p < 0.05), with 3 subjects reducing their insulin requirement to zero. Group I showed the expected rises in HbA$_{1c}$. No adverse hypoglycemic events were noted.

Conclusions: This study suggests that camel's milk is safe and efficacious in improving glycemic control in patients with type 1 diabetes, with a significant reduction in the dosage of insulin.

It had been previously observed by the same group that populations drinking camel's milk as part of their regular diet exhibited a low incidence of diabetes, and pilot intervention studies demonstrated improvements in diabetes control. This longer term RCT, albeit small, has indeed demonstrated significant effects on glycemic control parameters and reductions in insulin requirement actually to zero in 3/12 subjects. Camel's milk contains proteins which, being similar to insulin, may inhibit hepatic gluconeogenesis. Additionally it contains high concentrations of insulin, actually similar to human milk, but camel's milk does not undergo coagulation in the stomach thus making the insulin available for intestinal absorption. Whether there is mileage in exploring this effect further is unclear, but the principal lesson from this study is an exploration of the adaptation to the local environment and the design of a simple yet effective study design to investigate regional observations in greater depth. The good camel has now lost its hump! [29].

Follow-up on *Yearbooks 2010* and *2011*

The effect of oxandrolone on voice frequency in growth hormone-treated girls with Turner syndrome

Menke LA, Sas TC, van Koningsbrugge SH, de Ridder MA, Zandwijken GR, Boersma B, Dejonckere PH, de Muinck Keizer-Schrama SM, Otten BJ, Wit JM
Dutch Growth Research Foundation, Rotterdam, The Netherlands
l.a.menke@lumc.nl
J Voice 2011;25:602–610

Background: Previous studies published by this group have shown oxandrolone increases height gain, however it may also cause voice deepening in growth hormone (GH)-treated girls with Turner syndrome. This study also assessed the effect of oxandrolone on objective and subjective speaking voice frequency in GH-treated girls with Turner syndrome.
Methods: This multicenter, randomized, placebo-controlled, double-blind study enrolled 133 participants. Patients were randomized to treatment with GH (1.33 mg/m²/day) combined with either placebo, low-dose oxandrolone (0.03 mg/kg/day) or conventional-dose oxandrolone (0.06 mg/kg/day). Patients were treated from age 8 and estrogens were added from 12 years. Voices were recorded and subjective voice quality questionnaires were completed yearly from starting treatment until 6 months after discontinuing.
Results: Voice frequency standard deviation scores (SDS) were high for age at the baseline assessment (1.0 ± 1.2, p < 0.001) but normal for height. Compared with the placebo group, voices tended to become lower in the low-dose oxandrolone group (p = 0.09) and significantly lowered in the conventional-dose oxandrolone group (p = 0.007). At the final measurement, voice frequency SDS was still relatively high in the placebo group (0.6 ± 0.7, p = 0.002) but similar to healthy girls in both oxandrolone groups. Voice frequency became lower than –2 SDS in 1 patient (3%) on low-dose oxandrolone and 3 patients (11%) on conventional-dose oxandrolone. The percentage of patients reporting subjective voice deepening was similar between the dosage groups.
Conclusion: Untreated girls with Turner syndrome have relatively high-pitched voices. The addition of oxandrolone to GH decreases voice frequency in a dose-dependent way. Although most voice frequencies remain within the normal range, they may occasionally become lower than –2 SDS, especially on conventional doses of oxandrolone (0.06 mg/kg/day).

Safety and growth outcomes from this RCT have been reviewed in this chapter in 2010 and 2011 respectively [15, 30]. Last year we described this study as 'elegant, well designed and well conducted' and indeed this year's paper provides further evidence of the elegance of the design. It provides further information on the efficacy-to-safety ratio of oxandrolone by reporting the subjective and objective frequency of the speaking voice of participants. At baseline, voice frequency was found to be higher in participants, in comparison to chromosomally normal girls of the same age. This is particularly so for girls with monosomy or isochromosome karyotypes and girls who do not experience spontaneous puberty. The study confirmed that low-dose oxandrolone has a favorable efficacy/side effect profile, not only increasing final height, but resulting in a slight lowering of voice frequency to levels comparable to the general population. It also verified previous findings that conventional-dose oxandrolone can result in unfavorable side effect of significantly lowering voice (>–2 SDS in 11% of participants) as well as potentially causing virilization.

As clinicians, this is study is particularly useful as the results of all three resulting publications from this RCT help us to assist our patients and their families to make fully informed decisions about treatment. It provides evidence not only on outcomes we consider important, but also those valued by our patients.

References

1. Phillip M, Danne T, Shalitin S, Buckingham B, Laffel L, Tamborlane W, Battelino T, for the Consensus Forum Participants: Use of continuous glucose monitoring in children and adolescents. Pediatr Diabetes 2012;13:215–228.
2. Peters A, Laffel L: Diabetes care for emerging adults: recommendations for transition from pediatric to adult diabetes care systems: a position statement of the American Diabetes Association, with representation by the American College of Osteopathic Family Physicians, the American Academy of Pediatrics, the American Association of Clinical Endocrinologists, the American Osteopathic Association, the Centers for Disease Control and Prevention, Children with Diabetes, The Endocrine Society, the International Society for Pediatric and Adolescent Diabetes, Juvenile Diabetes Research Foundation International, the National Diabetes Education Program, and the Pediatric Endocrine Society (formerly Lawson Wilkins Pediatric Endocrine Society). Diabetes Care 2011;34:2477–2485.
3. Savendahl L, Maes M, Albertsson-Wikland K, Borgstrom B, Carel JC, et al: Long-term mortality and causes of death in isolated GHD, ISS, and SGA patients treated with recombinant growth hormone during childhood in Belgium, the Netherlands, and Sweden: preliminary report of three countries participating in the EU SAGhE Study. J Clin Endocrinol Metab 2012;97:E213–E217.
4. Carel JC, Ecosse E, Landier F, et al: Long-term mortality after recombinant growth hormone treatment for isolated growth hormone deficiency or childhood short stature: preliminary report of the French SAGhE Study. J Clin Endocrinol Metab 2012;97:416–425.
5. Gardner M, Sandberg DE: Growth hormone treatment for short stature: a review of psychosocial assumptions and empirical evidence. Pediatr Endocrinol Rev 2011;9:579–588.
6. Gold D: The clinical impact of vertebral fractures: quality of life in women with osteoporosis. Bone 1996;18:S185–S189.
7. Janz KF, Kwon S, Letuchy EM, Eichenberger Gilmore JM, Burns TL, Torner JC, et al: Sustained effect of early physical activity on body fat mass in older children. Am J Prev Med 2009;37:35–40.
8. Brage S, Wedderkopp N, Ekelund U, Franks PW, Wareham NJ, Andersen LB, et al: Features of the metabolic syndrome are associated with objectively measured physical activity and fitness in Danish children. Diabetes Care 2004;27:2141–2148.
9. Ekelund U, Anderssen S, Froberg K, Sardinha L, Andersen L, Brage S: Independent associations of physical activity and cardiorespiratory fitness with metabolic risk factors in children: the European Youth Heart Study. Diabetologia 2007;50:1832–1840.
10. Hudson LD, Court AJ: What paediatricians should know about eating disorders in children and young people. J Paediatr Child Health 2012 (E-pub ahead of print).
11. Jayasinghe Y, Grover SR, Zacharin M: Current concepts in bone and reproductive health in adolescents with anorexia nervosa. BJOG 2008;115:304–315.
12. Gordon CM, Grace E, Emans SJ, Feldman HA, Goodman E, Becker KA, et al: Effects of oral dehydroepiandrosterone on bone density in young women with anorexia nervosa: a randomized trial. J Clin Endocrinol Metab 2002;87:4935–4941.
13. Klibanski A, Biller B, Schoenfeld D, Herzog D, Saxe V: The effects of estrogen administration on trabecular bone loss in young women with anorexia nervosa. J Clin Endocrinol Metab 1995;80:898–904.
14. Grinspoon S, Thomas L, Miller K, Herzog D, Klibanski A: Effects of recombinant human IGF-I and oral contraceptive administration on bone density in anorexia nervosa. J Clin Endocrinol Metab 2002;87:2883–2891.
15. Butler G, Williams C, O'Riordan S: Evidence-based medicine in pediatric endocrinology; in Carel JC, Hochberg Z (eds): Yearbook of Pediatric Endocrinology 2011. Basel, Karger, 2011, pp 193–214.
16. Bergenstal RM, Tamborlane WV, Ahmann A, et al, for the STAR 3 Study Group: Effectiveness of sensor-augmented insulin-pump therapy in type 1 diabetes. N Engl J Med 2010;363:311–320.
17. Chiarelli F, Marcovecchio LM: Type 1 diabetes: clinical and experimental; in Carel JC, Hochberg Z (eds): Yearbook of Pediatric Endocrinology 2011. Basel, Karger, 2011, pp 121–140.
18. Nguyen B, McGregor KA, O'Connor J, Shrewsbury VA, Lee A, Steinbeck KS, et al: Recruitment challenges and recommendations for adolescent obesity trials. J Paediatr Child Health 2012;48:38–43.
19. Norman RJ, Dewailly D, Legro RS, Hickey TE: Polycystic ovary syndrome. Lancet 2007;370:685–697.
20. Vlasselaers D, Milants I, Desmet L, Wouters PJ, Vanhorebeek I, van den Heuvel I, et al: Intensive insulin therapy for patients in paediatric intensive care: a prospective, randomised controlled study. Lancet 2009;373:547–556.
21. Jeschke MG, Kulp GA, Kraft R, Finnerty CC, Mlcak R, Lee JO, et al: Intensive insulin therapy in severely burned pediatric patients: a prospective randomized trial. Am J Respir Crit Care Med 2010;182:351–359.
22. Diamanti-Kandarakis E, Christakou CD, Kandaraki E, Economou FN: Metformin – an old medication of new fashion: evolving new molecular mechanisms and clinical implications in polycystic ovary syndrome. Eur J Endocrinol 2010;162:193–212.
23. Wang DS, Jonker JW, Kato Y, Kusuhara H, Schinkel AH, Sugiyama Y: Involvement of organic cation transporter 1 in hepatic and intestinal distribution of metformin. J Pharmacol Exp Ther 2002;302:510–515.
24. Shaw RJ, Lamia KA, Vasquez D, Koo SH, Bardeesy N, DePinho RA, et al: The kinase LKB1 mediates glucose homeostasis in liver and therapeutic effects of metformin. Science 2005;310:1642–1646.
25. Barber T, Bennett A, Groves C, Sovio U, Ruokonen A, Martikainen H, et al: Association of variants in the fat mass and obesity associated (FTO) gene with polycystic ovary syndrome. Diabetologia 2008;51:1153–1158.

26. Xita N, Tsatsoulis A, Chatzikyriakidou A, Georgiou I: Association of the (TAAAA)n repeat polymorphism in the sex hormone-binding globulin (SHBG) gene with polycystic ovary syndrome and relation to SHBG serum levels. J Clin Endocrinol Metab 2003;88:5976–5980.
27. Ibáñez L, Ong KK, Mongan N, Jääskeläinen J, Marcos MV, Hughes IA, et al: Androgen receptor gene CAG repeat polymorphism in the development of ovarian hyperandrogenism. J Clin Endocrinol Metab 2003;88:3333–3338.
28. Juul A, Aksglaede L, Bay K, Grigor K Skakkebaek N (eds): Proceedings of the International Workshop on Klinefelter Syndrome 2010. Acta Paediatr 2011;100:791–792.
29. Kipling R: How the camel got his hump; in The Just So Stories. London, Macmillan, 1902.
30. Butler G: Evidence-based medicine in pediatric endocrinology; in Carel JC, Hochberg Z (eds): Yearbook of Pediatric Endocrinology 2010. Basel, Karger, 2010, pp 189–205.

Editor's Choice

Ken Ong and Ze'ev Hochberg

Optimizing therapy
Fluid resuscitation in severe infection

Mortality after fluid bolus in African children with severe infection

Maitland K, Kiguli S, Opoka RO, Engoru C, Olupot-Olupot P, Akech SO, Nyeko R, Mtove G, Reyburn H, Lang T, Brent B, Evans JA, Tibenderana JK, Crawley J, Russell EC, Levin M, Babiker AG, Gibb DM, Group FT
Kilifi Clinical Trials Facility, Kenya Medical Research Institute (KEMRI)-Wellcome Trust Research Programme, Kilifi, Kenya
kathryn.maitland@gmail.com
N Engl J Med 2011;364:2483–2495

Background: The study aimed to establish the role of fluid resuscitation in children with shock and life-threatening infections in resource-limited settings.
Methods: The authors randomized children with severe febrile illness and impaired perfusion to receive boluses of 20–40 ml/kg body weight of 5% albumin solution (albumin-bolus group) or 0.9% saline solution (saline-bolus group) or no bolus (control group) on admission to a hospital in Uganda, Kenya, or Tanzania (stratum A); children with severe hypotension were randomized to one of the bolus groups only (stratum B). All children received appropriate antimicrobial treatment, intravenous maintenance fluids, and supportive care, according to guidelines. Children with malnutrition or gastroenteritis were excluded. The primary endpoint was 48-hour mortality.
Results: Recruitment was halted after 3,141 of the projected 3,600 children in stratum A were enrolled. Malaria status (57% overall) and clinical severity were similar across groups. The 48-hour mortality was 10.6% (111 of 1,050 children), 10.5% (110 of 1,047 children), and 7.3% (76 of 1,044 children) in the albumin-bolus, saline-bolus, and control groups, respectively (relative risk for saline bolus vs. control, 1.44; 95% CI 1.09–1.90; p = 0.01; albumin bolus vs. saline bolus, 1.01; 0.78–1.29; p = 0.96; any bolus vs. control, 1.45; 1.13–1.86; p = 0.003). Regarding secondary outcomes, the 4-week mortality was 12.2, 12.0, and 8.7% in the three groups, respectively (p = 0.004 for any bolus vs. control). Neurologic sequelae occurred in 2.2, 1.9, and 2.0% in the respective groups (p = 0.92), and pulmonary edema or increased intracranial pressure occurred in 2.6, 2.2, and 1.7% (p = 0.17), respectively. In stratum B, 69% of the children (9 of 13) in the albumin-bolus group and 56% (9 of 16) in the saline-bolus group died (p = 0.45). The results did not differ between centers or across subgroups by severity of shock, malaria, coma, sepsis, acidosis, or severe anemia status.
Conclusions: Fluid boluses significantly increased 48-hour mortality in critically ill children with impaired perfusion in these resource-limited settings in Africa.

This paper, describing the Fluid Expansion as Supportive Therapy (FEAST) study, won the *BMJ* 2012 Paper of the Year award. The World Health Organization recommends reserving fluid resuscitation for children with advanced shock (characterized by a delayed capillary refill time of more than 3 s, weak and fast pulse, and cold extremities) in poor-resource settings, such sub-Saharan Africa, in which intensive care facilities are rarely available. These trial findings clearly show that earlier use of fluid resuscitation in such settings is not beneficial. The trial was discontinued early, on the recommendations of its data and safety monitoring committee, as both bolus therapy groups showed increased 48-hour mortality in the absence of features of fluid overload. The authors speculate that the vasoconstrictor response in shock may confer protection by reducing perfusion to nonvital tissues and that rapid reversal with fluid resuscitation is deleterious. Other possible adverse consequences of fluid boluses include reperfusion injury, subclinical effects on pulmonary compliance, myocardial function, or intracranial pressure. In these settings, and possibly in others, fluid bolus therapy should be reserved for children with clear signs of hypotension.

Effect of a dietary portfolio of cholesterol-lowering foods given at two levels of intensity of dietary advice on serum lipids in hyperlipidemia: a randomized controlled trial

Jenkins DJ, Jones PJ, Lamarche B, Kendall CW, Faulkner D, Cermakova L, Gigleux I, Ramprasath V, de Souza R, Ireland C, Patel D, Srichaikul K, Abdulnour S, Bashyam B, Collier C, Hoshizaki S, Josse RG, Leiter LA, Connelly PW, Frohlich J
Clinical Nutrition and Risk Factor Modification Center, St Michael's Hospital, Toronto, ON, Canada
cyril.kendall@utoronto.ca
JAMA 2011;306:831–839

Background: Combining foods with recognized cholesterol-lowering properties (dietary portfolio) effectively lowers serum cholesterol under metabolically controlled conditions. This study aimed to assess the effect of a dietary portfolio administered at two levels of intensity on change in low-density lipoprotein cholesterol (LDL-C) among participants following self-selected diets.

Methods: This parallel-design trial randomized 351 participants with hyperlipidemia from four participating academic centers across Canada (Quebec City, Toronto, Winnipeg, and Vancouver) to one of three treatments lasting 6 months. Those on 'control diet' received advice for 6 months on a low-saturated fat diet. The 'routine dietary portfolio' group received counseling at two clinic visits over 6 months on dietary incorporation of plant sterols, soy protein, viscous fibers, and nuts. The 'intensive dietary portfolio' group received the same counseling at seven clinic visits over 6 months. The primary outcome was % change in serum LDL-C.

Results: In the modified intention-to-treat analysis (n = 345), the overall attrition rate did not differ between treatments (18% for intensive dietary portfolio, 23% for routine dietary portfolio, and 26% for control; Fisher exact test, p = 0.33). The % LDL-C changes were −13.8% (95% CI −17.2 to −10.3%; p < 0.001) for the intensive dietary portfolio; −13.1% (−16.7 to −9.5%; p < 0.001) for the routine dietary portfolio, and −3.0% (95% CI −6.1 to 0.1%; p = 0.06) for the control diet. Among participants randomized to one of the dietary portfolio interventions, % reduction in LDL-C on the dietary portfolio was associated with dietary adherence (r = −0.34, n = 157, p < 0.001).

Conclusions: A dietary portfolio was more effective than low-saturated fat dietary advice in lowering LDL-C during 6 months of follow-up.

While there is increasing evidence to start using statins in children and adolescents with familial hypercholesterolemia, such very long-term treatments should only be given after a period of optimal dietary management, which usually involves advice to follow a low-saturated fat diet, whole-grain cereals, and plenty of fruits and vegetables. This clinical trial now shows that such typical dietary advice may have little effect on reducing LDL-C levels. Mean LDL-C at baseline in these participants was 171 mg/dl (4.4 mmol/l) and reduced by only −8 mg/dl (0.2 mmol/l) in those given routine low-saturated fat dietary advice. In contrast, average reductions in LDL-C were −26 mg/dl (−0.67 mmol/l) and −24 mg/dl (−0.62 mmol/l) in the intensive and routine dietary portfolio groups, which is around half of that observed with statins. Of note, all three diets were vegetarian, were weight-maintaining, and participants in all three arms showed equal mild weight loss, by on average of 1.5 kg over 6 months. These findings should encourage the incorporation of foods with active cholesterol-lowering properties, such as plant sterols (e.g. plant sterol ester-enriched margarines), viscous fibers (oats, barley, and psyllium), soy (soy milk, tofu, and soy meat analogues), and nuts (including tree nuts and peanuts).

The pendrin anion exchanger gene is transcriptionally regulated by uroguanylin: a novel enterorenal link

Rozenfeld J, Tal O, Kladnitsky O, Adler L, Efrati E, Carrithers SL, Alper SL, Zelikovic I
Laboratory of Developmental Nephrology, Department of Physiology and Biophysics, Haifa, Israel
Am J Physiol Renal Physiol 2012;302:F614–624

Background: The pendrin/SLC26A4 Cl^-/HCO_3^- exchanger, encoded by the PDS gene, is expressed in cortical collecting duct (CCD) non-A intercalated cells. Pendrin is essential for CCD bicarbonate secretion and is also involved in NaCl balance and blood pressure regulation. The intestinal peptide uroguanylin (UGN) is produced in response to oral salt load and can function as an 'intestinal natriuretic hormone'. This study aimed to investigate whether UGN modulates pendrin activity and to explore the underlying molecular mechanisms.

Results: Injection of UGN into mice resulted in decreased pendrin mRNA and protein expression in the kidney. UGN decreased endogenous pendrin mRNA levels in HEK293 cells. A 4.2-kb human PDS (hPDS) promoter sequence and consecutive 5' deletion products were cloned into luciferase reporter vectors and transiently transfected into HEK293 cells. Exposure of transfected cells to UGN decreased hPDS promoter activity. This UGN-induced effect on the hPDS promoter occurred within a 52-bp region encompassing a single heat-shock element (HSE). The effect of UGN on the promoter was abolished when the HSE located between nt −1119 and −1115 was absent or was mutated. Furthermore, treatment of HEK293 cells with heat-shock factor 1 (HSF1) small interfering RNA (siRNA) reversed the UGN-induced decrease in endogenous PDS mRNA level. In conclusion, pendrin-mediated Cl^-/HCO_3^- exchange in the renal tubule may be regulated transcriptionally by the peptide hormone UGN. UGN exerts its inhibitory activity on the hPDS promoter likely via HSF1 action at a defined HSE site.

Conclusions: These data define a novel signaling pathway involved in the enterorenal axis controlling electrolyte and water homeostasis.

> We were not aware of an 'entero-renal axis'. Here is an ancient dilemma: eating salt results in renal salt wasting even before intestinal salt is absorbed. How does the kidney know that salt was taken? It turns out that the intestinal peptide uroguanylin (UGN) is produced in response to oral salt load, travels to the kidneys and within minutes exerts its function as an 'intestinal natriuretic hormone'. UGN signaling involves an enhancing promoter activity of the pendrin gene PDS. We are familiar with pendrin mutations in the deafness-goiter syndrome Pendred. Yet pendrin is also expressed in the distal renal tubule where it exerts Cl^-/HCO_3^- exchange and responds the UGN by salt wasting.

Genetic defect in CYP24A1, the vitamin D 24-hydroxylase gene, in a patient with severe infantile hypercalcemia

Dauber A, Nguyen TT, Sochett E, Cole DE, Horst R, Abrams SA, Carpenter TO, Hirschhorn JN
Division of Endocrinology, Children's Hospital Boston, Clinical Investigator Training Program, Boston, MA, USA
andrew.dauber@childrens.harvard.edu
J Clin Endocrinol Metab 2012;97:E268–274

Background: Idiopathic infantile hypercalcemia (IIH) is a disorder, the genetic etiology and physiological basis of which are not well understood. The objective of the study was to describe the underlying physiology and genetic cause of hypercalcemia in an infant with severe IIH and to extend these genetic findings into an additional cohort of children with IIH.

Methods: This was an inpatient study of a single patient with consanguineous parents at an academic medical center with follow-up in a specialty clinic cohort. The patient population was 1 patient with severe IIH for gene discovery and physiological testing and 27 patients with idiopathic infantile hypercalcemia in the replication cohort. Interventions included a calcium isotopic absorption study as well as homozygosity mapping and whole-exome sequencing in a single patient followed up by gene sequencing in the replication cohort. Fractional absorption of calcium and genetic variants causing hypercalcemia were measured.

Results: Intestinal calcium absorption was extremely elevated (~90%). A rare homozygous deletion in the CYP24A1 gene was found, leading to the loss of a single highly conserved amino acid. In vivo functional studies confirmed decreased 24-hydroxylase activity because the subject had undetectable levels of 24,25-dihydroxyvitamin D. No coding variants in CYP24A1 were found in the 27 additional patients with IIH.

Conclusions: The study confirms that CYP24A1 plays a causal role in some but not all cases of IIH via markedly increased intestinal absorption of calcium, suggesting that genetic diagnosis could be helpful in a subset of IIH patients. This case demonstrates the power of an unbiased, genome-wide approach accompanied by informative physiological studies to provide new insights into human biology.

This year we learnt of a novel mechanism of hypercalcemia by loss of function of the vitamin D 24-hydroxylase enzyme, leading to defective detoxification mechanism of 1,25(OH)2D to 1,24,25(OH)3D. Similar reports were made by two other authors [1–3]. Interestingly, the severity of the hypercalcemia in the infants decreased or corrected with age. Despite the several reports from three groups in a single year, this is not a common mechanism for hypercalcemia. Those of you who can measure $1,24(OH)_2D$ can easily diagnose these rare cases.

A new double AKT
AKT1 and AKT2

A mosaic-activating mutation in AKT1 associated with the Proteus syndrome

Linchurst MJ, Sapp JC, Teer JK, Johnston JJ, Finn EM, Peters K, Turner J, Cannons JL, Bick D, Blakemore L, Blumhorst C, Erockmann K, Calder P, Cherman N, Deardorff MA, Everman DB, Golas G, Greenstein RM, Kato BM, Keppler-Noreuil KM, Kuznetsov SA, Miyamoto RT, Newman K, Ng D, O'Brien K, Rothenberg S, Schwartzentruber DJ, Singhal V, Tirabosco R, Upton J, Wientroub S, Zackai EH, Hoag K, Whitewood-Neal T, Robey PG, Schwartzberg PL, Darling TN, Tosi LL, Mullikin JC, Biesecker LG
National Human Genome Research Institute, Bethesda, MD, USA
N Engl J Med 2011;365:611–619

Background: The Proteus syndrome is characterized by the overgrowth of skin, connective tissue, brain, and other tissues, and is hypothesized to be caused by somatic mosaicism.

Methods: Exome sequencing was performed on DNA from biopsy samples obtained from patients with the Proteus syndrome. DNA sequences were compared between affected and unaffected tissues from the same patients. Findings were confirmed and extended, using a custom restriction-enzyme assay, by analyzing further DNA in 158 samples from 29 Proteus syndrome patients. Activation of the AKT protein in affected tissues was assayed using phosphorylation-specific antibodies on Western blots.

Results: 26 out of 29 patients with the Proteus syndrome had a somatic activating mutation (c.49G→A, p.Glu17Lys) in the oncogene AKT1, encoding the AKT1 kinase, an enzyme known to mediate processes such as cell proliferation and apoptosis. Tissues and cell lines from patients harbored admixtures of mutant alleles that ranged from 1% to approximately 50%. Mutant cell lines showed greater AKT phosphorylation than did control cell lines. A pair of single-cell clones that were established from the same starting culture and differed with respect to their mutation status had different levels of AKT phosphorylation.

Conclusions: The Proteus syndrome is caused by a somatic activating mutation in AKT1. These findings prove the hypothesis of somatic mosaicism and implicate activation of the PI3K-AKT pathway in overgrowth and tumor susceptibility in humans.

An activating mutation of AKT2 and human hypoglycemia

Hussain K, Challis B, Rocha N, Payne F, Minic M, Thompson A, Daly A, Scott C, Harris J, Smillie BJ, Savage DB, Ramaswami U, De Lonlay P, O'Rahilly S, Barroso I, Semple RK
Clinical and Molecular Genetics Unit, Developmental Endocrinology Research Group, Institute of Child Health, University College London, London, UK
Science 2011;334:474

Background and Methods: Pathological fasting hypoglycemia in humans is usually explained by excessive circulating insulin or insulin-like molecules or by inborn errors of metabolism impairing liver glucose production. The authors studied 3 unrelated children with unexplained, recurrent, and severe fasting hypoglycemia. One child also displayed asymmetrical growth.

Results: All 3 patients were found to carry the same de novo mutation, p.Glu17Lys, in the serine/threonine kinase AKT2, in 2 cases as heterozygotes and in 1 case in mosaic form. In heterologous cells, the mutant AKT2 was constitutively recruited to the plasma membrane, leading to insulin-independent activation of downstream signaling.

Conclusions: These findings show that constitutive, cell-autonomous activation of insulin signaling pathways causes severe fasting hypoglycemia with suppression of ketone bodies and branched chain amino acids in the absence of detectable circulating insulin levels.

I strongly encourage clinicians to read these two fascinating reports, which demonstrate the power of whole-exome sequencing to understand the basis on human disease and reveal new insights into human biology. Both insulin and insulin-like growth factor-1 (IGF-1) signal on the phosphoinositide 3-kinase (PI3K)/AKT/mTOR pathway, leading to activation of downstream metabolic and somatic pathways. The contrast between the largely metabolic phenotype of patients with germline or mosaic-activating mutations in AKT2 (Hussain et al.) and the marked somatic overgrowth due to mosaic-activating mutations in AKT1 (Lindhurst et al.) illustrates the distinct functions of AKT1 and AKT2 in humans.

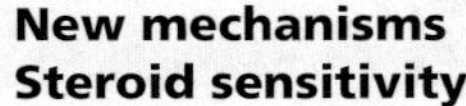

**New mechanisms
Steroid sensitivity**

Genome-wide association between GLCCI1 and response to glucocorticoid therapy in asthma

Tantisira KG, Lasky-Su J, Harada M, Murphy A, Litonjua AA, Himes BE, Lange C, Lazarus R, Sylvia J, Klanderman B, Duan QL, Qiu W, Hirota T, Martinez FD, Mauger D, Sorkness C, Szefler S, Lazarus SC, Lemanske RF Jr, Peters SP, Lima JJ, Nakamura Y, Tamari M, Weiss ST
Channing Laboratory, Brigham and Women's Hospital and Harvard Medical School, Boston, MA, USA
rekgt@channing.harvard.edu
N Engl J Med 2011;365:1173–1183

Background: The response to treatment for asthma is characterized by wide interindividual variability. A substantial number of patients show no response. The authors hypothesized that a genome-wide association study (GWAS) would reveal novel pharmacogenetic determinants of the response to inhaled glucocorticoids.

Methods: The authors performed a family-based GWAS of 534,290 single-nucleotide polymorphisms (SNPs) and selected a small number of statistically powerful variants for association with changes in lung function in response to inhaled glucocorticoids. A significant, replicated association was found, and its functional effects were characterized.

Results: A significant pharmacogenetic association at SNP rs37972, in the glucocorticoid-induced transcript 1 gene (GLCCI1), was replicated in four independent populations totaling 935 persons (p = 0.0007). rs37972 is in complete linkage disequilibrium with SNP rs37973 and both SNPs were associated with decrements in GLCCI1 expression. In isolated cell systems, rs37973 was associated with decreased luciferase reporter activity. Pooled data from treatment trials indicate reduced lung function in response to inhaled glucocorticoids in subjects with the variant allele (p = 0.0007). Overall, the mean (±SE) increase in forced expiratory volume in 1 s in the treated subjects who were homozygous for the rs37973 variant was only about one third of that seen in similarly treated subjects who were homozygous for the wild-type allele (3.2 ± 1.6 vs. 9.4 ± 1.1%), and their risk of a poor response was higher (OR 2.36; 95% CI 1.27–4.41). This genotype accounted for 6.6% of inhaled glucocorticoid response variability.

Conclusions: A functional GLCCI1 variant was associated with substantial decrements in the response to inhaled glucocorticoids in patients with asthma.

We all see patients with variable responses to glucocorticoid therapy resulting in either poor responses to treatment, variable risk of side effects, or both. This landmark study sheds light on the underlying genetic basis of interindividual differences in glucocorticoid sensitivity. GLCCI1 expression is enhanced by glucocorticoids, and the degree of induced GLCCI1 expression in B-cell lines was associated with the clinical response to inhaled glucocorticoids in the same subjects. The authors therefore surmise that patients with rs37972 and rs37973 variants have diminished clinical responses to inhaled gluco-corticoids, due to reduced GLCCI1 expression and consequently reduced inflammatory-cell apoptosis, a key mechanism through which glucocorticoids resolve lymphocytic and eosinophilic inflammation in asthma. Notably, GLCCI1 is expressed in lung cells and immune cells, which raises the strong possibility of tissue-specific steroid-sensitivity – patients with rs37972 and rs37973 variants who require higher steroid doses for asthma control may yet remain highly susceptible to glucocorticoid-induced adrenal suppression or growth-plate suppression.

New treatments
TSHR antagonists

Complete inhibition of rhTSH-, Graves' disease IgG-, and M22-induced cAMP production in differentiated orbital fibroblasts by a low-molecular-weight TSHR antagonist

Van Zeijl CJ, van Koppen CJ, Surovtseva OV, de Gooyer ME, Plate R, Conti P, Karstens WJ, Timmers M, Saeed P, Wiersinga WM, Miltenburg AM, Fliers E, Boelen A
Academic Medical Center, Department of Endocrinology, Amsterdam, The Netherlands
a.boelen@amc.uva.nl
J Clin Endocrinol Metab 2012;97:E781–785

Background: Autoimmune stimulation of the TSH receptor (TSHR) on orbital fibroblasts (OF) is a proposed mechanism underlying Graves' ophthalmopathy.

Methods: In cultured and differentiated OF from patients with severe Graves' ophthalmopathy undergoing orbital decompression surgery, the authors tested whether a novel low-molecular-weight (LMW) TSHR antagonist Org-274179-0 inhibits cAMP production induced by rhTSH, Graves' disease IgG (GD-IgG), or M22 (a potent human monoclonal TSHR stimulating antibody).

Results: cAMP production increased after incubation either with 10 mU/ml rhTSH (3-fold; ≤ 0.05), 1 mg/ml GD-IgG (2-fold; ≤ 0.05), or 500 ng/ml M22 (5-fold; ≤ 0.05). Incubation with the LMW TSHR antagonist dose dependently inhibited rhTSH, GD-IgG as well as the M22-induced cAMP production at nanomolar concentrations; complete blockade was affected at 10^{-6} M.

Conclusions: These findings suggest that the production of cAMP, stimulated by the Graves' disease antibodies GD-IgG and M22, is exclusively mediated via the TSHR.

LMW TSHR antagonists have been proposed as possible future therapeutic agents for Graves' hyperthyroidism, and particularly for Graves' ophthalmopathy for which there are limited treatment modalities. The TSH receptor (TSHR) is expressed on fibroblasts in orbital adipose/connective tissue and in extraocular muscles of patients, and the authors hypothesized that these receptors are an important target of autoimmunity. The new compound, Org-274179-0, appears to be far more potent than previously tested TSHR antagonists. Future studies are needed to test whether Org-274179-0 inhibits the production of glycosaminoglycan by the orbital tissues.

Intranasal insulin suppresses food intake via enhancement of brain energy levels in humans

Jauch-Chara K, Friedrich A, Rezmer M, Melchert UH, Scholand-Engler HG, Hallschmid M, Oltmanns KM
Department of Psychiatry and Psychotherapy, University of Lübeck, Lübeck, Germany
Diabetes 2012 (E-pub ahead of print)

Background: Cerebral insulin exerts anorexic effects in humans and animals through yet unknown mechanisms. Insulin facilitates glucose uptake by most tissues of the body and thereby promotes intracellular energy supply. Therefore, the authors hypothesized that intranasal insulin reduces food consumption by enhancing neuroenergetic levels.

Methods: In a double-blind, placebo-controlled, cross-over study, 15 healthy men (BMI 22.2 ± 0.37 kg/m^2) aged 22–28 years were given intranasal insulin 40 IU or placebo after an overnight fast. Cerebral energy metabolism was measured by ^{31}P magnetic resonance spectroscopy. At 100 min after the intranasal spray, participants consumed an ad libitum test buffet.

Results: Intranasal insulin increased brain energy (i.e. adenosine triphosphate and phosphocreatine levels). In the placebo arm, cerebral energy content correlated inversely with subsequent calorie intake. Moreover, the degree of rise in brain energy following intranasal insulin correlated with the subsequent reduction in calorie consumption.

Conclusions: The brain appears to regulate food intake behavior dependent on its current energetic status. Intranasal insulin seems a promising future treatment option in obesity to increase cerebral energy homeostasis and reduce free-choice food intake.

Effect of intranasal insulin on cognitive function: a systematic review

Shemesh E, Rudich A, Harman-Boehm I, Cukierman-Yaffe T
Goldman Medical School, Department of Clinical Biochemistry, Faculty of Health Sciences, Ben-Gurion University of the Negev, Beer-Sheva, Israel
J Clin Endocrinol Metab 2012;97:366–376

Background: Epidemiological and mechanistic studies suggest that insulin may influence cognitive function. The authors systematically reviewed clinical trials that tested the potential effects of intranasal insulin administration on cognitive functions.

Methods: Interventional studies published in English measuring changes in cognitive functions in response to intranasal insulin were included.

Results: Eight studies (328 participants) were included. Seven studies included healthy subjects' response to intranasal insulin, and three evaluated the cognitive effect among patients with. Among healthy people (7 studies), Cohen's effect size calculations suggest that only 160 IU/day intranasal insulin induced potential beneficial effects. Among patients with minimal cognitive impairment or overt Alzheimer's disease, only lower doses of insulin were assessed, and 20 IU revealed potential beneficial effects on cognitive functions. No significant side effects of intranasal insulin administration were reported.

Conclusions: The current limited clinical experience suggests potential beneficial cognitive effects of intranasal insulin. Analyses provide clinical considerations for future research aimed at elucidating whether intranasal insulin may be used to improve cognitive functions.

Intranasal insulin has been shown to induce immune tolerance to insulin in adults with established type 1 diabetes, and its efficacy to prevent diabetes is currently being tested in the Intranasal Insulin Trial (INIT II), in Australia and New Zealand.

These fascinating studies describe other potential future roles for intranasal insulin, a route of administration that is known to increase cerebrospinal fluid insulin levels and therefore achieve central actions, but without altering peripheral circulating insulin levels. A physiological postprandial rise in brain insulin may act as a relevant satiety signal and giving intranasal before meals to reduce meal calorie consumption, as studied by Jauch-Chara et al., or enhancing the meal-related signal by postprandial administration to reduce postmeal snacking, may both be considered as future therapeutic strategies.

Other central actions of insulin include neuronal maintenance and neurogenesis and this could explain why adult diabetic patients have faster rates of decline in cognitive function, and higher risk of dementia. In their systematic review, Shemesh et al. describe that much more evidence is needed to be able to robustly evaluate the potential therapeutic role for intranasal insulin to prevent or reverse cognitive decline.

New tests
β-Cell death

Detection of β-cell death in diabetes using differentially methylated circulating DNA

Akirav EM, Lebastchi J, Galvan EM, Henegariu O, Akirav M, Ablamunits V, Lizardi PM, Herold KC
Department of Immunobiology and Internal Medicine, Yale University School of Medicine, New Haven, CT, USA
Proc Natl Acad Sci USA 2011;108:19018–19023

Background: In diabetes mellitus, β-cell destruction is largely silent and can be detected only after significant loss of insulin secretion capacity.

Methods and Results: The authors developed a method for detecting β-cell death in vivo by amplifying and measuring the proportion of insulin 1 gene DNA from β cells in mouse serum. By using primers that are specific for DNA methylation patterns in β cells, circulating copies of β-cell-derived demethylated DNA were detected in serum of mice by quantitative PCR. Accordingly, there was a detectable increase of β-cell-derived DNA after induction of diabetes with streptozotocin and during development of diabetes in nonobese diabetic mice. The authors extended the use of this assay to measure β-cell-derived insulin DNA in human tissues and serum. Higher levels of demethylated insulin gene DNA were found in patients with new-onset type 1 diabetes compared with age-matched control subjects.

Conclusions: This novel method provides a noninvasive approach to detect β-cell death in vivo that may be used to track the progression of diabetes and guide its treatment.

It is estimated that over 90% of the β cell has already been silently destroyed by the time the patient presents with type 1 diabetes, which is probably far too late for successful preservation of β-cell function. These authors developed a novel method to identify and quantify circulating DNA that is released specifically from β cells when they die. A key role for genomic methylation is to control tissue-specific gene expression; as insulin is secreted exclusively by the pancreas, the authors correctly hypothesized that β-cell insulin gene DNA would have its own unique methylation pattern. The next challenge to overcome was to design an assay to detect these tiny amounts of DNA using methylation-sensitive primers. The authors discuss the many potential uses of such as assay, both for the prediction and monitoring of disease and interventions such as transplantation, and also for studying β-cell turnover during growth and development.

Bariatric surgery versus intensive medical therapy in obese patients with diabetes

Schauer PR, Kashyap SR, Wolski K, Brethauer SA, Kirwan JP, Pothier CE, Thomas S, Abood B, Nissen SE, Bhatt DL
Bariatric and Metabolic Institute, Cleveland Clinic M61, Cleveland, OH, USA
schauep@ccf.org
N Engl J Med 2012;366:1567–1576

Background: Observational studies have shown improved glycemic control in patients with type 2 diabetes mellitus (T2DM) after bariatric surgery.

Methods: This nonblinded, single-center trial randomized 150 obese patients with uncontrolled T2DM (mean age 49 ± 8 years, 66% women) to intensive medical therapy alone, or medical therapy plus Roux-en-Y gastric bypass or sleeve gastrectomy. At baseline, mean glycated hemoglobin level (HbA_{1c}) was 9.2 ± 1.5%. The primary endpoint was HbA_{1c} of 6.0% or less 12 months after treatment.

Results: 93% completed 12 months of follow-up. The proportion of patients with the primary endpoint was 12% (5 of 41) in the medical-therapy group, 42% (21 of 50) in the gastric-bypass group (p = 0.002), and 37% (18 of 49) in the sleeve-gastrectomy group (p = 0.008). Glycemic control improved in all three groups, with a mean HbA_{1c} 7.5 ± 1.8% in the medical-therapy group, 6.4 ± 0.9% in the gastric-bypass group (p < 0.001), and 6.6 ± 1.0% in the sleeve-gastrectomy group (p = 0.003). Weight loss was greater in the gastric-bypass group and sleeve-gastrectomy group (−29.4 ± 9.0 and −25.1 ± 8.5 kg, respectively) than in the medical-therapy group (−5.4 ± 8.0 kg) (p < 0.001 for both comparisons). The use of drugs to lower glucose, lipid, and blood-pressure levels decreased significantly in both surgical groups and increased in the intensive medical therapy group. Four patients required reoperation. There were no deaths or life-threatening complications.

Conclusions: In obese patients with uncontrolled T2DM, 12 months of medical therapy plus bariatric surgery was more effective than medical therapy alone to achieve glycemic control. Follow-up is needed to assess the durability of these results.

Bariatric surgery versus conventional medical therapy for type 2 diabetes

Mingrone G, Panunzi S, De Gaetano A, Guidone C, Iaconelli A, Leccesi L, Nanni G, Pomp A, Castagneto M, Ghirlanda G, Rubino F
Department of Internal Medicine, Università Cattolica S. Cuore, Rome, Italy
gmingrone@rm.unicatt.it
N Engl J Med 2012;366:1577–1585

Background: Roux-en-Y gastric bypass and biliopancreatic diversion can markedly ameliorate diabetes in morbidly obese patients, often resulting in diabetes remission.

Methods: This nonblinded, single-center trial, randomized 60 obese (BMI ≥ 35) patients (ages 30–60 years) with diabetes duration >5 years and glycated hemoglobin level (HbA_{1c}) of 7.0% or more, to conventional medical therapy or either gastric bypass or biliopancreatic diversion. At baseline, mean glycated hemoglobin level (HbA_{1c}) was 8.65 ± 1.45%. The primary endpoint was diabetes remission at 2 years (defined as fasting glucose <100 mg/dl (5.6 mmol/l) and HbA_{1c} <6.5% in the absence of pharmacologic therapy).

Results: At 2 years, diabetes remission had occurred in no patients in the medical-therapy group, 75% in the gastric-bypass group, and 95% in the biliopancreatic-diversion group (p < 0.001 for both comparisons). Age, sex, baseline BMI, duration of diabetes, and weight changes did not predict diabetes remission at 2 years or improvement in glycemia at 1 and 3 months. Glycemic control improved in all three groups; at 2 years mean HbA_{1c} was 7.69 ± 0.57% in the medical-therapy group, 6.35 ± 1.42% in the gastric-bypass group (p < 0.001), and 4.95 ± 0.49% in the biliopancreatic-diversion group. Two patients required reoperation, 1 for incisional hernia and 1 for intestinal obstruction. There were no deaths.

Conclusions: In severely obese patients with T2DM, bariatric surgery resulted in better glucose control than medical therapy. Preoperative BMI and weight loss did not predict the improvement in hyperglycemia after these procedures.

Is bariatric surgery no longer the last resort for obese adults with T2DM? These two trials report remarkable benefits of surgery on glycemic control and indeed very high rates of remission of T2DM in severely obese adults. It should be noted that both trials assessed highly invasive forms of surgery, rather than gastric banding, they were underpowered to robustly assess the risks of complications and side effects of treatment, and disappointingly using available baseline criteria they were unable to identify who would benefit the most. We should always take a cautious approach in translating new therapies from adults to children and adolescents, however the recently reported failure of conventional oral medication for T2DM in the latter group (see paper by the TODAY Study Group in the chapter 'Type 2 Diabetes, Metabolic Syndrome and Lipids') will increase the pressure to find effective alternative treatments.

Environmental concerns
Chemical obesity

Urinary bisphenol A (BPA) concentration associates with obesity and insulin resistance

Wang T, Li M, Chen B, Xu M, Xu Y, Huang Y, Lu J, Chen Y, Wang W, Li X, Liu Y, Bi Y, Lai S, Ning G
Key Laboratory for Endocrine and Metabolic Diseases of Ministry of Health, Shanghai Clinical Center for Endocrine and Metabolic Diseases, Shanghai Institute of Endocrine and Metabolic Diseases, Department of Endocrinology and Metabolism, Rui-Jin Hospital, Shanghai Jiao Tong University School of Medicine, Shanghai, China
J Clin Endocrinol Metab 2012;97:E223–227

Background: Bisphenol A (BPA) is one of the world's highest-volume chemicals in use today. Previous studies have suggested BPA disturbs body weight regulation and promotes obesity and insulin resistance. But epidemiological data in humans were limited.
Methods: To determine whether BPA associates with obesity and insulin resistance, the authors examined a cross-sectional study of 3,390 adults aged 40 years or older, in Songnan Community, Baoshan District, Shanghai, China. Questionnaire, clinical and biochemical measurements, and urinary BPA concentration were determined. Overweight was defined as a BMI of 24–28 kg/m^2 and obesity as a BMI of 28 kg/m^2 or higher. Abdominal obesity was defined as waist circumference at least 90 cm for men and 85 cm for women. Insulin resistance was defined using the index of homeostasis model assessment.
Results: Those in the highest quartile of BPA had the highest prevalence of obesity (OR 1.50; 95% CI 1.15–1.97), abdominal obesity (OR 1.28; 95% CI 1.03–1.60), and insulin resistance (OR 1.37; 95% CI 1.06–1.77). Among participants with a BMI <24 kg/m^2, compared with the lowest quartile, the highest quartile of BPA increased the prevalence of insulin resistance by 94% (OR 1.94; 95% CI 1.20–3.14), but this association was not observed in those with a BMI of 24 kg/m^2 or higher.
Conclusions: BPA was positively associated with obesity, abdominal obesity, and insulin resistance in middle-aged and elderly Chinese adults.

You would think that after a decade of scientific offense, bisphenol A (BPA) would disappear from our environmental, but it remains one of the world's highest-volume chemicals in use today. Among other untoward effects, BPA promotes obesity by its effects on adipocyte differentiation, lipid accumulation, insulin resistance, glucose transport, and adiponectin secretion (NHANES 2003–2004 and 2005–2006). The association is now confirmed: urinary BPA was associated with generalized obesity, abdominal obesity, and insulin resistance in middle-aged and elderly adult Chinese. Also this year, canned soup consumption increased urinary bisphenol [4].

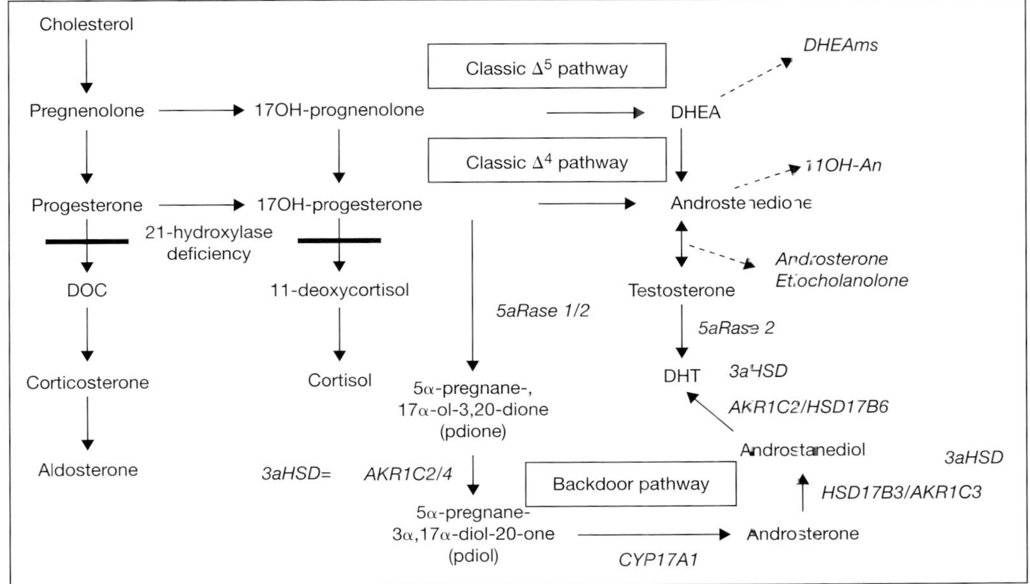

Fig.1. Pathways to androgen synthesis in 21-hydroxylase deficiency.

A new chapter in steroid metabolism
Infants take the backdoor

Increased activation of the alternative 'backdoor' pathway in patients with 21-hydroxylase deficiency: evidence from urinary steroid hormone analysis

Kamrath C, Hochberg Z, Hartmann MF, Remer T, Wudy SA
Division of Pediatric Endocrinology and Diabetology, Steroid Research and Mass Spectrometry Unit, Center of Child and Adolescent Medicine, Justus Liebig University, Giessen, Germany
Clemens.kamrath@paediat.med.uni-giessen.de

J Clin Endocrinol Metab 2012;97:E367–375

Background: 17-Hydroxyprogesterone (17-OHP) can be converted to dihydrotestosterone (DHT) via an alternative 'backdoor' route that bypasses the conventional intermediates androstenedione and testosterone. In this backdoor pathway, 17-OHP is converted to 5α-pregnane-3α,17α-diol-20-one (pdiol), which is an excellent substrate for the 17,20-lyase activity of CYP17A1 to produce androsterone.

Methods: To obtain evidence for the presence of the backdoor pathway in patients with 21-hydroxylase deficiency (21-OHD), the authors compared urinary steroid hormone profiles determined by gas chromatography-mass spectrometry of 142 untreated 21-OHD patients (age range 1 day to 25.4 years; 51 males) with 138 control subjects. The activity of the backdoor pathway was assessed using the ratios of the urinary concentrations of pdiol to those of the metabolites of the classic Δ⁴ and Δ⁵ pathways. In contrast to etiocholanolone, which originates almost exclusively from the classic pathways, androsterone may be derived additionally from the backdoor pathway. Therefore, the androsterone to etiocholanolone ratio can be used as an indicator for the presence of the backdoor pathway.

Results: Untreated 21-OHD subjects showed increased urinary ratios of pdiol to the Δ⁴ and Δ⁵ pathway metabolites and a higher androsterone to etiocholanolone ratio.

Conclusions: The elevated ratios of pdiol to the Δ⁴ and Δ⁵ pathway metabolites as well as the higher androsterone to etiocholanolone ratio in patients with 21-OHD indicate postnatal activity of the backdoor pathway with maximum activity during early infancy. These data provide new insights into the pathophysiology of androgen biosynthesis in 21-OHD.

This article was accompanied by an eye-opening editorial in *JCEM* [5]. In the presence of a block in 21-hydroxylation, 17-hydroxyprogesterone (17-OHP) accumulates. Textbooks claim that 17-OHP is the precursor for androstenedione, which was regarded as being an androgen as well as being a precursor of testosterone and DHT; the latter being the critical androgen for in utero virilization. Only that the human 17,20-lyase can hardly convert 17-OHP to androstenedione – the so-called Δ^4 pathway. Androstenedione is normally a product of DHEA through the Δ^5 pathway (fig. 1), yet the fetal adrenal normally produces abundant DHEA which converts to estriol in the placenta, defending the female fetus from virilization. This enigma is now solved with the demonstration of the 'backdoor pathway' – a new chapter to be learnt in steroid metabolism. They show that total flux to androgens through the classical Δ^4 and Δ^5 pathways is not elevated in 21-OHD children until after the first year of life, whereas 17OH-allopregnanolone (or Pdiol) is drastically elevated. Pdiol provides the entrance to the 'backdoor pathway', ultimately producing the nonaromatizable DHT as the source of virilization in utero and until age one. This solves another enigma: it is now appreciated that estrogens, not androgens advance bone age; why is it then that children with CAH rarely advance their bone ages during the first year of life? The answer lies in the nonaromatizable nature of DHT, the end-product of the backdoor pathway.

Stressful puberty

Individual differences in boys' and girls' timing and tempo of puberty: modeling development with nonlinear growth models

Marceau K, Ram N, Houts RM, Grimm KJ, Susman EJ
Department of Psychology, The Pennsylvania State University, University Park, PA, USA
kpm170@psu.edu

Dev Psychol 2011;47:1389–1409

Context: Pubertal development is a nonlinear process progressing from prepubescent beginnings through biological, physical, and psychological changes to full sexual maturity.
Aim: To tether theoretical concepts of puberty with sophisticated longitudinal, analytical models capable of articulating pubertal development more accurately, the authors used nonlinear mixed-effects models to describe both the timing and tempo of pubertal development in the sample of 364 white boys and 373 white girls measured across 6 years as part of the National Institute of Child Health and Human Development Study of Early Child Care and Youth Development. Individual differences in timing and tempo were extracted with models of logistic growth.
Outcomes: Differential relations emerged for how boys' and girls' timing and tempo of development were related to physical characteristics (body mass index, height, and weight) and psychological outcomes (internalizing problems, externalizing problems, and risky sexual behavior). Timing and tempo are associated in boys but not girls. Pubertal timing and tempo are particularly important for predicting psychological outcomes in girls but only sparsely related to boys' psychological outcomes.
Conclusions: Results highlight the importance of considering the nonlinear nature of puberty and expand the repertoire of possibilities for examining important aspects of how and when pubertal processes contribute to development.

Reported early family environment covaries with menarcheal age as a function of polymorphic variation in estrogen receptor-α

Manuck SB, Craig AE, Flory JD, Halder I, Ferrell RE
Behavioral Physiology Laboratory, University of Pittsburgh, Pittsburgh, PA, USA
manuck@pitt.edu

Dev Psychopathol 2011;23:69–83

Context: Age at menarche, a sentinel index of pubertal maturation, was examined in relation to early family relationships (conflict, cohesion) and polymorphic variation in the gene encoding estrogen receptor-α (ESR1) in a midlife sample of 455 European-American women.

Outcomes: Consistent with prior literature, women who reported being raised in families characterized by close interpersonal relationships and little conflict tended to reach menarche at a later age than participants reared in families lacking cohesion and prone to discord. Moreover, this association was moderated by ESR1 variation, such that quality of the family environment covaried positively with menarcheal age among participants homozygous for minor alleles of the two ESR1 polymorphisms studied here (rs9304799, rs2234693), but not among women of other ESR1 genotypes. In addition, (a) family relationship variables were unrelated to ESR1 variation, and (b) genotype-dependent effects of childhood environment on age at menarche could not be accounted for by personality traits elsewhere shown to explain heritable variation in reported family conflict and cohesion.

Conclusions: These findings are consistent with theories of differential susceptibility to environmental influence, as well as the more specific hypothesis (by Belsky) that girls differ genetically in their sensitivity to rearing effects on pubertal maturation.

The attachment theory claims that growing in an insecure environment during the transition from infancy to childhood and from childhood to juvenility programs a person to an insecure reproductive strategy: early puberty, multiple sexual partners, early fecundity, and many offspring from several partners. Such individuals will also provide insecure attachment for their many offspring [6]. In a previous study from the same database, Belsky et al. showed that individuals who had been insecure as infants initiated and completed pubertal development earlier and had an earlier age of menarche compared with individuals who had been secure infants, even after accounting for age of menarche in the infants' mothers [7]. A second genetic possibility is suggested by accumulating evidence of gene-environment interaction, in which DNA polymorphisms have been found to modify environmental influences on behavioral phenotypes as childhood temperament, early cognitive abilities, juvenile and adult antisocial behavior, and depression. Recently, common polymorphisms of the ESR1 gene have been associated with menarche ages of adolescent girls in Greece [8]. The present article shows that the quality of the family environment covaried positively with menarche age among subjects homozygous for minor alleles of the two ESR1 polymorphisms, but not among women of other ESR1 genotypes. The family relationship variables were unrelated to ESR1 variation. To what extent do these observations reflect an interaction of genetic and environmental variation? Genotype-dependent associations of early family environment with menarche age in the present study could conceivably entail interactive effects involving other genes, strictly environmental factors (gene-environment interaction), or both.

Psychosocial risk and correlates of early menarche in Mexican-American girls

Jean RT, Wilkinson AV, Spitz MR, Prokhorov A, Bondy M, Forman MR
Department of the Army, Office of the Surgeon General, Pharmacovigilance Center, Silver Spring, MD, USA
Rosenie.Thelus.ctr@us.army.mil
Am J Epidemiol 2011;173:1203–1210

Context: Mexican-American girls have one of the fastest rates of decline in age at menarche.

Aim: To study the role of psychosocial factors on age at menarche in this population.

Methods: Using data from a longitudinal cohort of Mexican-American girls from the Houston, Texas, metropolitan area recruited in 2005, the authors investigated associations between family life and socioeconomic environment and age at menarche in 523 girls.

Outcomes: After adjusting for maternal age at menarche, daughter's age, and body mass index at baseline, perception of family life environment as conflict-prone was significantly associated with an earlier age at menarche (<11 years). Additionally, there was a 2-fold higher risk (OR 2.22; 95% CI 1.12, 4.40) of early menarche among daughters of mothers who were single parents compared with those who were not. Furthermore, girls who matured early had a 2.5-fold increased risk (OR 2.69; 95% CI 1.04, 6.96) of experimenting with cigarettes compared with those who had an average-to-late age at menarche (≥11 years).

Conclusion: This study provides important information regarding the role of family life environment and single parenting on age at menarche in Mexican-Americans. Awareness of the impact of the family life environment and fathers' absence during the early years should be emphasized when addressing early age at menarche across cultures.

This study adds to the previous two: caregiving behaviors of parents are predictive indicators of the security of their environment. The biological rationale is that in stressful conditions, parenting becomes less sensitive; the child experiences psychosocial stress and adaptively responds in an adaptive reproductive strategy. This article provides important information regarding the role of family life environment and single parenting on the timing and duration of puberty. When addressing a child, be aware of the impact of the family life environment and fathers' absence during the early years.

References
1. Schlingmann KP, Kaufmann M, Weber S, Irwin A, Goos C, John U, et al: Mutations in CYP24A1 and idiopathic infantile hypercalcemia. N Engl J Med 2011;365:410–421.
2. Tebben PJ, Milliner DS, Horst RL, Harris PC, Singh RJ, Wu Y, et al: Hypercalcemia, hypercalciuria, and elevated calcitriol concentrations with autosomal dominant transmission due to CYP24A1 mutations: effects of ketoconazole therapy. J Clin Endocrinol Metab 2012;97:E423–E427.
3. Raja-Khan N, Kunselman AR, Demers LM, Ewens KG, Spielman RS, Legro RS: A variant in the fibrillin-3 gene is associated with TGF-β and inhibin B levels in women with polycystic ovary syndrome. Fertil Steril 2010;94:2916–2919.
4. Carwile JL, Ye X, Zhou X, Calafat AM, Michels KB: Canned soup consumption and urinary bisphenol A: a randomized crossover trial. JAMA 2011;306:2218–2220.
5. Auchus RJ, Miller WL: Congenital adrenal hyperplasia – more dogma bites the dust. J Clin Endocrinol Metab 2012;97:772–775.
6. Belsky J, Fearon RM: Early attachment security, subsequent maternal sensitivity, and later child development: does continuity in development depend upon continuity of caregiving? Attach Hum Dev 2002;4:361–387.
7. Belsky J, Houts RM, Fearon RM: Infant attachment security and the timing of puberty: testing an evolutionary hypothesis. Psychol Sci 2010;21:1195–1201.
8. Stavrou I, Zois C, Chatzikyriakidou A, Georgiou I, Tsatsoulis A: Combined estrogen receptor α and estrogen receptor β genotypes influence the age of menarche. Hum Reprod 2006;21:554–557.

Science and Medicine

Ze'ev Hochberg and Ken Ong

Aussies out of Africa

An Aboriginal Australian genome reveals separate human dispersals into Asia

Rasmussen M, Guo X, Wang Y, Lohmueller KE, Rasmussen S, Albrechtsen A, Skotte L, Lindgreen S, Metspalu M, Jombart T, Kivisild T, Zhai W, Eriksson A, Manica A, Orlando L, De La Vega FM, Tridico S, Metspalu E, Nielsen K, Avila-Arcos MC, Moreno-Mayar JV, Muller C, Dortch J, Gilbert MT, Lund O, Wesolowska A, Karmin M, Weinert LA, Wang B, Li J, Tai S, Xiao F, Hanihara T, van Driem G, Jha AR, Ricaut FX, de Knijff P, Migliano AB, Gallego Romero I, Kristiansen K, Lambert DM, Brunak S, Forster P, Brinkmann B, Nehlich O, Bunce M, Richards M, Gupta R, Bustamante CD, Krogh A, Foley RA, Lahr MM, Balloux F, Sicheritz-Ponten T, Villems R, Nielsen R, Wang J, Willerslev E
Centre for GeoGenetics, Natural History Museum of Denmark, Copenhagen, Denmark
Science 2011;334:94–98

Background and Methods: This study reports an Aboriginal Australian genomic sequence obtained from a 100-year-old lock of hair donated by an Aboriginal man from southern Western Australia in the early 20th century.
Results: The authors detected no evidence of European admixture and estimated contamination levels to be below 0.5%. They found that Aboriginal Australians are descendants of an early human dispersal into eastern Asia, possibly 62,000–75,000 years ago. This dispersal is separate from the one that gave rise to modern Asians 25,000–38,000 years ago. They also found evidence of gene flow between populations of the two dispersal waves prior to the divergence of Native Americans from modern Asian ancestors.
Conclusions: The findings support the hypothesis that present-day Aboriginal Australians descended from the earliest humans to occupy Australia, likely representing one of the oldest continuous populations outside of Africa.

In *Yearbook 2011* we highlighted the sequencing of the Neanderthal genome, which suggested that Europeans and Asians have inherited 2–6% of their genomes from Neanderthals. The current paper is an interesting report of genomic sequencing based on DNA extracted from a lock of hair collected 100 years ago on an Australian train, from what the collector described as a pure-blood native Aboriginal Australian. The findings show that people living in Southeast Asia and Australian Aboriginals inherited about 5% of their DNA from the Denisovans (linked only to a cave in southern Siberia), as well as 4–6% from Neanderthals, but that they mostly descend from the first humans who ventured out of Africa more than 60,000 years ago. It suggests at least two waves of human migration into Asia: early migrants that included the ancestors of contemporary Aboriginal Australians, New Guineans and some other Oceanians, followed by a second wave that gave rise to the present residents of mainland Asia. Some members of the two waves exchanged genes before the Denisovans vanished.

Discovery of sexual dimorphisms in metabolic and genetic biomarkers

Mittelstrass K, Ried JS, Yu Z, Krumsiek J, Gieger C, Prehn C, Roemisch-Margl W, Polonikov A, Peters A, Theis FJ, Meitinger T, Kronenberg F, Weidinger S, Wichmann HE, Suhre K, Wang-Sattler R, Adamski J, Illig T
Unit of Molecular Epidemiology, Helmholtz Center Munich, German Research Center for Environmental Health, Neuherberg, Germany
PLoS Genet 2011;7:e1002215

Background: Metabolomic profiling and the integration of genome-wide association study (GWAS) data is a powerful tool to comprehensively explore gene regulatory networks and to investigate the effects of genetic variation at the molecular level. Serum metabolite concentrations allow a direct readout of biological processes, and specific metabolomic signatures have been associated with complex diseases, such as Alzheimer's disease and cardiovascular and metabolic disorders. There are well-known differences between the sexes in the incidence, prevalence, age of onset, symptoms, and severity of many diseases, as well as drug responses. However, most of the studies published so far did not analyze their data stratified by gender.
Methods: This study investigated sex-specific differences in serum metabolite concentrations and their underlying genetic determination. Discovery and replication stages were based on over 3,300 independent individuals from KORA F3 and F4 with measurements of 131 metabolites, including amino acids, phosphatidylcholines, sphingomyelins, acylcarnitines, and C6 sugars.
Results: Significant differences in concentrations between males and females were found for 102/131 metabolites (p values $<3.8 \times 10^{-4}$; Bonferroni-corrected threshold). Sex-specific GWAS showed genome-wide significant differences in β estimates between SNPs in the CPS1 locus (carbamoyl-phosphate synthase 1, p $<3.8 \times 10^{-10}$) and glycine concentrations. The metabolite profiles of males and females were differed significantly and specific genetic variants in metabolism-related genes depicted sexual dimorphism.
Conclusions: This study provides new important insights into sex-specific differences in cell regulatory processes and underscores that studies should consider sex-specific effects in design and interpretation.

The new science of metabolomics addresses the entire metabolic tree, or at least large groups of metabolites, rather than each metabolite on its own. Thus, each individual has his/her own fingerprint metabolomic profile. Here is a no-surprise for a pediatric endocrinologist: the serum metabolomic profile shows significant differences between men and women, for 101 of the 131 metabolites, mostly in lipid and amino acid species. The same is true for people with different body composition patterns. Therefore, any analysis of metabolomic profiles must be normalized with respect to gender and body composition. It also means that gender-specific therapies may be required for diseases with an important metabolic component.

A nuclear-receptor-dependent phosphatidylcholine pathway with antidiabetic effects

Lee JM, Lee YK, Mamrosh JL, Busby SA, Griffin PR, Pathak MC, Ortlund EA, Moore DD
Program in Developmental Biology, Baylor College of Medicine, Houston, TX, USA
Nature 2011;474:506–510

Background: Nuclear hormone receptors regulate diverse metabolic pathways and the orphan nuclear receptor LRH-1 (also known as NR5A2) regulates bile acid biosynthesis. Structural studies have identified phospholipids as potential LRH-1 ligands, but their functional relevance is unclear. Here, the authors show that an unusual phosphatidylcholine species with two saturated 12 carbon fatty acid acyl side chains (dilauroyl phosphatidylcholine (DLPC)) is an LRH-1 agonist ligand in vitro.

Methods and Results: DLPC treatment induced bile acid biosynthetic enzymes in mouse liver, increased bile acid levels, and lowered hepatic triglycerides and serum glucose. DLPC treatment also decreased hepatic steatosis and improved glucose homeostasis in two mouse models of insulin resistance. Both the antidiabetic and lipotropic effects were lost in liver-specific *Lrh-1* knockouts.
Conclusions: These findings identify an LRH-1-dependent phosphatidylcholine signaling pathway that regulates bile acid metabolism and glucose homeostasis.

It is known that bile acids ward off fatty liver disease and maintain stable blood sugar levels. Therefore, it would be helpful if we could enhance the production of bile acids. To explore this possibility, Lee et al. investigated the liver receptor homolog-1 (LRH-1) protein, which maintains bile acid excretion. They found that a dilauroyl phosphatidylcholine (DLPC), a trace component of lecithin, activated both the mouse and human forms of the protein and mildly increased bile acid levels in the blood, which in turn reduced fat generation by the liver, reduced fatty liver disease, and improved glucose tolerance and insulin sensitivity. It is a fairly small compound and hopefully it will not be long before it is tested in obese patients with fatty liver disease.

Light relief

UVA phototransduction drives early melanin synthesis in human melanocytes

Wicks NL, Chan JW, Najera JA, Ciriello JM, Oancea E
Department of Molecular Pharmacology, Physiology and Biotechnology, Brown University, Providence, RI, USA
Curr Biol 2011;21:1906–1911

Background: Exposure of human skin to solar ultraviolet radiation (UVR), a powerful carcinogen comprising ~95% ultraviolet A (UVA) and ~5% ultraviolet B (UVB) at the Earth's surface, promotes melanin synthesis in epidermal melanocytes, which protects skin from DNA damage. UVB causes DNA lesions that lead to transcriptional activation of melanin-producing enzymes, resulting in delayed skin pigmentation within days. In contrast, UVA causes primarily oxidative damage and leads to immediate pigment darkening (IPD) within minutes, via an unknown mechanism. No receptor protein directly mediating phototransduction in skin has been identified.
Methods and Results: The authors demonstrate that exposure of primary human epidermal melanocytes (HEMs) to UVA causes calcium mobilization and early melanin synthesis. Calcium responses were abolished by treatment with G protein or phospholipase C (PLC) inhibitors or by depletion of intracellular calcium stores. They show that the visual photopigment rhodopsin is expressed in HEMs and contributes to UVR phototransduction. Upon UVR exposure, significant melanin production was measured within 1 h; cellular melanin continued to increase in a retinal- and calcium-dependent manner up to fivefold after 24 h.
Conclusions: The findings identify a novel UVA-sensitive signaling pathway in melanocytes that leads to calcium mobilization and melanin synthesis and may underlie the mechanism of IPD in human skin.

Surprisingly, the photosensitive receptor rhodopsin, previously thought to exist only in the eye, is also expressed in melanocyte skin cells in response to UV irradiation, where it triggers the generation of melanin (tanning) – the natural sunscreen that protects us from UVB-induced DNA damage. The fine balance between too little UVB exposure, that will cause vitamin D deficiency, and too much UVB, and the ensuing folic acid deficiency, turns out to use rhodopsin activation not by an enzymatic reaction but by a photosensitive mechanism – just like photosynthesis in plants.

A cardiac microRNA governs systemic energy homeostasis by regulation of MED13

Grueter CE, van Rooij E, Johnson BA, DeLeon SM, Sutherland LB, Qi X, Gautron L, Elmquist JK, Bassel-Duby R, Olson EN
Department of Molecular Biology, University of Texas Southwestern Medical Center, Dallas, TX, USA
Cell 2012;149:671–683

Background: Obesity, type 2 diabetes, and heart failure are associated with aberrant cardiac metabolism. *Methods and Results:* The paper shows that the heart regulates systemic energy homeostasis via MED13, a subunit of the Mediator complex, which controls transcription by thyroid hormone and other nuclear hormone receptors. MED13, in turn, is negatively regulated by a heart-specific microRNA, miR-208a. Cardiac-specific overexpression of MED13 or pharmacologic inhibition of miR-208a in mice confers resistance to high-fat diet-induced obesity and improves systemic insulin sensitivity and glucose tolerance. Conversely, genetic deletion of MED13 specifically in cardiomyocytes enhances obesity in response to high-fat diet and exacerbates metabolic syndrome. The metabolic actions of MED13 result from increased energy expenditure and regulation of numerous genes involved in energy balance in the heart. *Conclusions:* These findings reveal a role of the heart in systemic metabolic control and point to MED13 and miR-208a as potential therapeutic targets for metabolic disorders.

The ultimate complication of obesity, the metabolic syndrome and type 2 diabetes is cardiac disease. Research has focused on metabolic aberrations and how they compromise the cardiovascular system. Grueter et al. suggest that the heart itself may regulate whole-body metabolism. Their work focuses on MED13, a regulatory subunit of Mediator (a protein complex bridging transcription factors and RNA polymerase). Cardiac-specific overexpression of MED13 results in an increase in energy expenditure and resistance to diet-induced obesity and metabolism by altering expression of genes controlled by the thyroid hormone receptor. Another important aspect of this paper is that cardiac expression of MED13 is negatively regulated by a microRNA that is encoded by an intron of a cardiac-specific myosin gene. Promising direction inhibition of this miRNA in wild-type mice on a high-fat diet slowed both weight gain and the development of glucose intolerance.

Expressed by training

Acute exercise remodels promoter methylation in human skeletal muscle

Barres R, Yan J, Egan B, Treebak JT, Rasmussen M, Fritz T, Caidahl K, Krook A, O'Gorman DJ, Zierath JR
Department of Molecular Medicine and Surgery, Karolinska University Hospital, Karolinska Institutet, Stockholm, Sweden
Cell Metab 2012;15:405–411

Background: DNA methylation is a covalent biochemical modification controlling chromatin structure and gene expression. Exercise elicits gene expression changes that trigger structural and metabolic adaptations in skeletal muscle. *Methods and Results:* This work aimed to determine whether DNA methylation plays a role in exercise-induced gene expression. Whole genome methylation was decreased in skeletal muscle biopsies obtained from healthy sedentary men and women after acute exercise. Exercise induced a dose-dependent expression of PGC-1α, PDK4, and PPAR-δ, together with a marked hypomethylation on each respective promoter. Similarly, promoter methylation of PGC-1α, PDK4, and PPAR-δ was markedly decreased in mouse soleus muscles 45 min after ex-vivo contraction. In L6 myotubes, caffeine exposure induced gene hypomethylation in parallel with an increase in the respective mRNA content.

Conclusions: These results provide evidence that acute gene activation is associated with a dynamic change in DNA methylation in skeletal muscle and suggest that DNA hypomethylation is an early event in contraction-induced gene activation.

Epigenetic changes are much faster that we hitherto believed; transient promoter methylation occurs after an acute exercise. The same effect was achieved by ex-vivo muscle contraction and caffeine-mediated DNA hypomethylation in myocytes, implicating a role for Ca^{2+} release. Thus, genes can be activated by contraction, and this is preceded by their demethylation.

The sirtuin SIRT6 regulates lifespan in male mice

Kanfi Y, Naiman S, Amir G, Peshti V, Zinman G, Nahum L, Bar-Joseph Z, Cohen HY
The Mina & Everard Goodman Faculty of Life Sciences, Bar-Ilan University, Ramat-Gan, Israel
Nature 2012;483:218–221

Background: The significant increase in human lifespan during the past century confronts us with great medical challenges. To meet these challenges, the mechanisms that determine healthy aging must be understood. Sirtuins are highly conserved deacetylases that have been shown to regulate lifespan in yeast, nematodes and fruit flies. However, the role of sirtuins in regulating worm and fly lifespan has recently become controversial. Moreover, the role of the seven mammalian sirtuins, SIRT1 to SIRT7 (homologues of the yeast sirtuin Sir2), in regulating lifespan is unclear.
Methods and Results: This study shows that male, but not female, transgenic mice overexpressing Sirt6 have a significantly longer lifespan than wild-type mice. Gene expression analysis revealed significant differences between male Sirt6-transgenic mice and male wild-type mice: transgenic males displayed lower serum levels of insulin-like growth factor 1 (IGF1), higher levels of IGF-binding protein 1 and altered phosphorylation levels of major components of IGF1 signaling, a key pathway in the regulation of lifespan.
Conclusions: This study shows the regulation of mammalian lifespan by a sirtuin family member and has important therapeutic implications for age-related diseases.

Mammals have 7 deacetylases that are labeled sirtuins (Sir1–Sir7). These are highly conserved NAD^+-dependent deacetylases that regulate lifespan in several organisms. Increasing the sirtuin level through genetic manipulation extends the lifespan of yeast, nematodes and flies. Some mammalian sirtuins regulate age-related diseases, but mice that overexpress SIRT1 have the same lifespan as control WT mice. We now learn that it is Sirt6 that prolongs life in mice; transgenic males displayed lower serum IGF1 and higher IGFBP1. What comes to mind next are the therapeutic implications for age-related diseases. And why do females not respond? Mice with a fat-specific insulin receptor gene knockout have been shown to have an increased mean lifespan of similar magnitude to that of SIRT6e, demonstrating the central role of fat in regulating lifespan.

Clearance of p16Ink4a-positive senescent cells delays aging-associated disorders

Baker DJ, Wijshake T, Tchkonia T, LeBrasseur NK, Childs BG, van de Sluis B, Kirkland JL, van Deursen JM
Department of Pediatric and Adolescent Medicine, Mayo Clinic College of Medicine, Rochester, MN, USA
Nature 2011;479:232–236

Background: Advanced age is the main risk factor for most chronic diseases and functional deficits in humans, but the fundamental mechanisms that drive aging remain largely unknown, impeding the development of interventions that might delay or prevent age-related disorders and maximize healthy lifespan. Cellular senescence, which halts the proliferation of damaged or dysfunctional cells, is an important mechanism to constrain the malignant progression of tumor cells. Senescent cells accumulate in various tissues and organs with aging and have been hypothesized to disrupt tissue structure and function because of the components they secrete.
Methods: This study examined whether senescent cells are causally implicated in age-related dysfunction and whether their removal is beneficial. To address these fundamental questions, they made use of a biomarker for senescence, p16Ink4a, to design a novel transgene, INK-ATTAC, for inducible elimination of p16Ink4a-positive senescent cells upon administration of a drug.
Results: In the BubR1 progeroid mouse background, INK-ATTAC removed p16Ink4a-positive senescent cells upon drug treatment. In tissues, such as adipose tissue, skeletal muscle and eye, in which p16Ink4a contributes to the acquisition of age-related pathologies, life-long removal of p16Ink4a-expressing cells delayed onset of these phenotypes. Furthermore, late-life clearance attenuated progression of already established age-related disorders.
Conclusions: Cellular senescence is causally implicated in generating age-related phenotypes and removal of senescent cells can prevent or delay tissue dysfunction and extend health span.

After dividing a limited number of times, cells enter a senescent nonproliferative phase. Baker et al. used genetic engineering to eliminate ensuing senescent cells. Mice with no senescent cells did not live longer than normal, but they lived better; they showed delayed onset of cataracts, fat accumulation, and muscle weakness, they could run for a longer time on a treadmill and perform more strenuous workouts – we remain hopeful for drug that will eliminate our own senescent cells.

Linking long-term dietary patterns with gut microbial enterotypes

Wu GD, Chen J, Hoffmann C, Bittinger K, Chen YY, Keilbaugh SA, Bewtra M, Knights D, Walters WA, Knight R, Sinha R, Gilroy E, Gupta K, Baldassano R, Nessel L, Li H, Bushman FD, Lewis JD
Division of Gastroenterology, Perelman School of Medicine, University of Pennsylvania, Philadelphia, PA, USA
gdwu@mail.med.upenn.edu
Science 2011;334:105–108

Background: Diet strongly affects human health, partly by modulating gut microbiome composition.
Methods: The authors used diet inventories and 16S rDNA sequencing to characterize fecal samples from 98 individuals.
Results: Fecal communities clustered into enterotypes distinguished primarily by levels of *Bacteroides* and *Prevotella*. Enterotypes were strongly associated with long-term diets, particularly protein and animal fat *(Bacteroides)* versus carbohydrates *(Prevotella)*. A controlled-feeding study of 10 subjects showed that microbiome composition changed detectably within 24 h of initiating a high-fat/low-fiber or low-fat/high-fiber diet, but that enterotype identity remained stable during the 10-day study.
Conclusions: Alternative enterotype states are associated with long-term diet.

The microbiome has been the focus of much interest and hope, particularly in the field of obesity. More recently the practice of fecal (microbiome) transplantation has been revived and received scientific evidence in the cure of broad-spectrum antibiotic-induced enteropathy [1]. The multispecies microbiome was classified, to include three enterotypes, named *Bacteroides*, *Prevotella*, and *Ruminococcus*. These enterotypes correlate with long-term diet, but not with age, weight, sex, or country; they can differ even between twin siblings. *Bacteroides* grow on high-meat diets; *Prevotella* on vegetarian food. But changes in the microbiome do not occur fast; Wu et al. show that 10 days of a dietary change makes no difference to your enterotype, suggesting that they are more influenced by long-term eating trends.

In utero epigenomic programming

Epigenetic mechanism underlying the development of polycystic ovary syndrome-like phenotypes in prenatally androgenized rhesus monkeys

Xu N, Kwon S, Abbott DH, Geller DH, Dumesic DA, Azziz R, Guo X, Goodarzi MO
Division of Endocrinology, Diabetes and Metabolism, Department of Medicine, Cedars-Sinai Medical Center, Los Angeles, CA, USA
PLoS One 2011;6:e27286

Context: The pathogenesis of polycystic ovary syndrome (PCOS) is poorly understood. PCOS-like phenotypes are produced by prenatal androgenization (PA) of female rhesus monkeys.

Hypothesis: Perturbation of the epigenome, through altered DNA methylation, is one of the mechanisms whereby PA reprograms monkeys to develop PCOS.

Methods: Infant and adult visceral adipose tissues (VAT) harvested from 15 PA and 10 control monkeys were studied. Bisulfite-treated samples were subjected to genome-wide CpG methylation analysis, designed to simultaneously measure methylation levels at 27,578 CpG sites. Analysis was carried out using Bayesian Classification with Singular Value Decomposition (BCSVD), testing all probes simultaneously in a single test. Stringent criteria were then applied to filter out invalid probes due to sequence dissimilarities between human probes and monkey DNA, and then mapped to the rhesus genome.

Outcomes: This yielded differentially methylated loci between PA and control monkeys, 163 in infant VAT, and 325 in adult VAT (BCSVD p < 0.05). Among these two sets of genes, we identified several significant pathways, including the antiproliferative role of TOB in T-cell signaling and transforming growth factor-β (TGF-β) signaling.

Conclusions: PA may modify DNA methylation patterns in both infant and adult VAT. This pilot study suggests that excess fetal androgen exposure in female nonhuman primates may predispose to PCOS via alteration of the epigenome, providing a novel avenue to understand PCOS in humans.

PCOS-like phenotypes are produced by prenatal androgenization (PA) of rhesus monkeys, sheep, rats and mice, including hyperandrogenism, oligomenorrhea, polyfollicular ovaries, increased adiposity, insulin resistance and impaired insulin secretion. Does this indicate that the intrauterine environment plays a role in the etiology of PCOS? The current study performed a genome-wide site-specific methylation array of visceral adipose tissue (VAT) from PA female rhesus monkeys. They report differentially methylated loci between PA and control monkeys' VAT. Among these are the antiproliferative T-cell signaling and TGF-β signaling, a pathway currently implicated in the pathogenesis of PCOS in women by genetic epidemiologic evidence [3]. Once again, epigenomics may be more relevant to diseases of modern civilization than genetics.

Transgenerational epigenetic instability is a source of novel methylation variants

Schmitz RJ, Schultz MD, Lewsey MG, O'Malley RC, Urich MA, Libiger O, Schork NJ, Ecker JR
Plant Biology Laboratory, The Salk Institute for Biological Studies, La Jolla, CA, USA
Science 2011;334:369–373

Background: Epigenetic information, which may affect an organisms' phenotype, can be stored and stably inherited in the form of cytosine DNA methylation. Changes in DNA methylation can produce meiotically stable epialleles that affect transcription and morphology, but the rates of spontaneous gain or loss of DNA methylation are unknown.
Methods: The authors examined spontaneously occurring variation in DNA methylation in *Arabidopsis thaliana* plants propagated by single-seed descent for 30 generations.
Results: 114,287 CG single methylation polymorphisms (SMPs) and 2,485 CG differentially methylated regions (DMRs) were identified, both of which showed patterns of divergence compared to the ancestral state.
Conclusions: Transgenerational epigenetic variation in DNA methylation can generate new allelic states that alter transcription providing a mechanism for inheritance of phenotypic diversity in the absence of genetic mutation.

But how can epigenetic variation lead to stable epimutations and gene sequence variants? See below.

Methylation stabilizes the genome

Genomic hypomethylation in the human germline associates with selective structural mutability in the human genome

Li J, Harris RA, Cheung SW, Coarfa C, Jeong M, Goodell MA, White LD, Patel A, Kang SH, Shaw C, Chinault AC, Gambin T, Gambin A, Lupski JR, Milosavljevic A
Bioinformatics Research Laboratory, Epigenome Center, Baylor College of Medicine, Houston, TX, USA
PLoS Genet 2012;8:e1002692

Background: The hotspots of structural polymorphisms and structural mutability in the human genome remain to be explained mechanistically. The authors examined associations between structural mutability and germline DNA methylation and with nonallelic homologous recombination (NAHR) mediated by low-copy repeats (LCRs).
Methods and Results: Combined evidence from four human sperm methylome maps, human genome evolution, structural polymorphisms in the human population, and previous genomic and disease studies consistently points to a strong association between germline hypomethylation and genomic instability. Specifically, methylation deserts, the ~1% fraction of the human genome with the lowest methylation in the germline, show tenfold enrichment for structural rearrangements that occurred in the human genome since the branching of chimpanzee and are highly enriched for fast-evolving loci that regulate tissue-specific gene expression. Analysis of copy number variants (CNVs) from 400 human samples identified using a custom-designed array comparative genomic hybridization (aCGH) chip, combined with publicly available structural variation data, indicates that association between structural mutability and germline hypomethylation is comparable in magnitude to the association between structural mutability and LCR-mediated NAHR. Moreover, rare CNVs occurring in the genomes of individuals diagnosed with schizophrenia, bipolar disorder, and developmental delay and de novo CNVs occurring in those diagnosed with autism are significantly more concentrated within hypomethylated regions.
Conclusions: These findings suggest a new connection between the epigenome, selective mutability, evolution, and human disease.

Approximately 10% of the human genome is structurally polymorphic at the submicroscopic scale (<4 Mb), a much larger fraction than affected by single nucleotide polymorphisms (SNPs). Structural mutations that occur in a number of well-studied unstable loci cause disease. The discovery of these structurally mutable disease-associated loci gave rise to the concept of genomic disorders. This excessive mutability has also accelerated evolution. Lack of methylation (hypomethylation) of genomic DNA has been previously associated with high structural mutability in cancer cells, and in this paper Li et al. related hypomethylation to structural mutability in the human germline. They confirm the role of low-copy repeats (LCRs) in promoting structural mutability on the genome scale and also reveal a surprisingly strong association between genomic instability and hypomethylation; the ~1% fraction of the human genome with the lowest methylation in human sperm harbors a tenfold higher number of structural mutations than the genome-wide average. This suggests a new connection between adaptive plasticity responses to the environment and heritable changes in gene sequence, which provide long-term evolutionary variation.

Unsilencing father's methylation

Topoisomerase inhibitors unsilence the dormant allele of Ube3a in neurons

Huang HS, Allen JA, Mabb AM, King IF, Miriyala J, Taylor-Blake B, Sciaky N, Dutton JW, Jr, Lee HM, Chen X, Jin J, Bridges AS, Zylka MJ, Roth BL, Philpot BD
Department of Cell and Molecular Physiology, University of North Carolina School of Medicine, Chapel Hill, NC, USA
Nature 2012;481:185–189

Background: Angelman syndrome is a severe neurodevelopmental disorder caused by deletion or mutation of the maternally-inherited ubiquitin protein ligase E3A gene (UBE3A). The paternal allele of UBE3A is intact but is epigenetically silenced, raising the possibility that Angelman syndrome could be treated if the silenced allele could be activated to restore functional UBE3A protein.

Methods and Results: The authors used an unbiased, high-content drug screen, in primary cortical neurons from mice, and identified twelve topoisomerase I inhibitors and four topoisomerase II inhibitors that unsilenced the paternal Ube3a allele. These drugs included topotecan, irinotecan, etoposide and dexrazoxane (ICRF-187). At nanomolar concentrations, topotecan upregulated catalytically active UBE3A in neurons from maternal Ube3a-null mice. Topotecan downregulated expression of the Ube3a antisense transcript that overlaps the paternal copy of Ube3a. When administered in vivo, topotecan unsilenced the paternal Ube3a allele in neurons in the hippocampus, neocortex, striatum, cerebellum and spinal cord. Paternal Ube3a expression remained elevated in a subset of spinal cord neurons for at least 12 weeks after cessation of topotecan treatment.

Conclusions: These results indicate that topotecan unsilences Ube3a in cis by reducing transcription of an imprinted antisense RNA, and suggest a therapeutic strategy for reactivating the dormant but functional allele of Ube3a in patients with Angelman syndrome.

Angelman syndrome (AS) is often widely taught as the exemplar of imprinted gene disorders, as it is caused by the specific loss of the maternally-inherited UBE3A gene. Conversely, defects in the corresponding paternally-inherited gene region cause Prader-Willi syndrome. The frequent outbreaks of laughter and jerky movements characteristic of AS gave it the eponym 'happy puppet syndrome'. However the condition is far from a happy one, being usually marked by seizures, sleep disturbance and severe learning difficulties and, like many inherited neurological disorders, no effective treatment strategies exist. The authors explored the intriguing possibility that the intact but dormant paternal UBE3A allele might be awakened. To do this, they screened 2,306 drug-like molecules using a primary mouse cortical neuron assay that linked paternal Ube3a to a yellow fluorescent protein. Their findings showed that transient topoisomerase inhibition, using drugs that are currently used in treating cancer, has lasting effects on paternal Ube3a gene expression and therefore may have potential benefits for patients with AS.

Accelerated recruitment of new brain development genes into the human genome

Zhang YE, Landback P, Vibranovski MD, Long M
Department of Ecology and Evolution, The University of Chicago, Chicago, IL, USA
PLoS Biol 2011;9:e1001179

Background: How the human brain evolved has attracted tremendous interest for decades.

Methods: Motivated by case studies of primate-specific genes implicated in brain function, the authors examined whether the young genes, those emerging genome-wide in the lineages specific to the primates or rodents, showed distinct spatial and temporal patterns of transcription compared to old genes, which had existed before primates and rodents split.

Results: The authors found consistent patterns across different sources of expression data: there were significantly larger proportions of young genes expressed in the fetal or infant brains of humans than of the mouse, and more young genes in humans have expression biased toward early developing brains than old genes. Most of these young genes are expressed in the evolutionarily newest part of human brain, the neocortex. Remarkably, they also identified a number of human-specific genes expressed in the prefrontal cortex, which is implicated in complex cognitive behaviors. The young genes upregulated in the early developing human brain have diverse functions, with a significant enrichment of transcription factors. Genes originating from different mechanisms show a similar expression bias in the developing brain. Moreover, the young genes upregulated in early brain development showed rapid protein evolution compared to old genes also expressed in the fetal brain. Strikingly, genes expressed in the neocortex arose soon after its morphological origin.

Conclusions: These four lines of evidence suggest that positive selection for brain function may have contributed to the origins of young genes expressed in the developing brain. These data demonstrate a striking recruitment of new genes into the early development of the human brain.

MicroRNA-driven developmental remodeling in the brain distinguishes humans from other primates

Somel M, Liu X, Tang L, Yan Z, Hu H, Guo S, Jiang X, Zhang X, Xu G, Xie G, Li N, Hu Y, Chen W, Paabo S, Khaitovich P
Key Laboratory of Computational Biology, CAS-MPG Partner Institute for Computational Biology, Chinese Academy of Sciences, Shanghai, China
PLoS Biol 2011;9:e1001214

Background: While many studies have reported the accelerated evolution of brain gene expression in the human lineage, the mechanisms underlying such changes are unknown.

Methods: The authors address this issue from a developmental perspective by analyzing mRNA and microRNA (miRNA) expression in two brain regions within macaques, chimpanzees, and humans throughout their lifespan.

Results: Constitutive gene expression divergence (differences between species independent of age) is comparable between humans and chimpanzees. However, humans display a 3–5 times faster evolutionary rate in divergence of developmental patterns, compared to chimpanzees. Such accelerated evolution of human brain developmental patterns (i) cannot be explained by life-history changes among species, (ii) is twice as pronounced in the prefrontal cortex than the cerebellum, (iii) preferentially affects neuron-related genes, and (iv) unlike constitutive divergence does not depend on *cis*-regulatory changes, but might be driven by human-specific changes in expression of *trans*-acting regulators. Developmental profiles of miRNAs, as well as their target genes, showed the fastest rates of human-specific evolutionary change. Using a combination of computational and experimental methods, the authors identified miR-92a, miR-454, and miR-320b as possible regulators of human-specific neural development.

Conclusions: Different mechanisms underlie adaptive and neutral transcriptome divergence. Changes in the expression of a few key regulators may have been a major driving force behind rapid evolution of the human brain.

Human evolution is dominated by investment in big brains with unique cognitive abilities. While there have been no major genome-wide changes in the coding regions of brain-related genes, changes in the regulation of these genes have played a key role. Zhang et al. examined the expression profile of genes in both fetal and adult brains in the human and mouse, and discovered that an excess of recently evolved genes are expressed in the early (fetal or infant) developing human brain compared with those in mouse brain. Apparently, evolutionary change in the development of the human brain happened at the protein level by gene origination and also via evolution of regulatory networks. Somel et al. compared gene-expression patterns in the brains of humans, chimpanzees and rhesus, and show that human brains showed many more differences in gene-expression patterns as newborns developed into adults, particularly in cognition-specific regions. Genes that encode miRNAs were among those whose expression varied. Somel et al. suggest that a small number of miRNAs and proteins controlling brain development could have driven the evolution of the human brain.

Electrifying embryology

Transmembrane voltage potential controls embryonic eye patterning in *Xenopus laevis*

Pai VP, Aw S, Shomrat T, Lemire JM, Levin M
Department of Biology and Tufts Center for Regenerative and Developmental Biology, Tufts University, Medford, MA, USA
Development 2012;139:313–323

Background: Uncovering the molecular mechanisms of eye development is crucial for understanding the embryonic morphogenesis of complex structures, as well as for the establishment of novel biomedical approaches to address birth defects and injuries of the visual system. During normal embryogenesis, a striking hyperpolarization demarcates a specific cluster of cells in the anterior neural field.
Methods and Results: To characterize change in transmembrane voltage potential (V_{mem}) as a novel biophysical signal for eye induction in *Xenopus laevis*. Depolarizing the dorsal lineages in which these cells reside results in malformed eyes. Manipulating V_{mem} of non-eye cells induces well-formed ectopic eyes that are morphologically and histologically similar to endogenous eyes. Remarkably, such ectopic eyes can be induced far outside the anterior neural field. A Ca^{2+} channel-dependent pathway transduces the V_{mem} signal and regulates patterning of eye field transcription factors.
Conclusions: These data reveal a new, instructive role for membrane voltage during embryogenesis and demonstrate that V_{mem} is a crucial upstream signal in eye development. Learning to control bioelectric initiators of organogenesis offers significant insight into birth defects that affect the eye and might have significant implications for regenerative approaches to ocular diseases.

Complex body structures arise from simple early embryonic structure by timed action of a relatively small 'tool box' of two dozen transcription factors. Pai et al. show how bioelectrical communications among cells specify the type of new organ to be created at a particular location. Manipulation of membrane voltage in *Xenopus* embryos caused the frog to grow eyes in the back and tail. By RNA encoding of ion channels, the researchers changed the membrane potential of these cell, causing abnormalities to occur. It seems that for every structure in the body there is a specific membrane voltage range that drives organogenesis.

Ecological specialization in fossil mammals explains Cope's rule

Raia P, Carotenuto F, Passaro F, Fulgione D, Fortelius M
Dipartimento di Scienze della Terra, Università degli Studi Federico II, Napoli, Italy
pascuale.raia@unina.it
Am Nat 2012;179:328–337

Background: Cope's rule is the trend toward increasing body size in a lineage over geological time. The rule has been explained either as passive diffusion away from a small initial body size or as an active trend upheld by the ecological and evolutionary advantages that large body size confers.
Methods: An explicit and phylogenetically informed analysis of body size evolution in Cenozoic mammals.
Results: Results show that body size increases significantly in most inclusive clades. This increase occurs through temporal substitution of incumbent species by larger-sized close relatives within the clades. These late-appearing species have smaller spatial and temporal ranges and are rarer than the incumbents they replace, traits that are typical of ecological specialists. Overlain on a net trend toward average size increase, significant pulses in origination of large-sized species are concentrated in periods of global cooling.
Conclusions: Cope's rule appears to derive mainly from increasing ecological specialization and clade-level niche expansion rather than from active selection for larger size. Cooling pulses plausibly record direct selection for larger body size according to Bergmann's rule, which thus appears to be independent of but concomitant with Cope's.

As much as hominids grew strategically from Lucy's 105 cm to present-day females' 165 cm, increasing body size in a lineage over geological time periods is common: members of most lineages get bigger over time deep time. The authors of this paper composed phylogenetic trees of 554 mammal species and confirm the rule: most have become bigger: small and unspecialized species are 'replaced' by larger species. Most of the peaks in body size increase occur alongside changes in the climate; drop in temperature resulted in an increase in size.

Evolution of the earliest horses driven by climate change in the Paleocene-Eocene thermal maximum

Secord R, Bloch JI, Chester SG, Boyer DM, Wood AR, Wing SL, Kraus MJ, McInerney FA, Krigbaum J
Department of Earth and Atmospheric Sciences, University of Nebraska, Lincoln, NE, USA
rsecord2@unl.edu
Science 2012;335:959–962

Background: Body size plays a critical role in mammalian ecology and physiology. Previous research has shown that many mammals became smaller during the Paleocene-Eocene thermal maximum (PETM), the period of profound global warming, but the timing and magnitude of that change relative to climate change are unclear.
Methods and Results: A high-resolution record of continental climate and equid body size change shows a directional decrease in size of ~30% over the first ~130,000 years of the PETM, followed by a ~76% increase during the recovery phase of the PETM. These size changes are negatively correlated with temperature, as inferred from oxygen isotopes in mammal teeth, and were probably driven by shifts in temperature and possibly high atmospheric CO_2 concentrations.
Conclusions: These findings could be important for understanding mammalian evolutionary responses to future global warming.

Body size sets the energetic demands of organisms; big animals consume more energy than small animals. Children in underprivileged nutritional environments are not 'stunted', but are adequately adapted to low energy cues. Yet, the survival and fitness advantage of being big make animals, including humans, grow bigger over evolutionary time for as long as energy is available. Thus, the body sizes of mammal lineages have varied greatly over evolutionary history. The extinction of dinosaurs ~65.5 million years ago eliminated big animals, but at the same time enhanced ecological (and therefore phenotypic) diversification, which ultimately led to size increases to current magnitudes. Secord et al. illustrate the well-known 'Bergmann's rule' – the critical role of temperature in driving body size evolution; larger sizes are found in colder environments, and smaller sizes in warmer areas. Body size decreased by ~30% at the start of the PETM, and increased abruptly by more than 75% at its end. Recent global warming has already led to changes in the distribution and morphology of species.

Change and variability in Plio-Pleistocene climates: modeling the hominin response

Grove M
School of Archaeology, Classics and Egyptology, University of Liverpool, Liverpool, UK
J Arch Sci 2011:38:3038–3047

Background: Research into the links between climatic change and hominin evolution has generated numerous hypotheses. In recent years, methodological refinement of, and increased research effort directed towards, reliable proxies for paleoclimatic change have provided a growing body of data with which to test such hypotheses. Whilst many archaeologists are aware of these data, few are cognizant of the wealth of techniques developed by theoretical biologists over the last half century to explicitly address the evolutionary consequences of adaptation to temporally heterogeneous environments.
Methods: This study expands and adapts one such technique for use with empirical data, and applies it to a global paleoclimatic record spanning the last 5 million years, in order to discern the potential impact of environmental heterogeneity on hominin evolution during this period. Of particular interest are the contributions of climatic change, associated with directional selection, and climatic variability, associated with selection for phenotypic plasticity.
Results: At this macro-scale, the author finds an early peak in selection for plasticity at approximately 2–2.7 million years ago (mya), combined with three major shifts in directional selection at approximately 3.3–3.4, 1.4–1.5, and 0.5–0.6 mya.
Conclusions: These results link the fossil and archaeological records to a number of environmental hypotheses of human evolution. In particular, it is argued that the origins of the genus *Homo* and the spread of Oldowan technology are associated not with a major turnover pulse, but with a period of selection for phenotypic plasticity.

Climatic changes are among the most powerful forces directing evolutionary events. Among such events are (1) hominids' trend to become bigger in size over the last 4.5 million years, and (2) a very marked plasticity of hominids enabling us to adapt to various conflicting environmental cues. This article calls for a distinction between climatic change and climatic variability. Whereas climatic change results in directional selection, such as progressive growth when the earth cools, climatic variability selects for plasticity. The results suggest that selection for plasticity increased 2.3–2.5 million years ago. This date range coincides with the evolution of *Homo* and the spread of the Oldowan. Plasticity is a fundamental requirement for the unique human adaptability, enabling *Homo sapiens* to live in Greenland and the Sahara, in the Himalaya and the Dead Sea.

A small puzzle solved

LB1 and LB6 *Homo floresiensis* are not modern human (*Homo sapiens*) cretins

Brown P
Palaeoanthropology, Faculty of Arts and Sciences, University of New England, Armidale, NSW, Australia
pbrown3@une.edu.au
J Hum Evol 2012;62:201–224

Background: Excavations in the late Pleistocene deposits at Liang Bua cave, Flores, have uncovered the skeletal remains of several small-bodied and small-brained hominins in association with stone artifacts and the bones of Stegodon. Due to their combination of plesiomorphic, unique and derived traits, they were ascribed to a new species, *Homo floresiensis*, which, along with Stegodon, appears to have become extinct ~17 ka (thousand years ago). However, recently it has been argued that several characteristics of *H. floresiensis* were consistent with dwarfism and evidence of delayed development in modern human (*Homo sapiens*) myxedematous endemic (ME) cretins.

Methods and Results: This research compared the skeletal and dental morphology in *H. floresiensis* with the clinical and osteological indicators of cretinism, and the traits that have been argued to be associated with ME cretinism in LB1 and LB6. Contrary to published claims, morphological and statistical comparisons did not identify the distinctive skeletal and dental indicators of cretinism in LB1 or LB6 *H. floresiensis*. Brain mass, skeletal proportions, epiphyseal union, orofacial morphology, dental development, size of the pituitary fossa and development of the paranasal sinuses, vault bone thickness and dimensions of the hands and feet all distinguish *H. floresiensis* from modern humans with ME cretinism.

Conclusions: The research team responsible for the diagnosis of ME cretinism had not examined the original *H. floresiensis* skeletal materials, and perhaps, as a result, their research confused taphonomic damage with evidence of disease, and thus contained critical errors of fact and interpretation. Behavioral scenarios attempting to explain the presence of cretinous *H. sapiens* in the Liang Bua Pleistocene deposits, but not unaffected *H. sapiens*, are both unnecessary and not supported by the available archaeological and geochronological evidence from Flores.

Yearbook has followed the saga of the hobbits from the Indonesian island Flores from its first publication (*Yearbook 2005*). With an average height of <1 m, a weight of 1 kg and brain weight of 380 g, it was debated whether these people who roamed the island 18,000 years ago were short-statured *H. sapiens*, or a new species. It evoked then the phenomenon of insular dwarfism, the phenomenon of plants and animals growing short when resources are limited and when there is no need to grow big for lack of predators. Others suggested that these were cretins or Laron dwarfs. Over the years the Flores hobbits were a matter of much debate and ugly politics of science. From available archaeological and geochronological evidence from Flores it is now clear that these were members of a new species, now labeled *H. floresiensis*. This is even more exciting, and the origin of this species is yet to be deciphered.

Last but not least

Phenotypic correlates of male reproductive success in western gorillas

Breuer T, Robbins AM, Boesch C, Robbins MM
Department of Primatology, Max Planck Institute for Evolutionary Anthropology, Leipzig, Germany, and Mbeli Bai Study. Wildlife Conservation Society, Congo Program, Brazzaville, PR Congo
J Hum Evol 2012;62:466–472

Background: Sexual selection is thought to drive the evolution of sexually dimorphic traits that increase male reproductive success. Despite a large degree of sexual dimorphism among haplorhine primates, phenotypic traits that may influence the reproductive success of males are largely unstudied due to their long lifespans and the difficulties in quantifying such traits noninvasively.

Methods: The authors employed digital photogrammetry of body length and crest size, as well as ranking of the gluteal muscle size, to test whether these sexually dimorphic traits are associated with long-term measures of male reproductive success in western gorillas.

Results: Among 19 adult male gorillas monitored for up to 12.5 years, all three physical traits were positively correlated with the average number of mates per male, but only crest size and gluteal muscle size were significantly correlated with offspring survival and the annual rate of siring offspring that survive to weaning age.

Conclusions: The authors discuss why such sexually dimorphic traits might be under ongoing selection in gorillas and other species.

Examination of morphological and behavioral features of great apes provides insights into the group structure, and social behavior of our ancestors. Gorilla males are twice as large in mass as females, and have markedly larger gluteus muscles. When it comes to sexual selection, longer males are preferred by females. Yet it is only the gluteus mass that predicts better survival of the offspring. Female gorillas look at the wrong trait: they find long males to be attractive, but crest size and gluteus musculature may be imperative; they correlate with the ability of the male to provide protection to offspring.

References
1. Kau AL, Ahern PP, Griffin NW, Goodman AL, Gordon JI: Human nutrition, the gut microbiome and the immune system. Nature 2011;474:327–336.
2. Hammer MF, Woerner AE, Mendez FL, Watkins JC, Wall JD: Genetic evidence for archaic admixture in Africa. Proc Natl Acad Sci USA 2011;108:15123–15128.
3. Reich D, Patterson N, Kircher M, Delfin F, Nandineni MR, Pugach I, Ko AM, Ko YC, Jinam TA, Phipps ME, Saitou N, Wollstein A, Kayser M, Paabo S, Stoneking M: Denisova admixture and the first modern human dispersals into Southeast Asia and Oceania. Am J Hum Genet 2011;89:516–528.

Carré, A. 29
Carrithers, S.L. 211
Casanova, J.L. 62, 100
Casas, R. 145
Cascón, A. 109
Casey, S. 82
Castagneto, M. 217
Castanet, M. 29
Castano, L. 87, 145
Castetbon, K. 153
Censi, L. 93
Ceolotto, G. 114
Cermakova, L. 210
Cetin, A.H. 10
Chabot, J.A. 40
Chabre, O. 126
Chabrier, G. 126
Chakrabarti, B. 7
Chakravarty, D. 40
Challis, B. 213
Chamberlain, C. 68
Chambon, C. 107
Chan, J.W. 225
Chan, L. 3
Channon, S. 29
Chanseaume, E. 162
Chanson, P. 61
Chao, M.V. 101
Charlet, A. 10
Charmandari, E. 99
Charolidi, N. 15
Chatterjee, K. 35
Chauvet, N. 18
Chavakis, T. 139
Chazot, F.B. 125
Chen, B. 218
Chen, H.C. 4
Chen, J. 92, 228
Chen, J.J. 4
Chen, W. 156, 232
Chen, X. 231
Chen, Y. 218
Chen, Y.Y. 228
Chen, Z. 77
Cherman, N. 68, 212
Chester, S.G. 234
Cheung, M. 156
Cheung, S.W. 230
Chevrier, L. 1
Chiarelli, F. 135, 196
Chiesa, A. 127
Child, C.J. 176
Childs, B.G. 228
Chinault, A.C. 230
Chiuri, R.M. 196
Chiusano, E. 29
Chng, K. 3
Choi, C.S. 9
Choi, J.H. 163

Choi, Y.H. 161
Chong, W. 68
Chopra, A. 205
Choquet, H. 166
Christian, H. 18
Christodoulou, C. 39
Chrysis, D. 70
Chuang, C.H. 99
Chuang, J. 169
Chung, S.A. 164
Cianfarani, S. 45
Cicala, M.V. 114
Cinti, S. 163
Ciriello, J.M. 225
Clark, A.J. 99
Clarke, I.J. 3
Clauser, E. 61
Clauss, L. 193
Cleary, P.A. 142
Clément, K. 160, 161
Cleveland, R.H. 74
Closa-Monasterolo, R. 204
Cloutier, J. 175
Cnop, M. 149
Coarfa, C. 230
Coats, J.K. 6
Codner, E. 127
Cognet, C. 100
Cohen, D.E. 165
Cohen, H.Y. 227
Cohn, D.H. 62
Colaianni, G. 65
Colao, A. 22
Cole, D.E. 211
Cole, T.J. 82
Cole, T.R. 103
Colli, M.L. 149
Collier, C. 210
Collins, F. 103
Collins, M. 68
Colombani, P. 40
Colton, C.K. 139
Comino-Méndez, I. 109
Conejero, G. 18
Coney, P. 197
Connelly, P.W. 210
Connolly, L.P. 164
Connor, K.L. 94
Conti, P. 214
Cooney, R.E. 91
Cooper, C. 158
Cooper, D.S. 42
Cooper, O. 22
Cooper, T.G. 121
Coopmans, W. 201
Copeland, K. 177
Copin, B. 26
Cordella, D. 34
Cormier-Daire, V. 62

Cortas, N.K. 76
Costagliola, S. 38
Coste, J. 46
Coste, O. 183
Costigan, C. 99
Cote, G.J. 126
Cotterill, A. 136
Cottrell, E.C. 102
Couch, R. 113
Coughlan, M.T. 151
Coupe, B. 8
Coutant, R. 124
Couture, C. 17
Couvineau, A. 61
Cox, C.L. 122
Cragun, D.L. 103
Craig, A.E. 220
Craig, S. 74
Cranley, W.R. 74
Crawley, J. 209
Crine, P. 74
Crofton, P.M. 119
Crozier, S.R. 158
Cuervo, A.M. 8
Cukierman-Yaffe, T. 215
Cuny, A. 119
Cutfield, W.S. 23, 93
Cutler Jr, G.B. 176
Cuttler, L. 177
Cypess, A.M. 164

D

Dackiw, A.P. 40
Daher, R.T. 76
Dahl, R.E. 92
Dahlqvist, P. 106
Daifotis, A.G. 191
Daley, G. 194
Dan, E. 204
Dall'Amico, D. 29
Day, A. 213
Dance, M. 53
Daniels, S.R. 156
Danielsson, A. 137
Danne, T. 194
Darling, T.N. 212
Dattani, M. 35
Dattani, M.T. 13, 15, 103
Dauber, A. 211
Daunay, A. 147
Davey-Smith, G. 154
Davidson, H.W. 138
Davies, T.F. 65
Davis, J.R. 20
Davis, P.H. 156
Davis, S.N. 194
Day, R. 103
Day, S. 128